LAMINATE VENEERS

Evidenced-Based Clinical Protocols

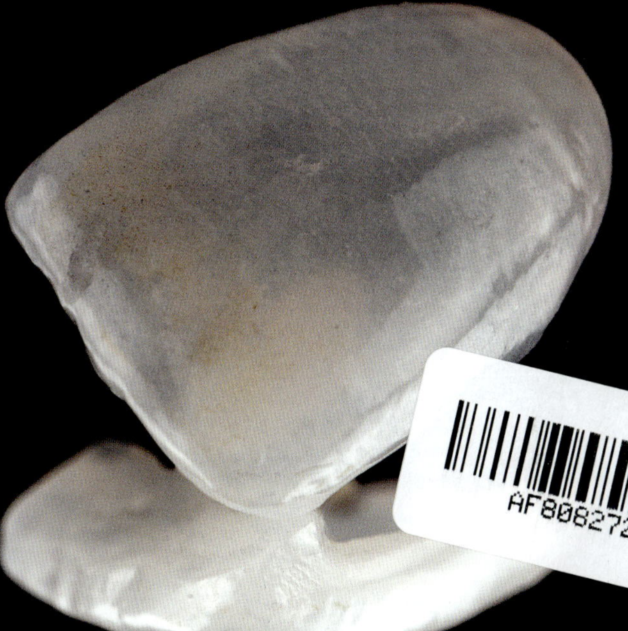

Markus B. Blatz

QUINTESSENCE PUBLISHING

Berlin | Chicago | Tokyo
Barcelona | London | Milan | Paris | Prague | Seoul | Warsaw
Beijing | Istanbul | Sao Paulo | Sydney | Zagreb

One book, one tree: In support of reforestation worldwide and to address the climate crisis, for every book sold Quintessence Publishing will plant a tree (https://onetreeplanted.org/).

QUINTESSENCE PUBLISHING
DEUTSCHLAND

Quintessenz Verlags-GmbH
Ifenpfad 2–4
12107 Berlin
Germany
www.quintessence-publishing.com

Quintessence Publishing Co Ltd
Grafton Road, New Malden
Surrey KT3 3AB
United Kingdom
www.quintessence-publishing.com

Editing, production, and reproduction: Quintessenz Verlags-GmbH, Berlin, Germany
ISBN 978-1-78698-142-4

Printed and bound in Croatia by Grafički zavod Hrvatske d.o.o.

CO-AUTHORS

Ulrike Blatz
José Ayub
Julian Conejo
Paco Rojas
Luis Quintero

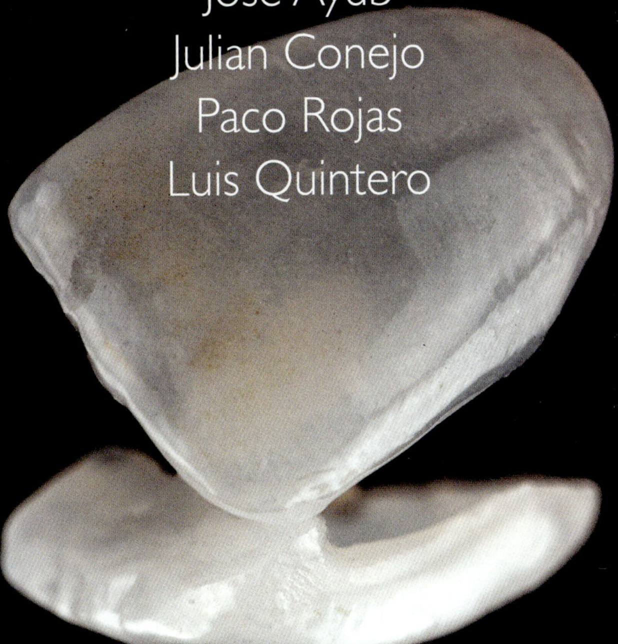

with contributions from

Ralph Georg
Miladinov Milos

EVIDENCE-BASED CLINICAL PROTOCOLS

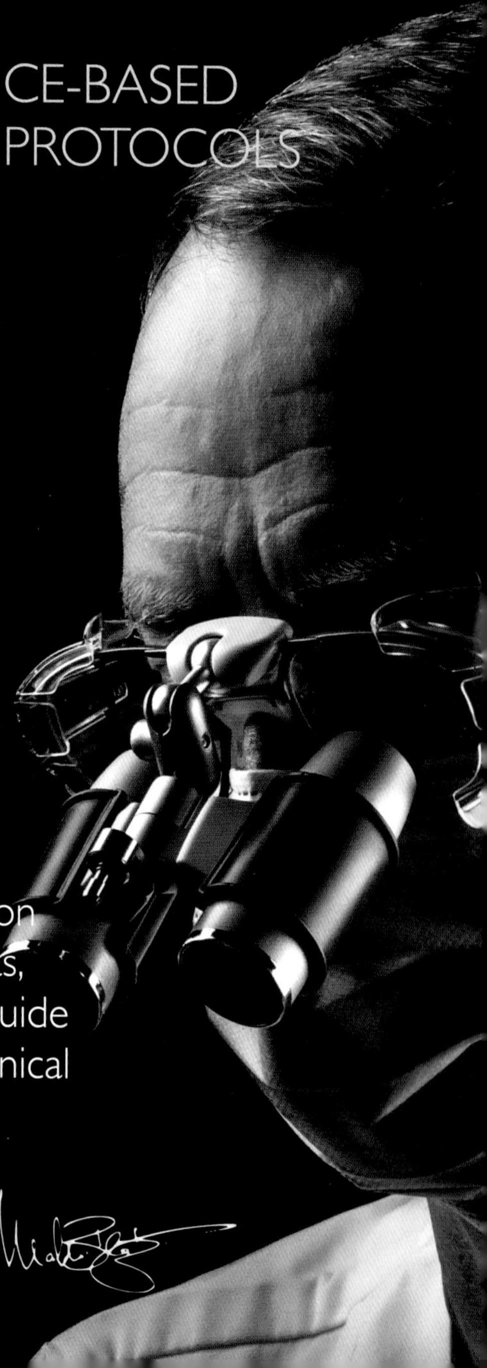

This series of pocketbooks, based on my social media posts, serves as a concise guide for contemporary clinical protocols and the supporting scientific evidence

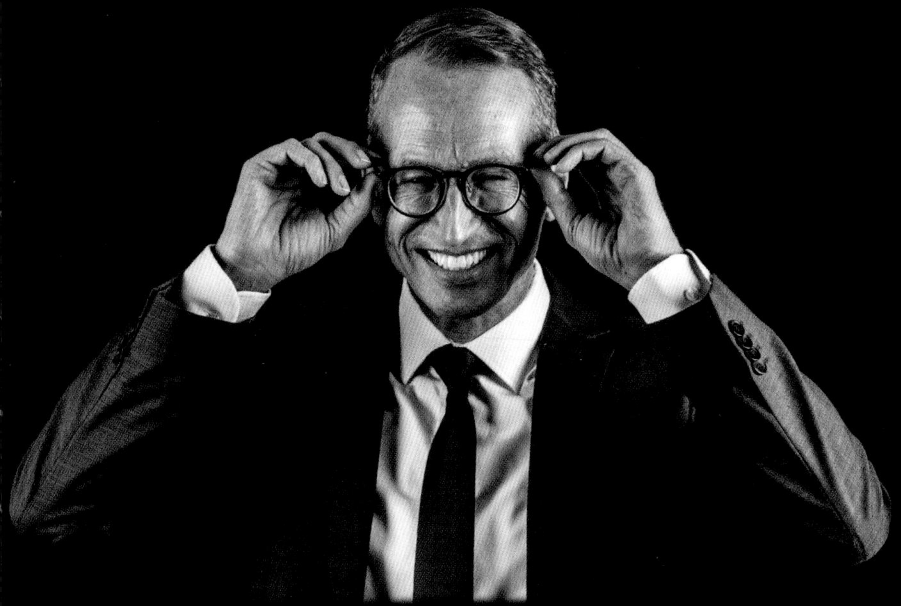

Prof Dr med dent habil Markus B. Blatz (DMD, PhD) is Professor of Restorative Dentistry, Chairman of the Department of Preventive and Restorative Sciences, and Assistant Dean for Digital Innovation and Professional Development at the University of Pennsylvania School of Dental Medicine in Philadelphia, Pennsylvania, USA. He graduated from the University of Freiburg, Germany, and received an additional Doctorate degree, Prosthodontics certificate, and the academic titles of Privatdozent and Professor from the same university. Prof Blatz has published and lectured extensively and is involved in numerous scientific dental journals as Editor-in-Chief, Associate Editor, and Editorial Board Member.

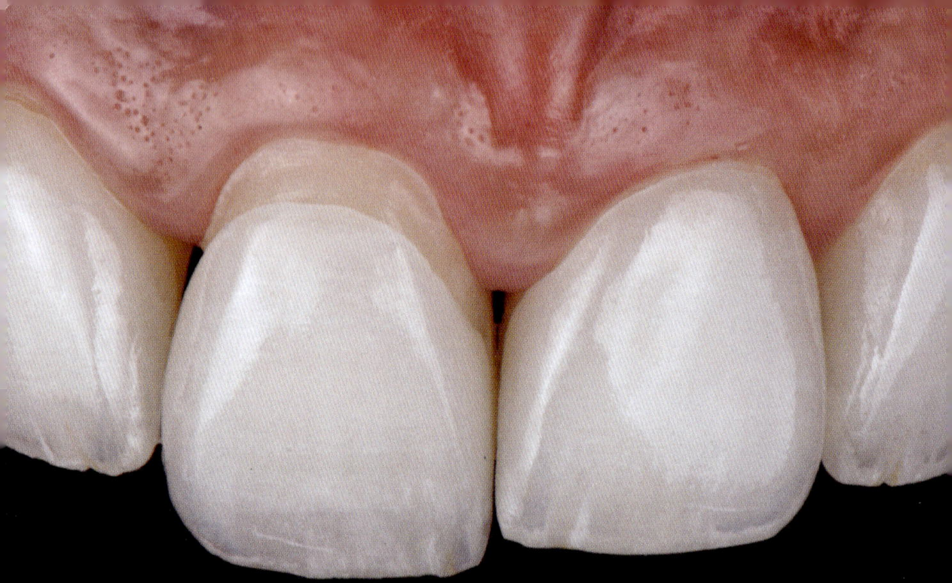

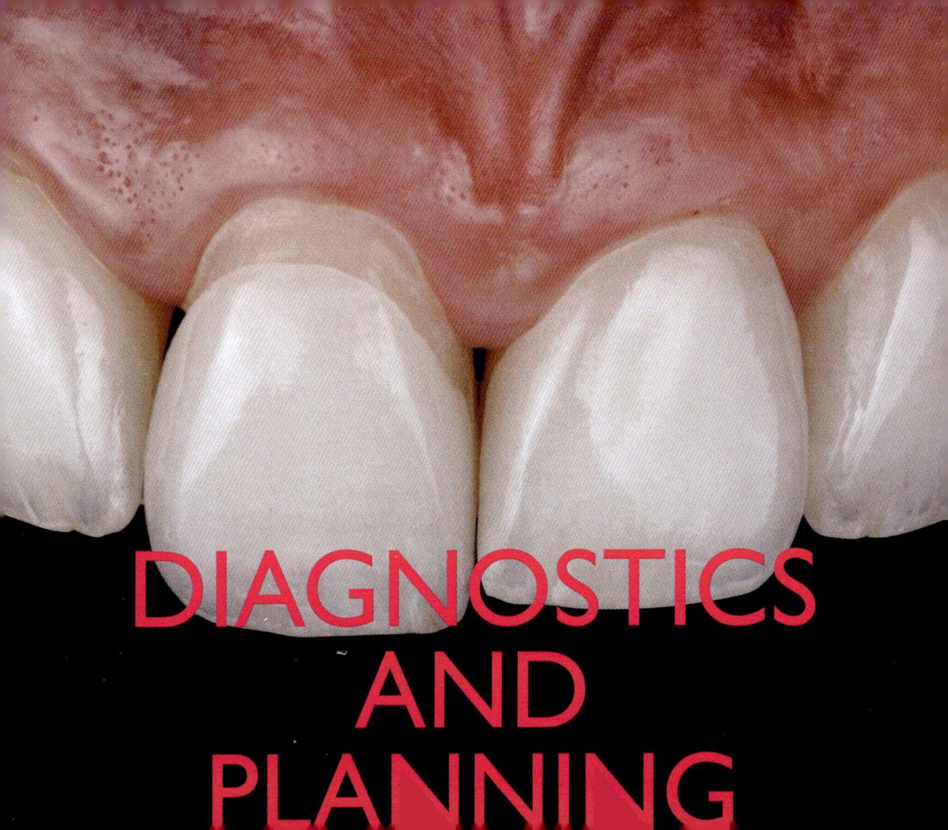

DIAGNOSTICS AND PLANNING

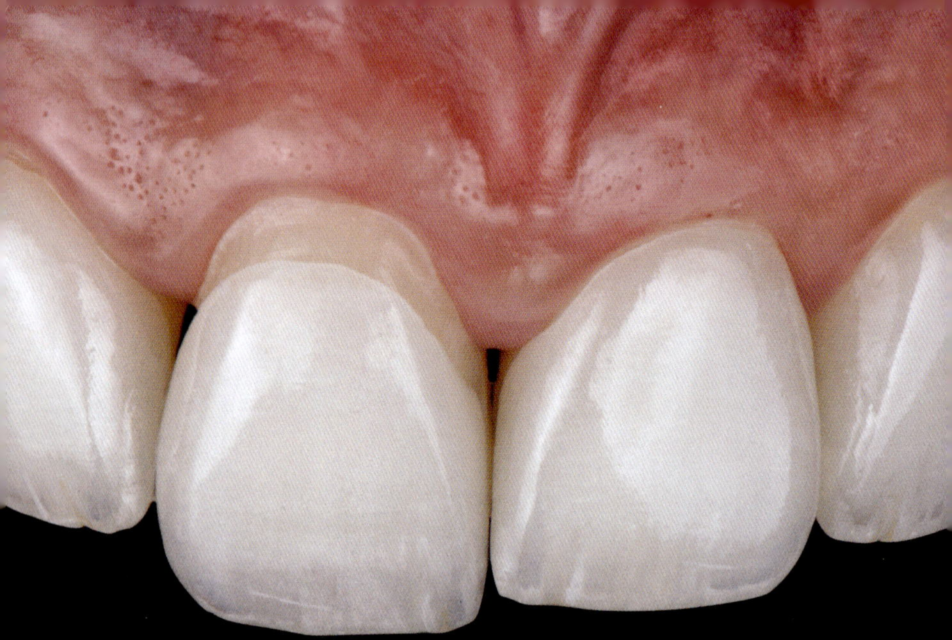

Our main responsibility as dentists is to help our patients keep their natural teeth as long as possible

For that, we have to be

MINIMALLY INVASIVE

MINIMALLY INVASIVE

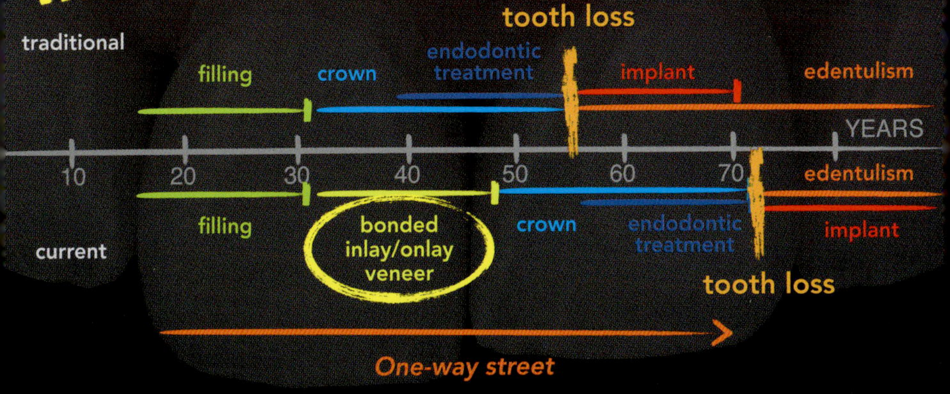

This graph illustrates the life cycle of a tooth undergoing restorative treatment

To move the "tooth loss" bar to the right, we must perform every step as minimally invasively as possible and apply current adhesive dentistry protocols and materials to stop the progression or "buy time" until the next, more invasive treatment step

Note that this is a one-way street

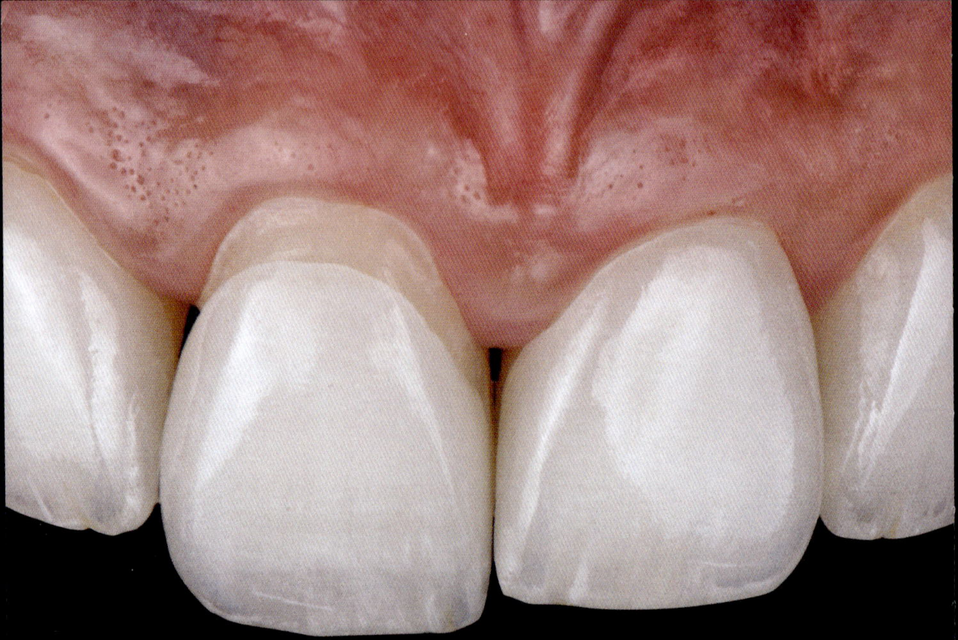

Resin-bonded laminate veneers are indicated when the possibilities of direct composite restorations are exceeded and a full-coverage crown is not (yet) needed

Their excellent clinical long-term success has been documented in numerous scientific studies and shown to largely depend on the clinician's expertise, technique, and handling

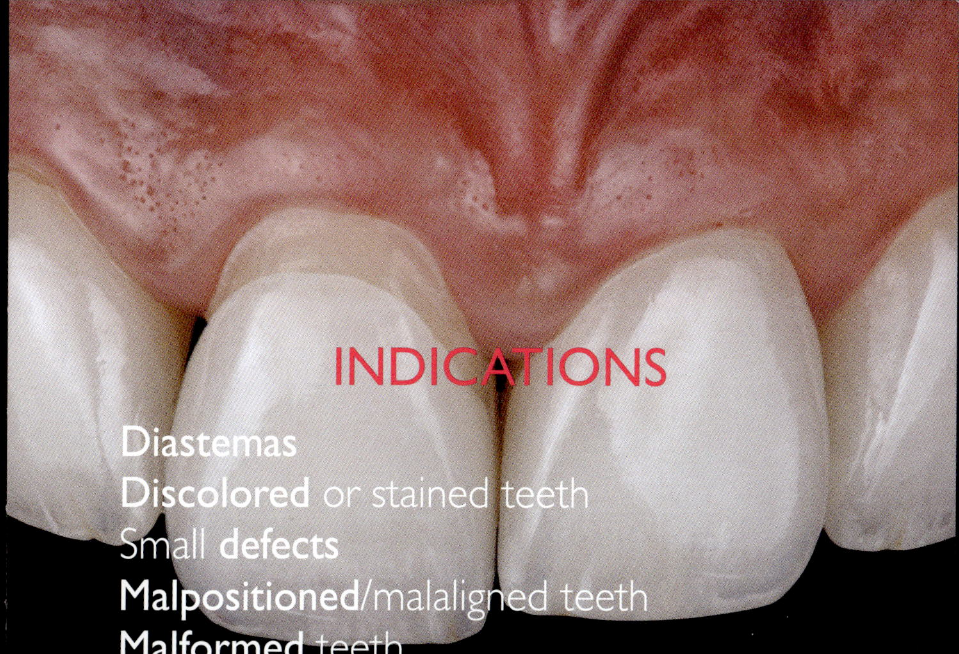

INDICATIONS

Diastemas
Discolored or stained teeth
Small **defects**
Malpositioned/malaligned teeth
Malformed teeth

CONTRAINDICATIONS

Heavy **bruxism**
Insufficient or **inadequate enamel**
Heavily **damaged** or **short** teeth
Oral **habits/malocclusion**
Severe **crowding** or malpositioning

Severely **malpositioned** teeth may require (prior) **orthodontic treatment**
Severely **discolored** teeth may require prior **tooth bleaching/whitening**

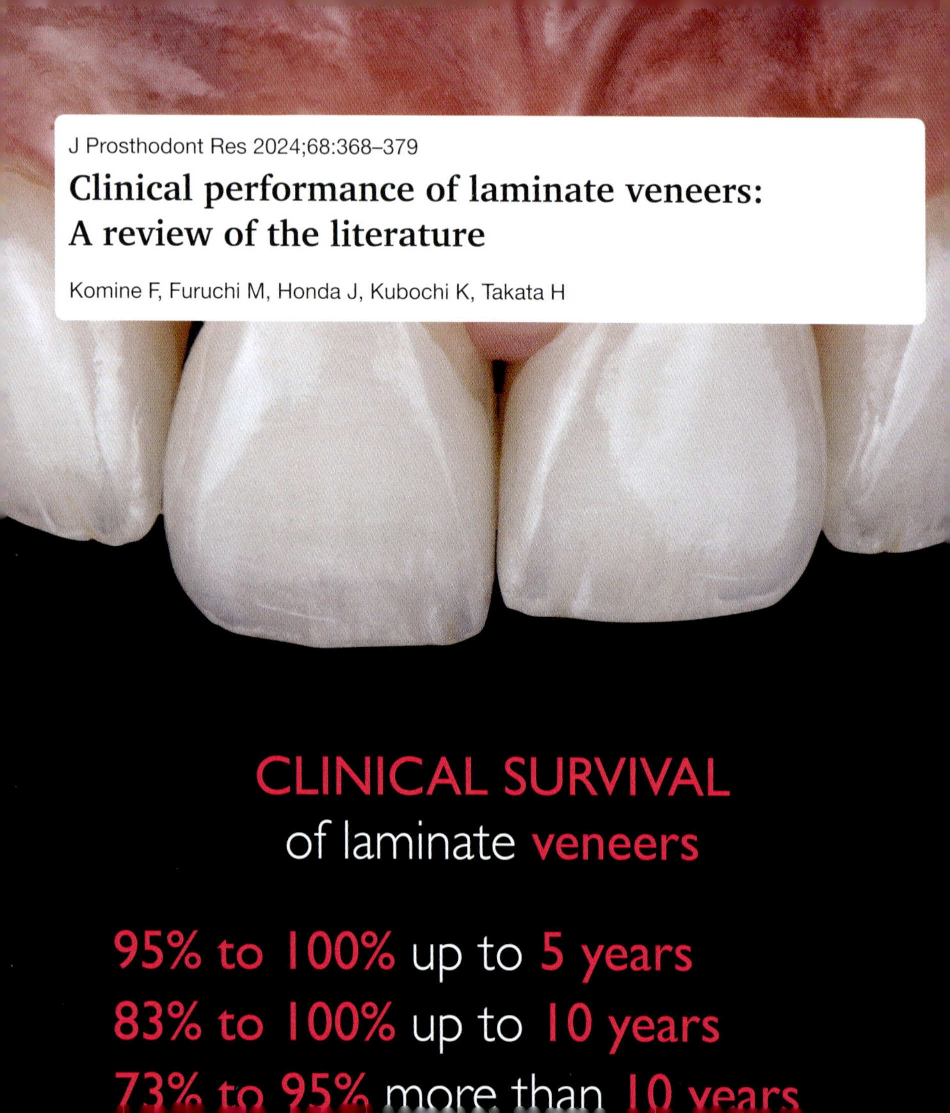
J Prosthodont Res 2024;68:368–379
Clinical performance of laminate veneers: A review of the literature
Komine F, Furuchi M, Honda J, Kubochi K, Takata H
CLINICAL SURVIVAL
of laminate veneers
95% to 100% up to 5 years
83% to 100% up to 10 years
73% to 95% more than 10 years

J Clin Med 2021;10:1074

Long-term survival and complication rates of porcelain laminate veneers in clinical studies: A systematic review

Alenezi A, Alsweed M, Alsidrani S, Chrcanovic BR

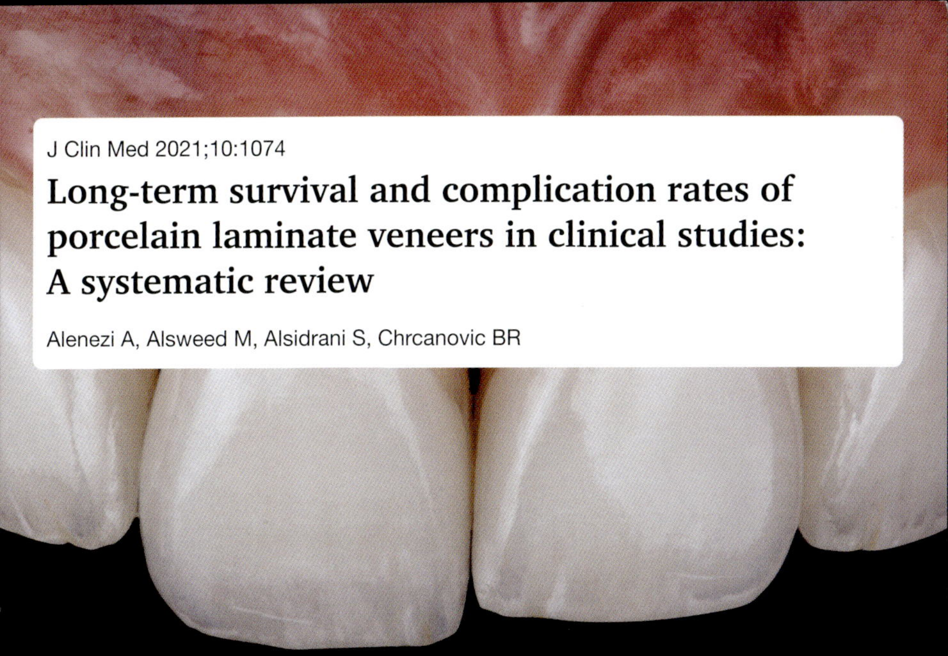

CLINICAL SURVIVAL
of laminate veneers

The 10-year estimated cumulative survival rate was 95.5%

J Dent Res 2019;98:1294–1304

Evolution of aesthetic dentistry

Blatz MB, Chiche G, Bahat O, Roblee R, Coachman C, Heymann H

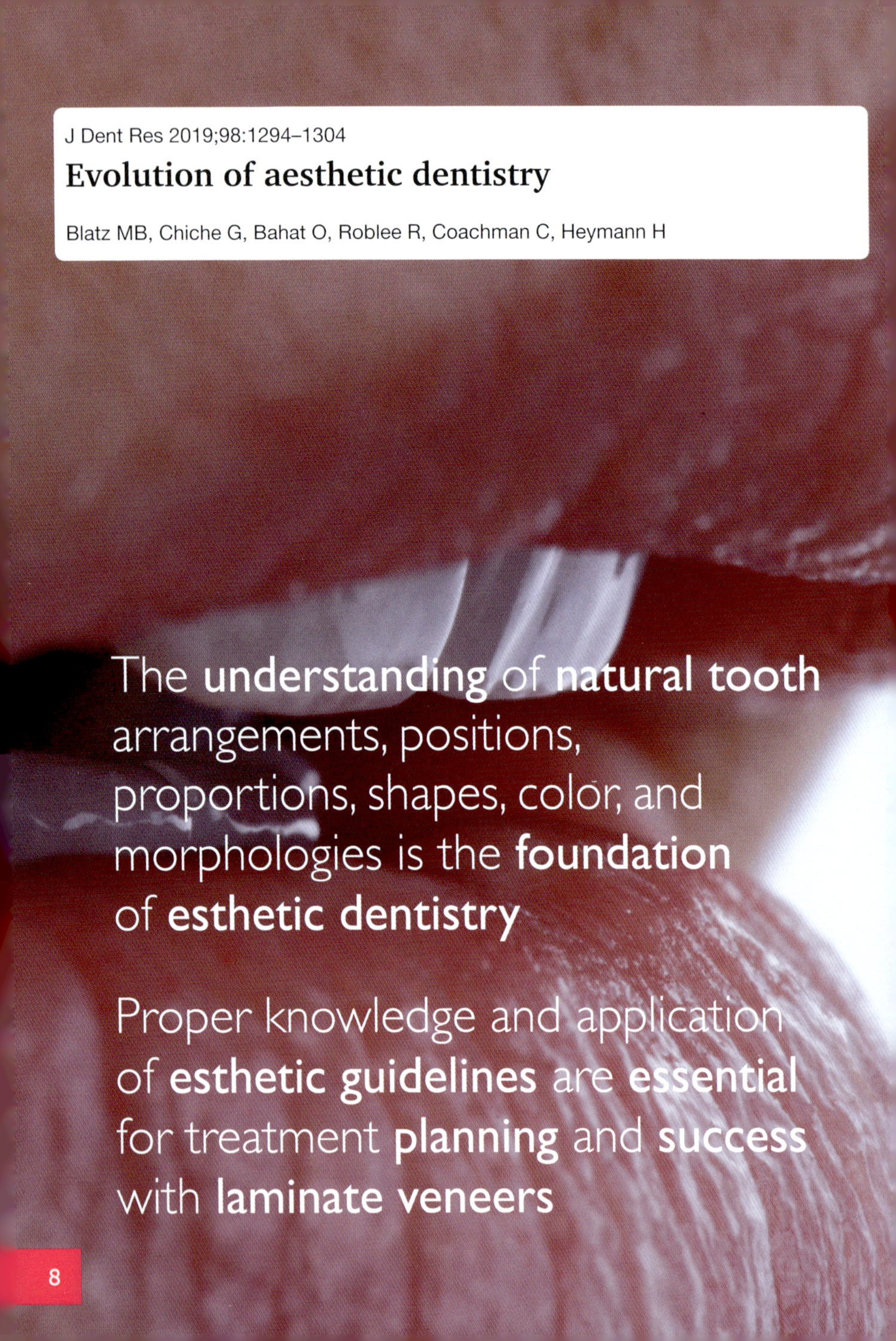

The **understanding** of **natural tooth** arrangements, positions, proportions, shapes, color, and morphologies is the **foundation** of **esthetic dentistry**

Proper knowledge and application of **esthetic guidelines** are **essential** for treatment **planning** and **success** with **laminate veneers**

Int J Periodontics Restorative Dent 2014;34:623–629

Analysis of select facial and dental esthetic parameters

Nold SL, Horvath SD, Stampf S, Blatz MB

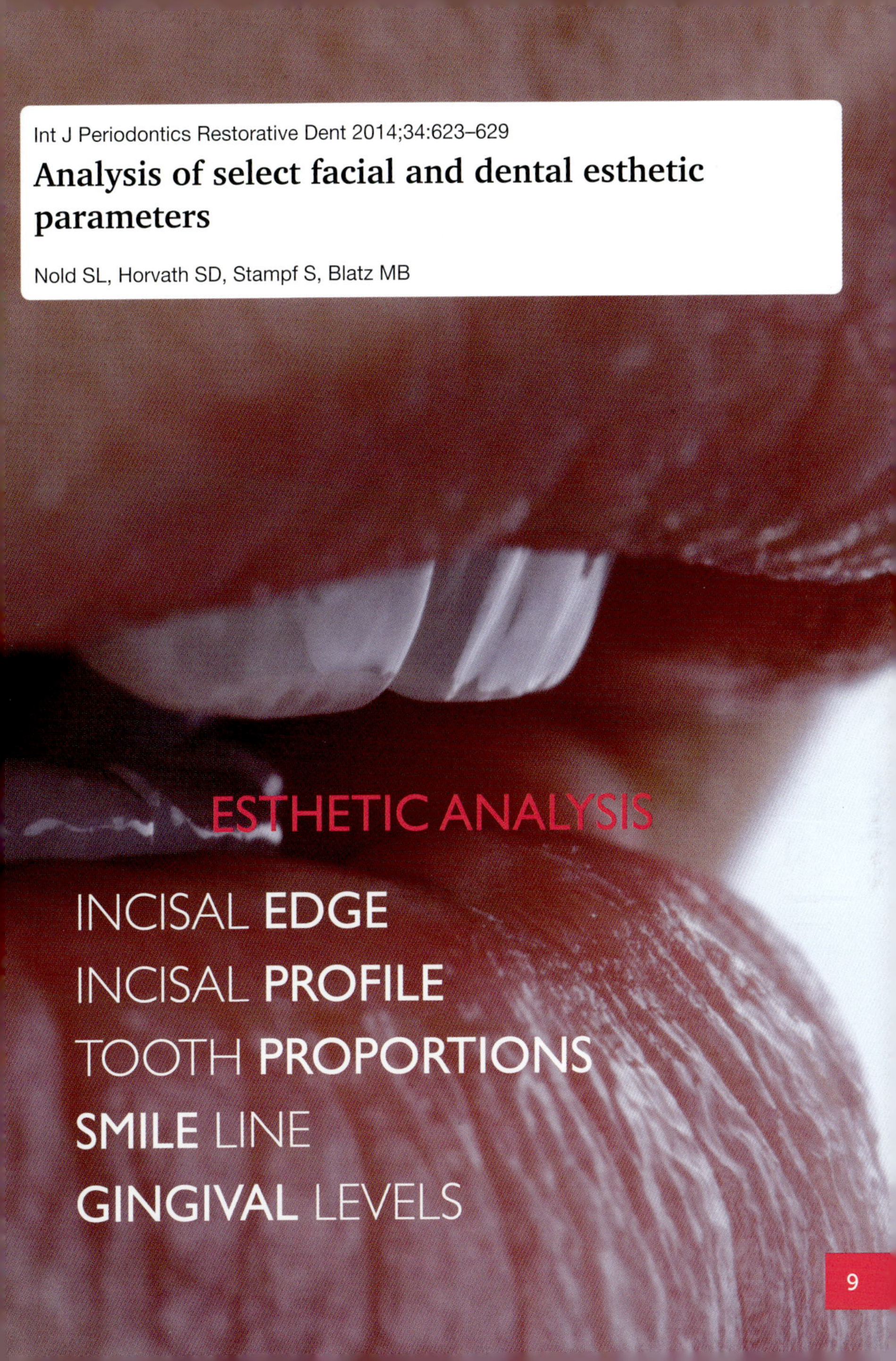

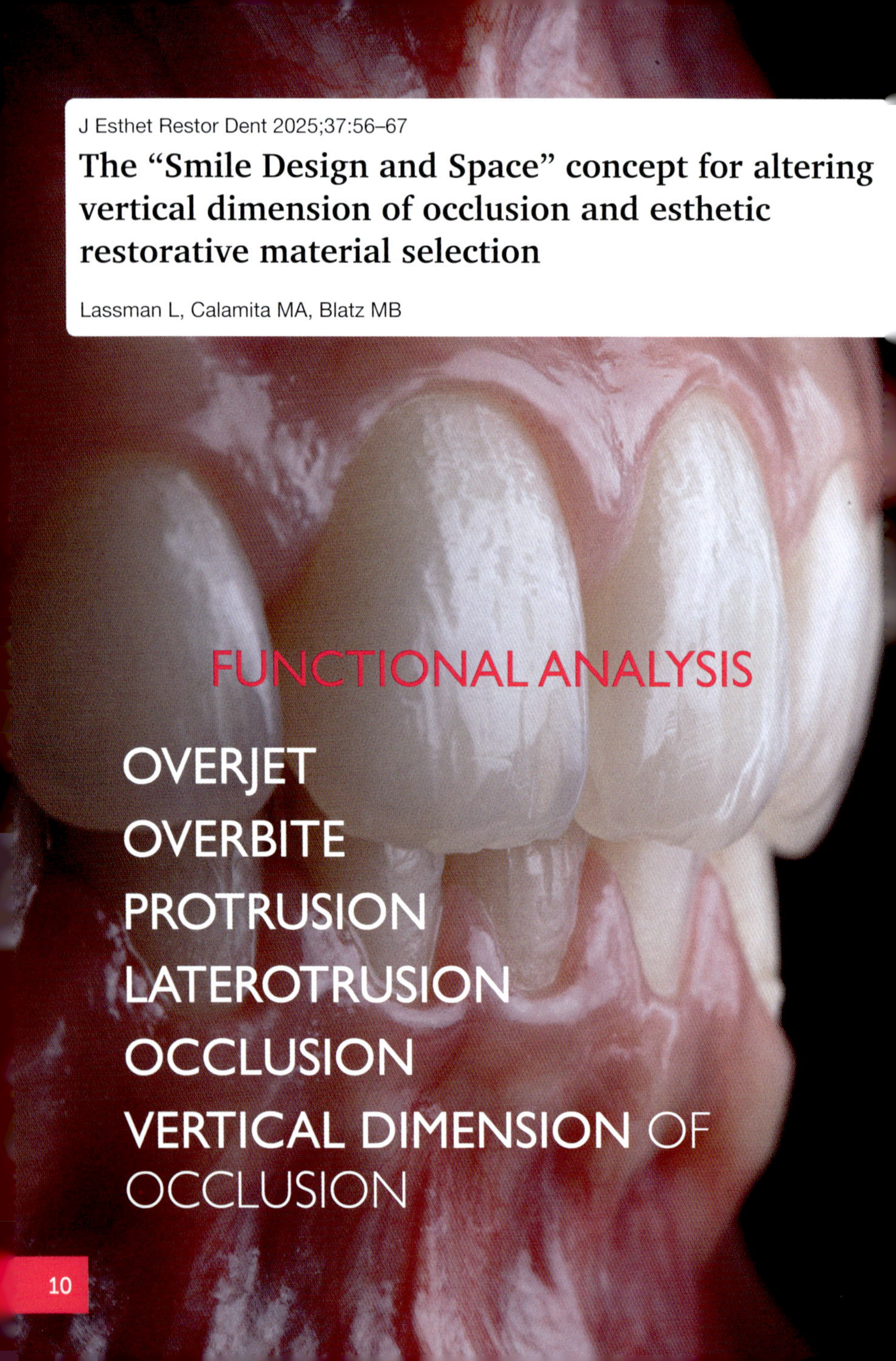

J Esthet Restor Dent 2025;37:56–67

The "Smile Design and Space" concept for altering vertical dimension of occlusion and esthetic restorative material selection

Lassman L, Calamita MA, Blatz MB

FUNCTIONAL ANALYSIS

OVERJET
OVERBITE
PROTRUSION
LATEROTRUSION
OCCLUSION
VERTICAL DIMENSION OF OCCLUSION

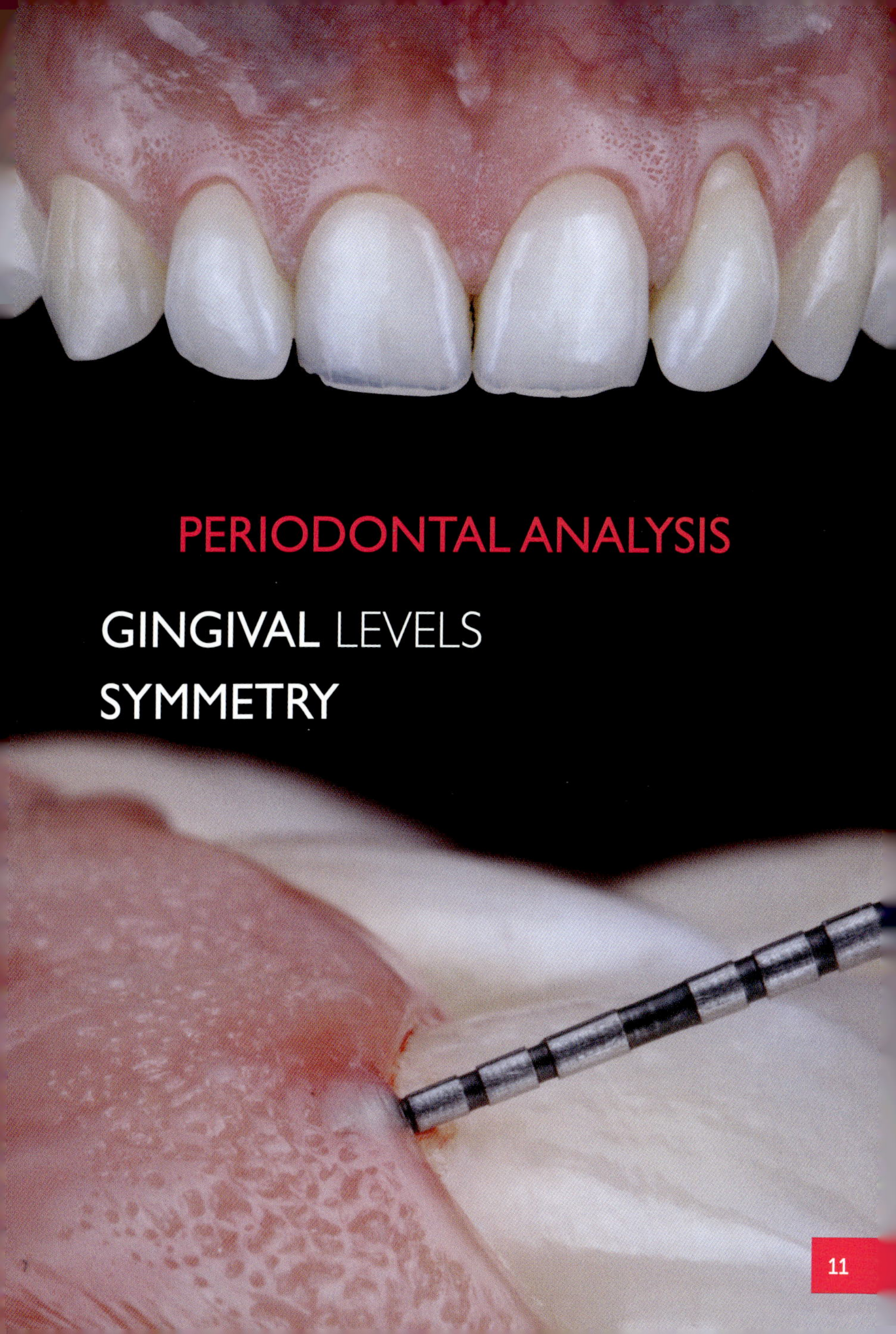

PERIODONTAL ANALYSIS

GINGIVAL LEVELS
SYMMETRY

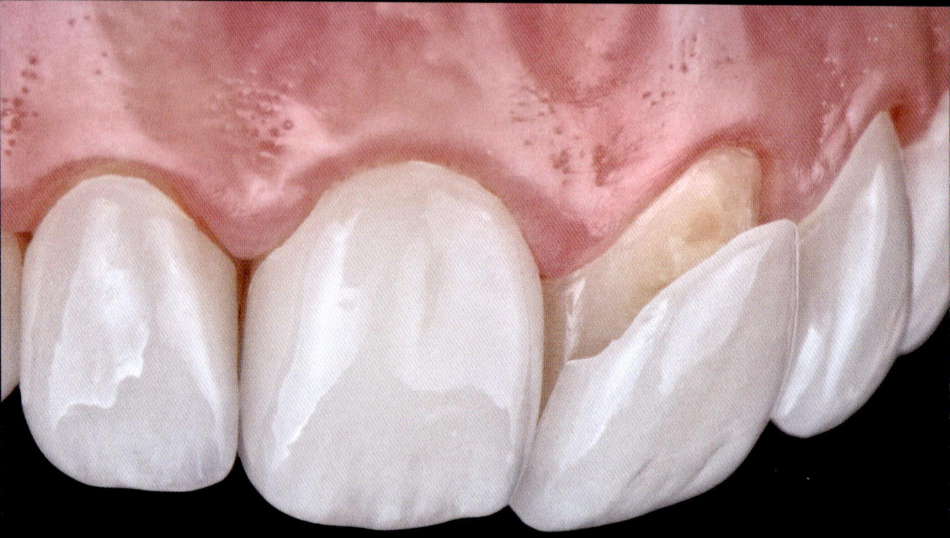

Detailed analyses and diagostics are essential for treatment planning and success with laminate veneers

The patient may require treatment before veneer restorations such as orthodontics, tooth whitening, periodontal surgery, and an increase of the vertical dimension of occlusion

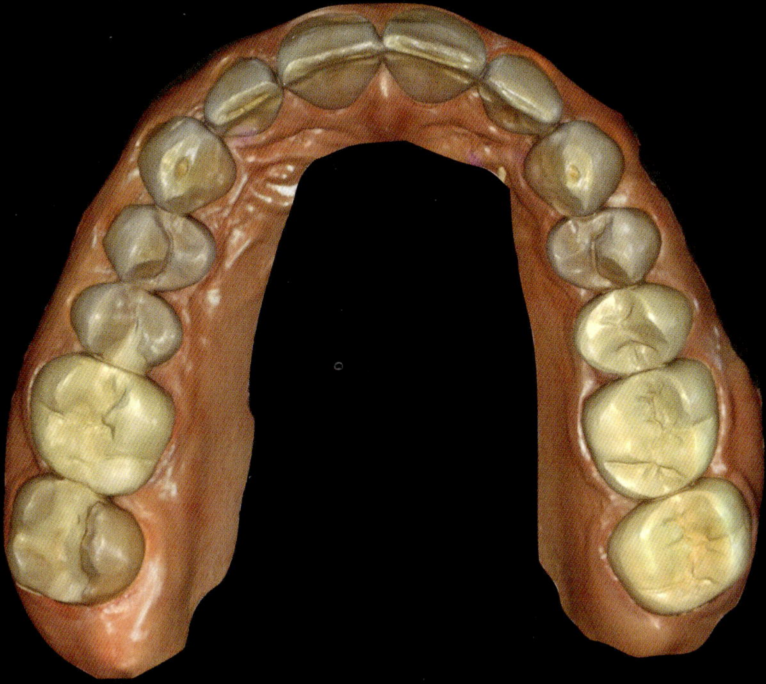

After thorough clinical and radiographic evaluations, preliminary impressions and fabrication of a digital or analog wax-up are indispensable

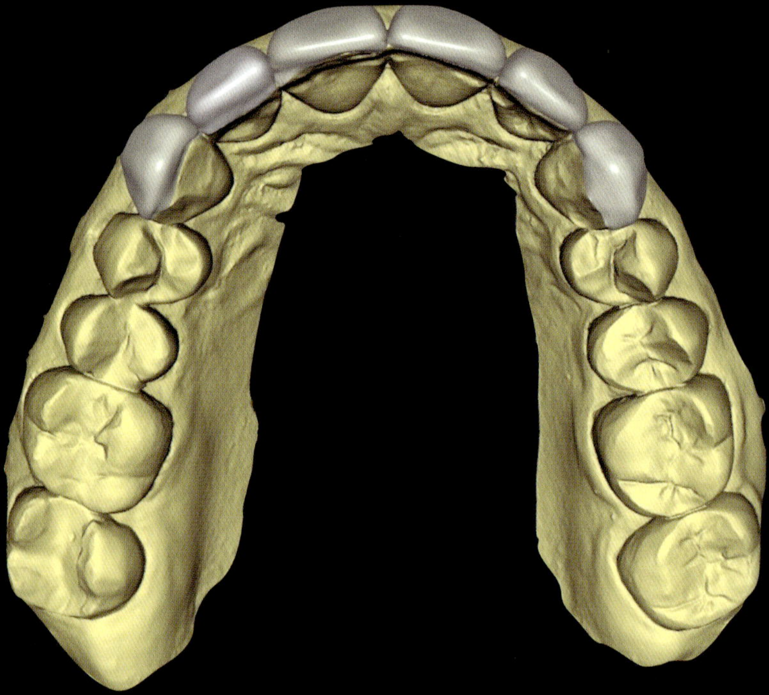

The wax-up determines the functional and esthetic tooth design and material selection for the definitive restorations as well as the amount of necessary tooth preparation

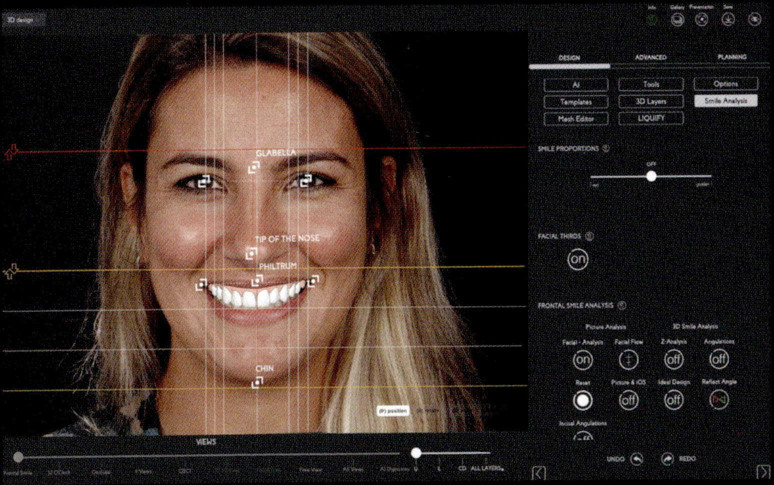

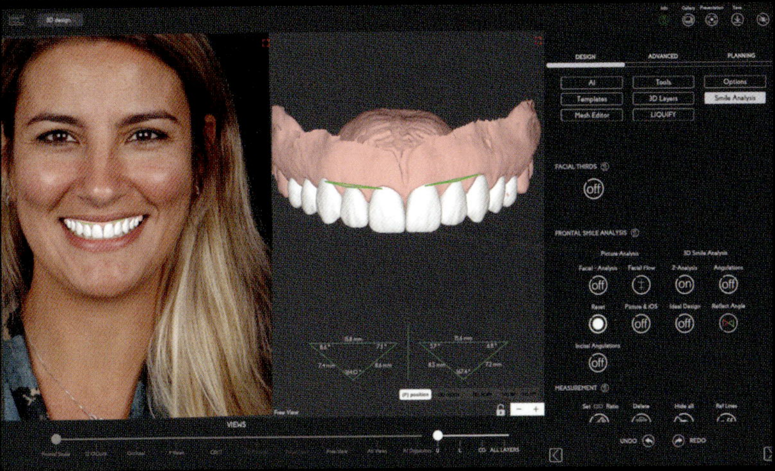

Digital Smile Design software, powered by **artificial intelligence**, facilitates precise **esthetic** and **functional analyses** and **planning**

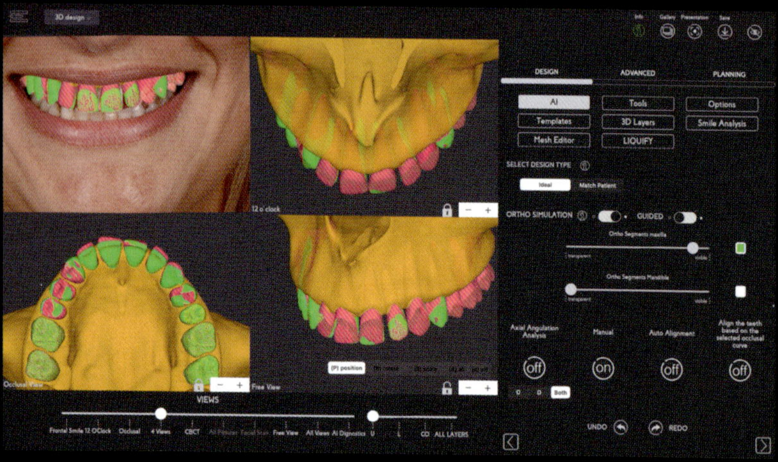

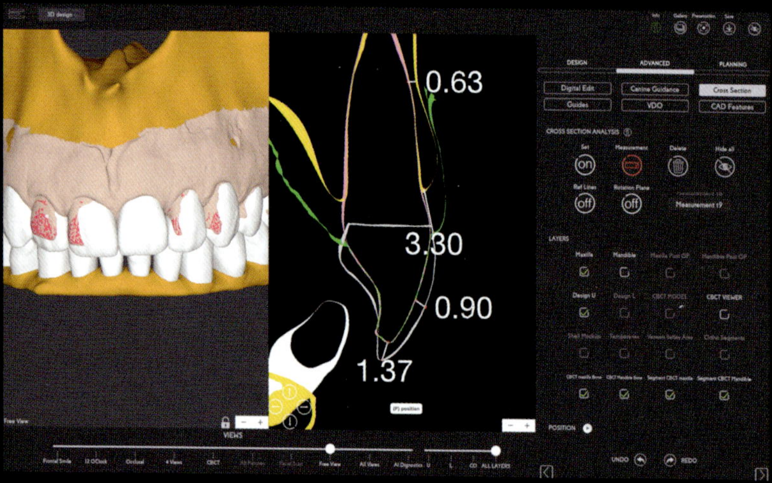

Possible **orthodontic** treatment and required **restoration dimensions** can be **precisely calculated** and **determined**

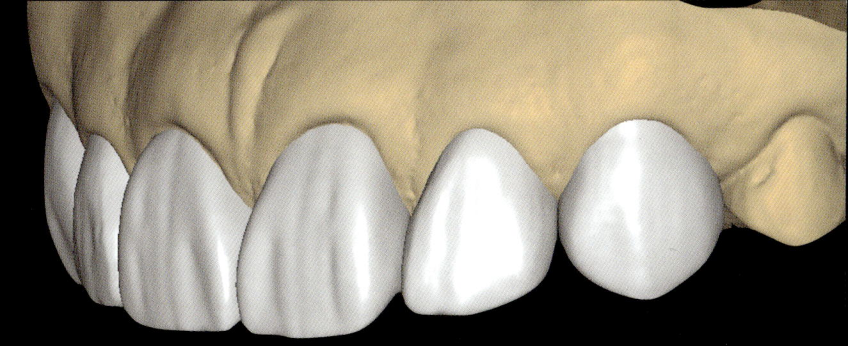

The **wax-up**, analog or digital, must be **tried in** with a **mock-up**, and all **esthetic** and **functional** parameters **verified in the mouth before** proceeding with **treatment**

The optimized **wax-up** serves as a **preparation guide** and **blueprint** for the **definitive restorations**

For **subtractive** cases that require **substantial changes**, an **additive "motivational" mock-up** may be made to give the patient "an idea"

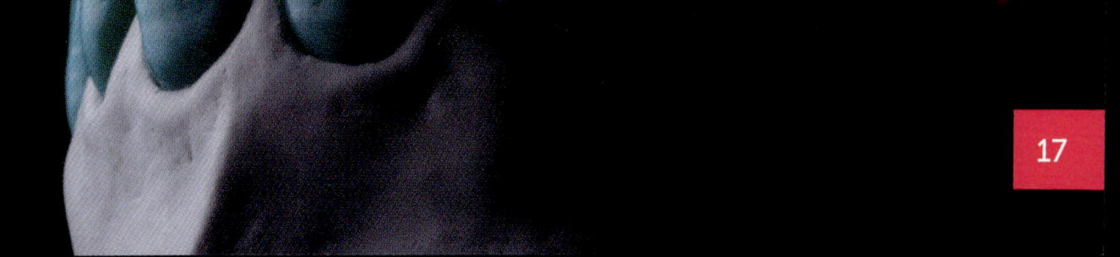

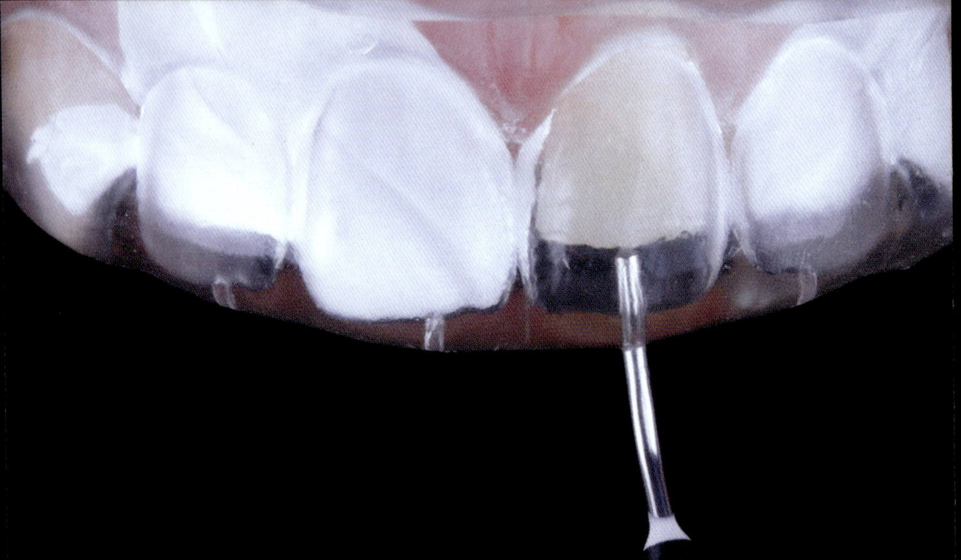

MOCK-UP TYPES

Indirect: handmade, milled or 3D-printed in the laboratory

Direct: injection technique or applied directly on the teeth with a polyvinyl siloxane (PVS) index or clear retainer

Materials: acrylics, BisGMA, (flowable) resin-based composites

Select the type of mock-up based on the **duration of the trial phase** (for one appointment or a longer time?)

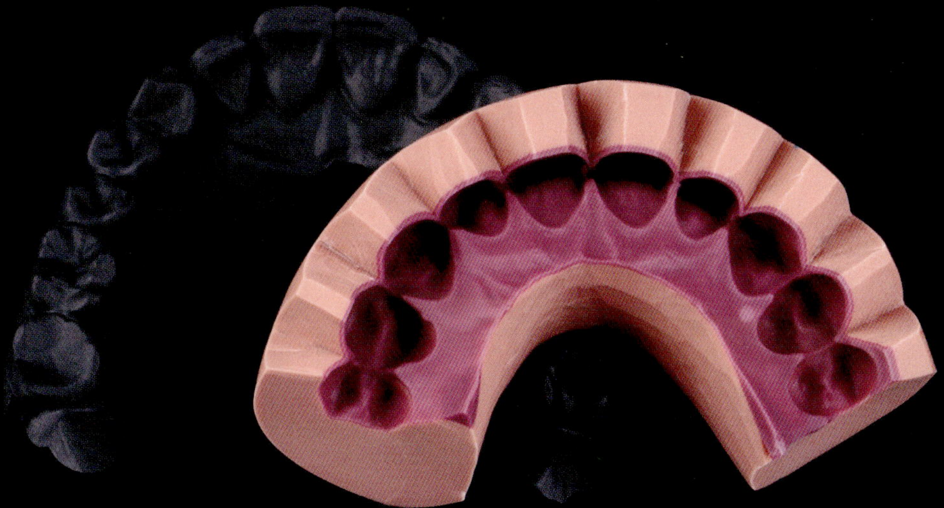

DIRECT MOCK-UP with INDEX

Make a **stone cast** or **3D-printed model** from the wax-up and a **PVS index**

Cut the index along the **gingival margins** for easy **removal** of excess material after intraoral placement

Fill the **PVS index** with a material of your choice (acrylic, BisGMA, composite) and **insert it over the teeth** to make an intraoral **mock-up**

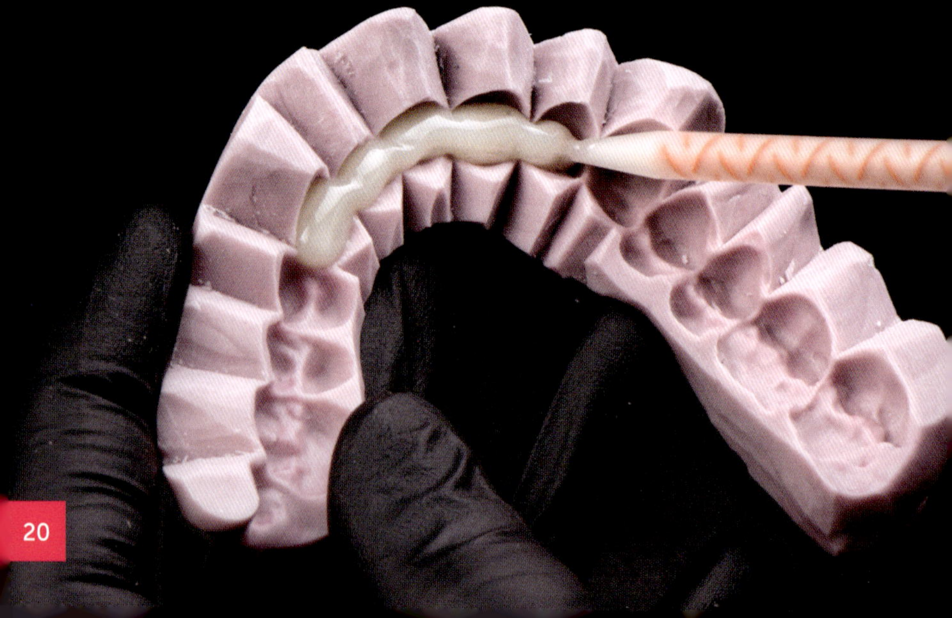

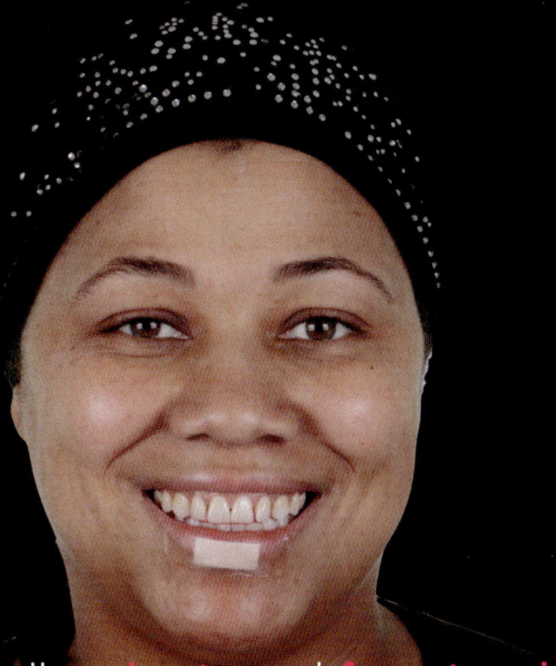

Verify all esthetic and functional parameters with a mock-up

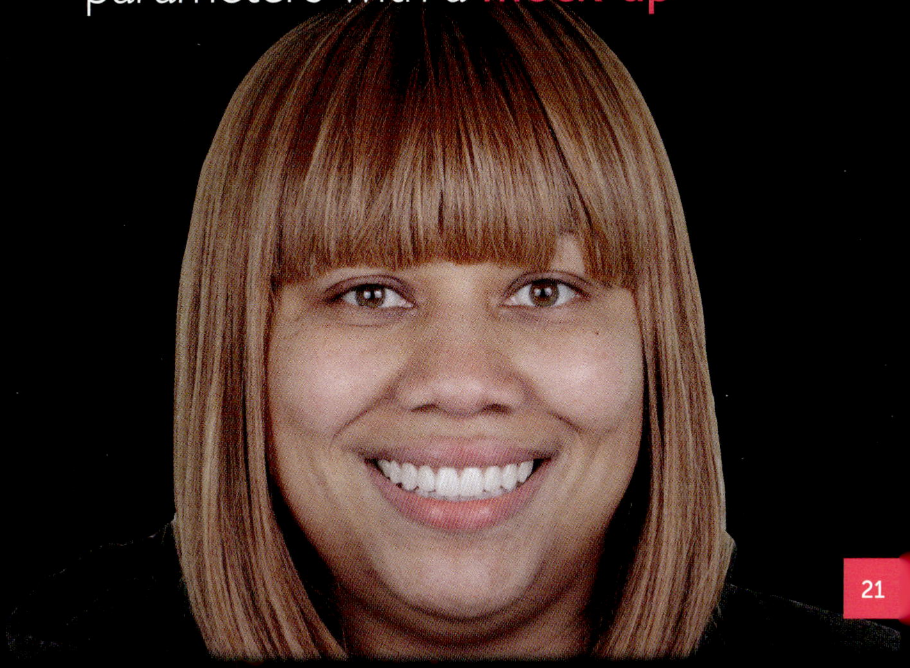

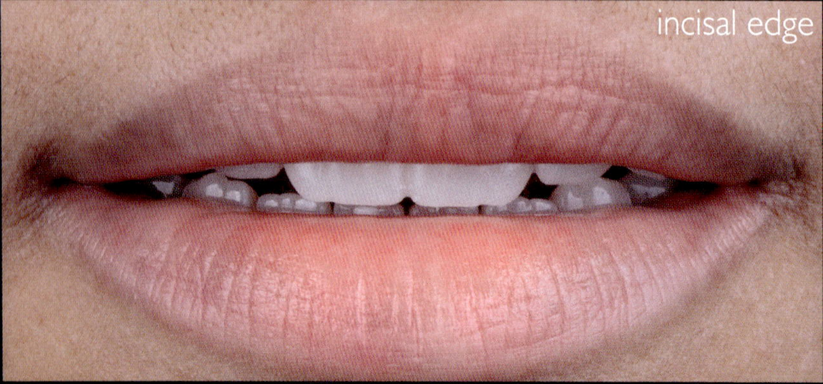

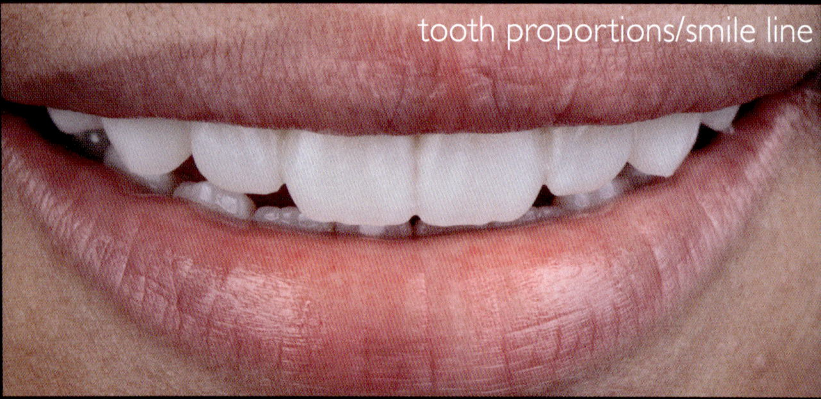

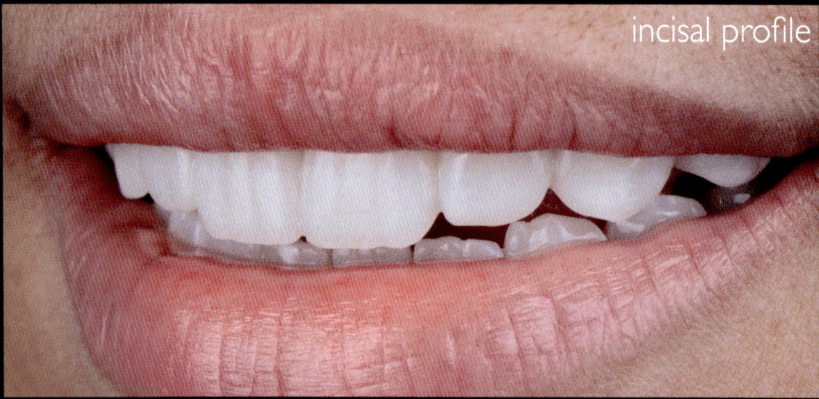

Verify **esthetics and function**

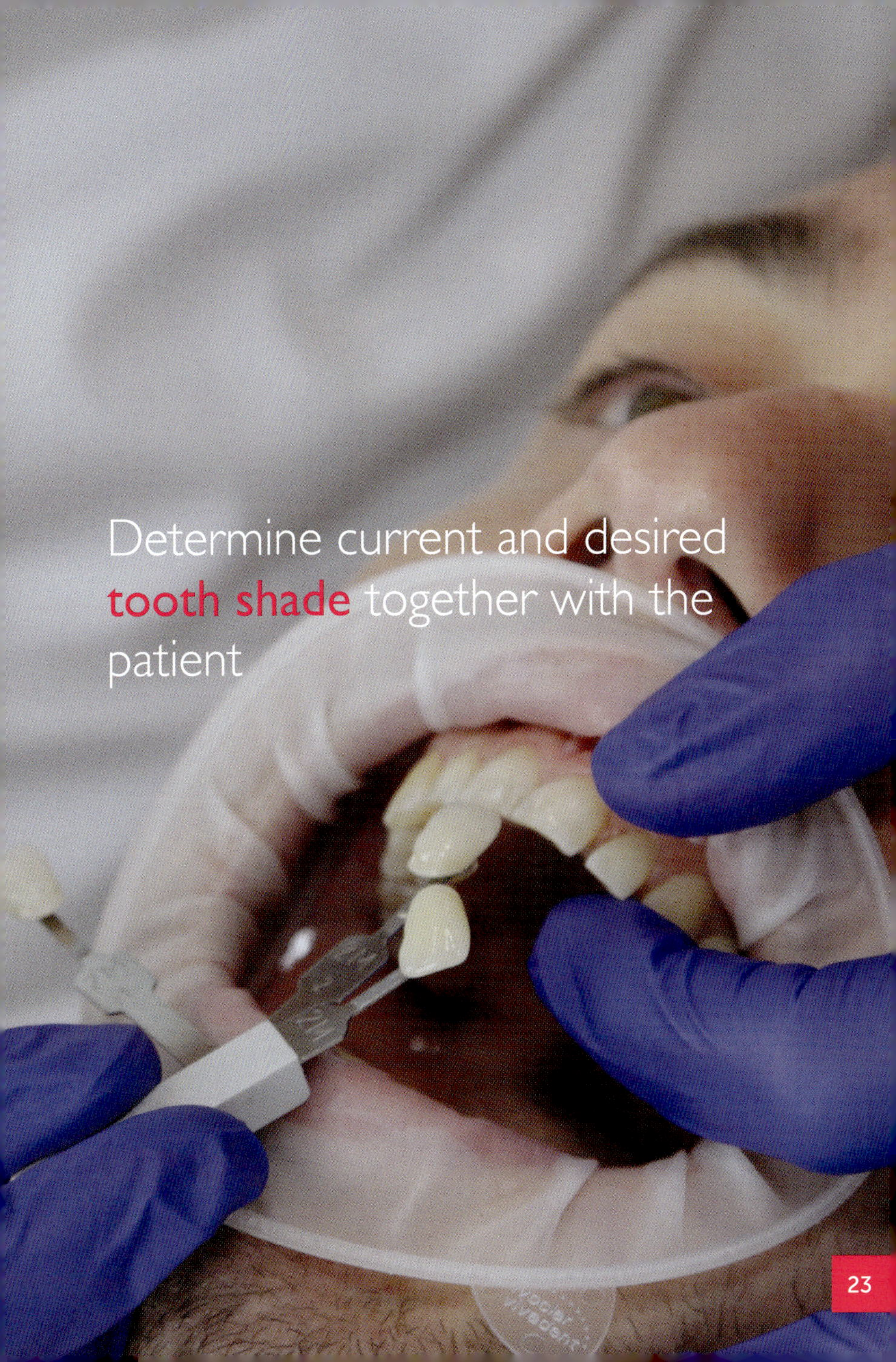

Determine current and desired **tooth shade** together with the patient

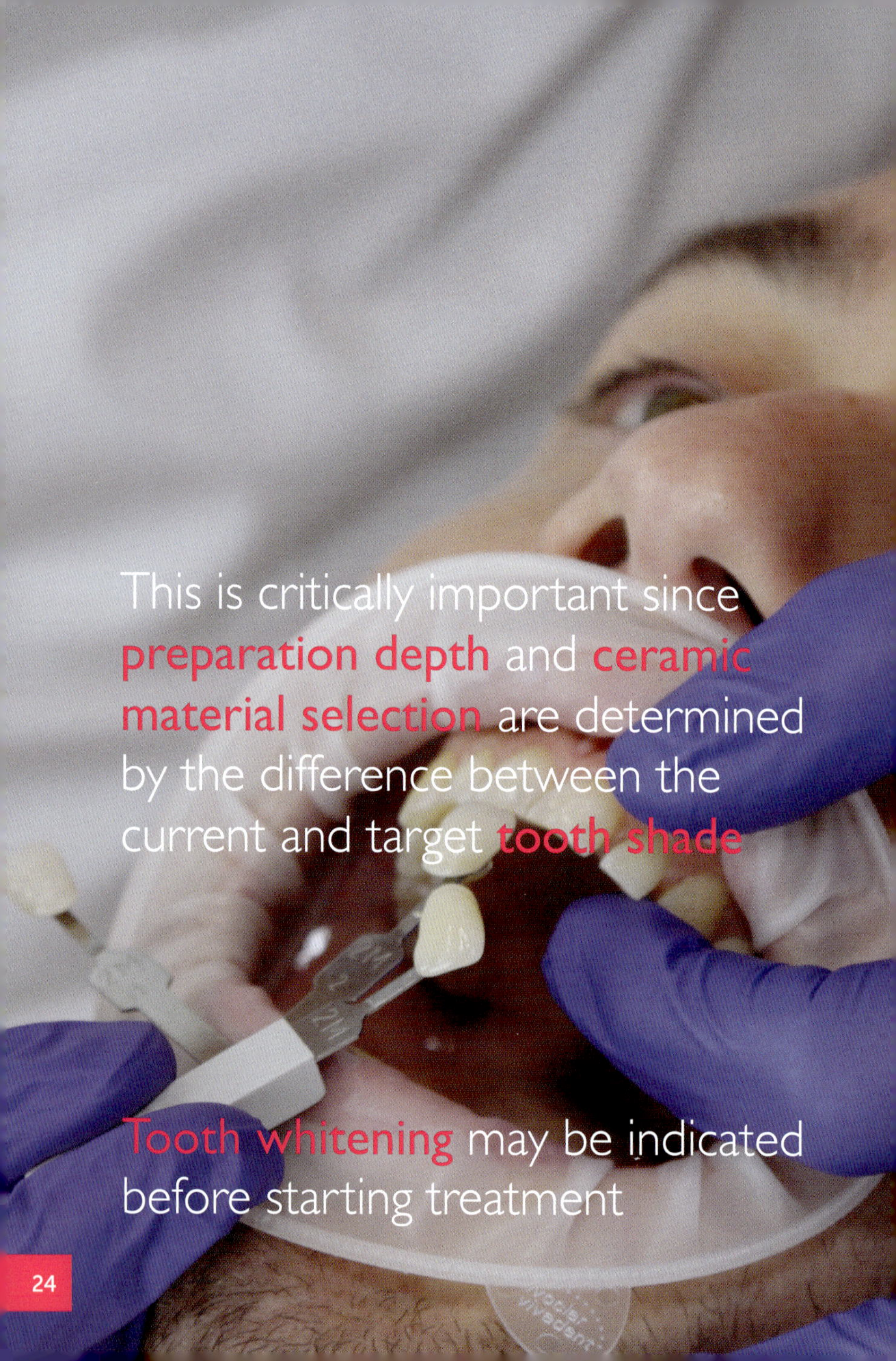

This is critically important since **preparation depth** and **ceramic material selection** are determined by the difference between the current and target **tooth shade**

Tooth whitening may be indicated before starting treatment

DIAGNOSTICS AND PLANNING

CHEAT SHEET

1. Clinical and radiographic evaluation and diagnostics
2. Esthetic and functional analyses
3. Preliminary intraoral scans or conventional impressions
4. Digital Smile Design or analog wax-up
5. Try-in of the digital or analog wax-up with the mock-up
   Verify esthetics and function
6. Determine current and desired tooth shade

PREPARATION AND IMPRESSION

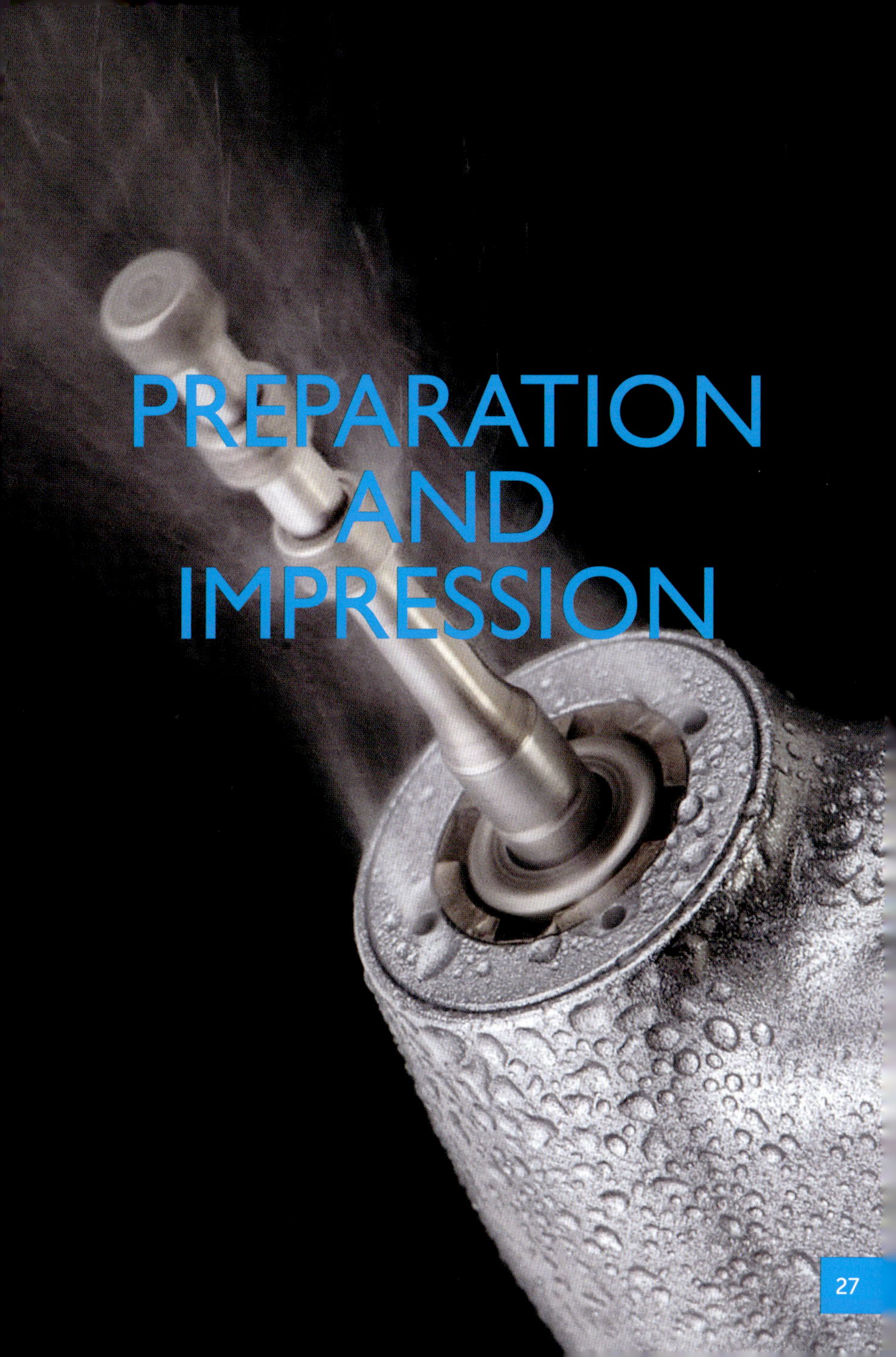

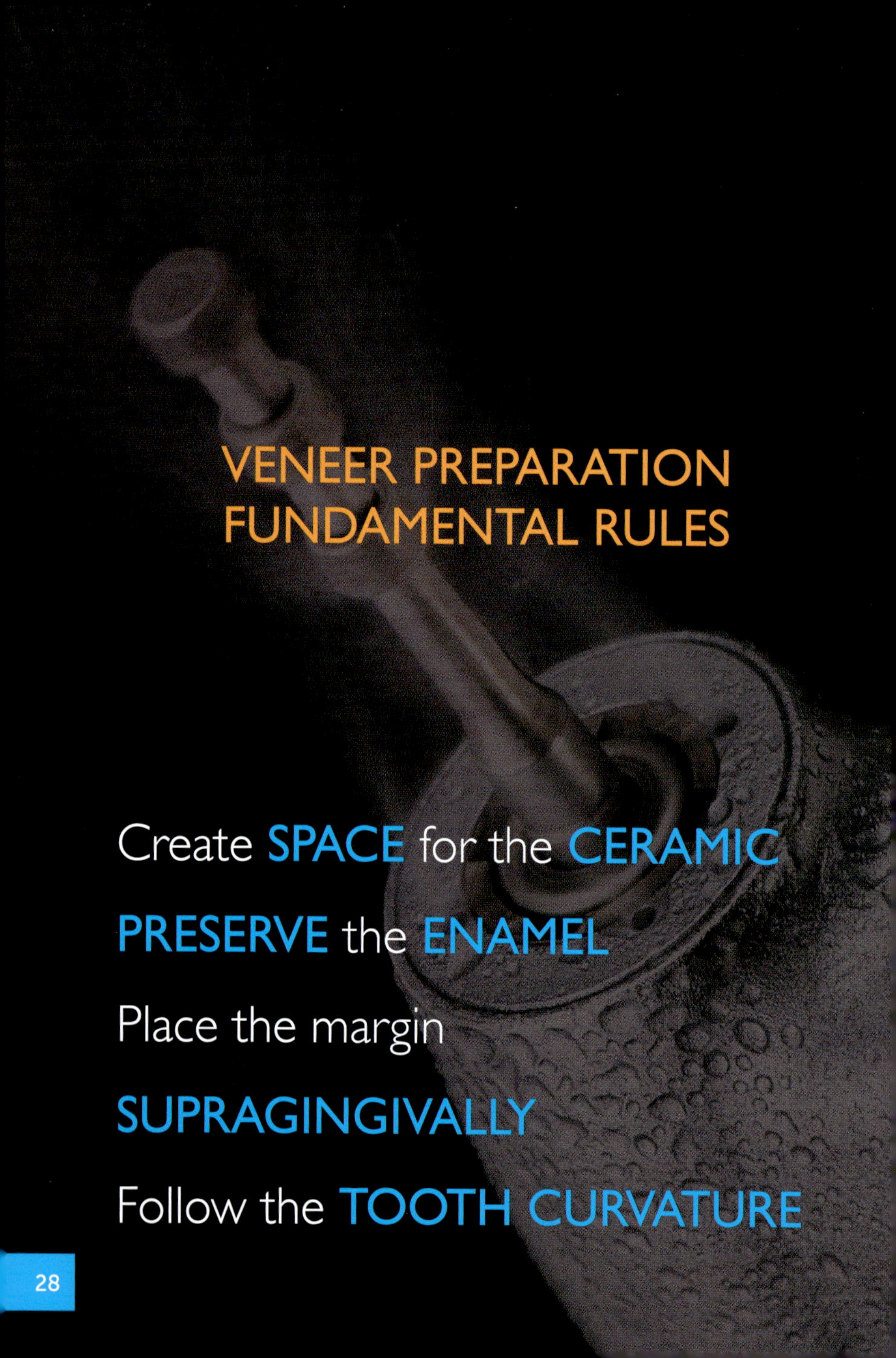

VENEER PREPARATION FUNDAMENTAL RULES

Create SPACE for the CERAMIC

PRESERVE the ENAMEL

Place the margin

SUPRAGINGIVALLY

Follow the TOOTH CURVATURE

The primary purpose of veneer preparation is to create space for the ceramic (or other indirect material) and to remove undercuts to facilitate the insertion of an indirect restoration

Unless you have a (3D-printed) preparation guide from your wax-up, start by preparing with a depth cutting bur into a mock-up (from the wax-up) to preserve as much enamel as possible, and remove tooth structure only where necessary

Some teeth may need only limited or no preparation, depending on the smile design, planned tooth size, shade, and morphology as well as minimum thickness requirements for the selected ceramic material

The typical space needed for feldspathic ceramics is 0.6 to 0.7 mm
Be sure to follow manufacturer instructions for minimum thickness requirements for other ceramic materials

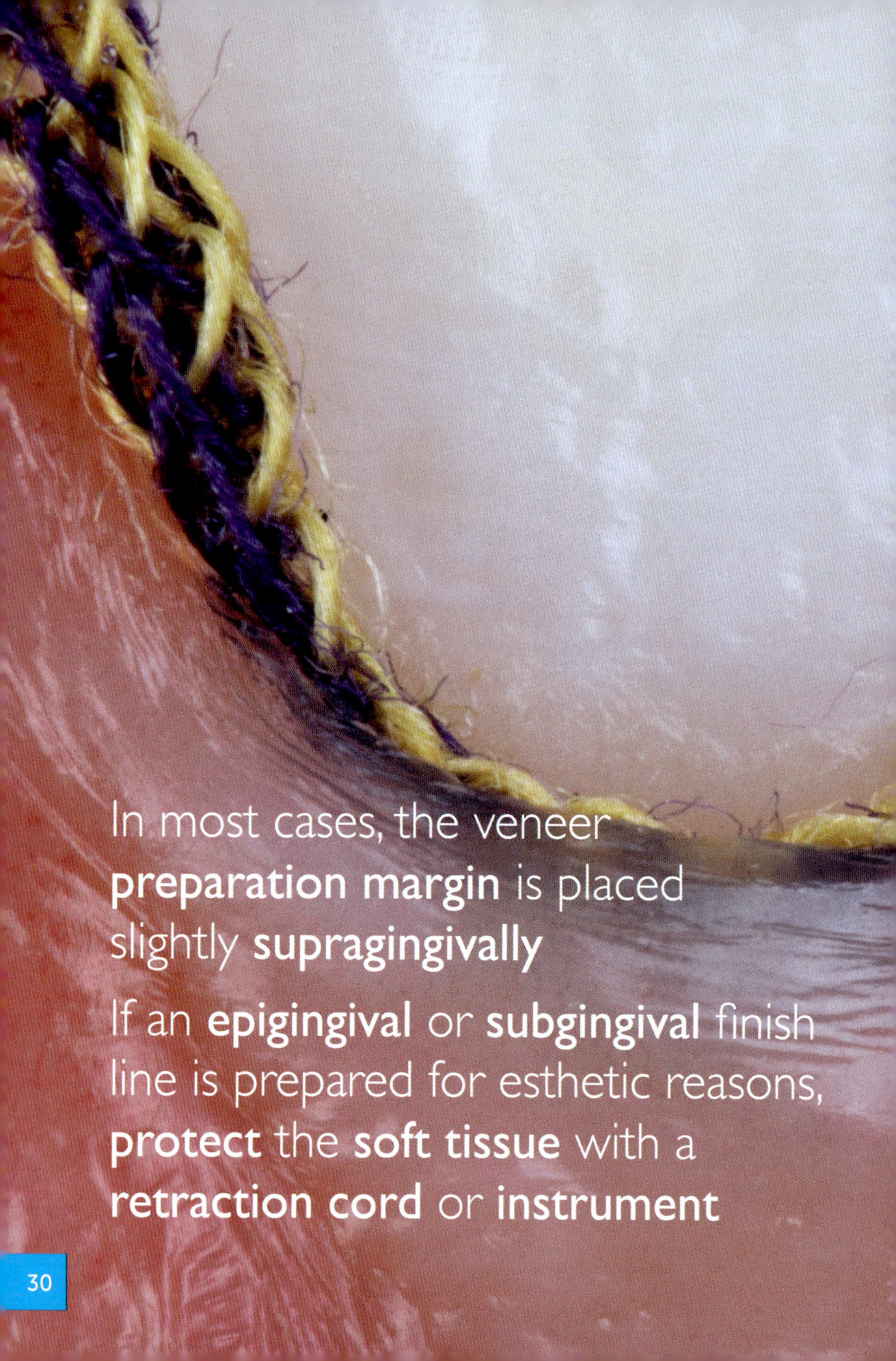

In most cases, the veneer **preparation margin** is placed slightly **supragingivally**

If an **epigingival** or **subgingival** finish line is prepared for esthetic reasons, **protect** the **soft tissue** with a **retraction cord** or **instrument**

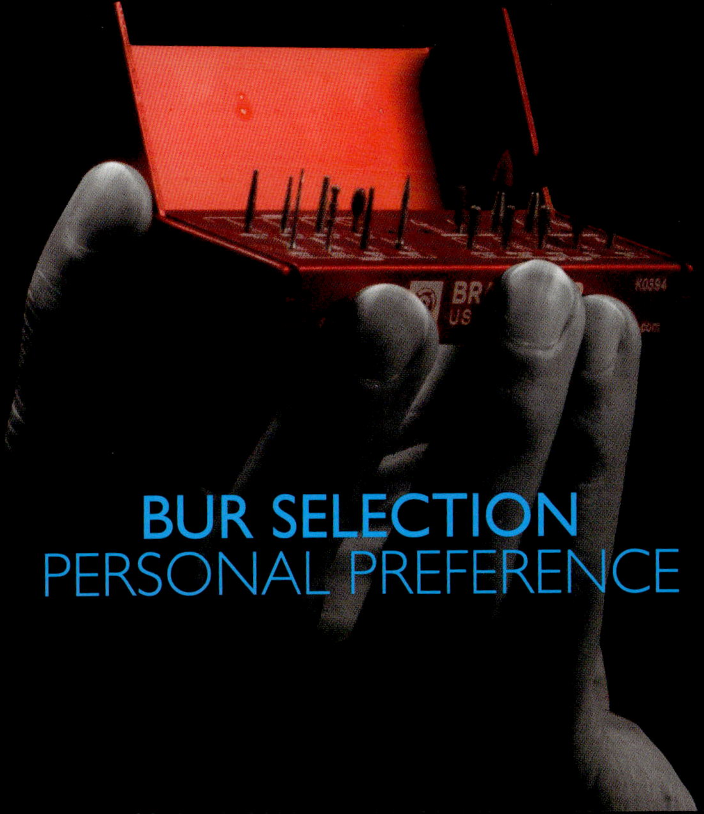

BUR SELECTION
PERSONAL PREFERENCE

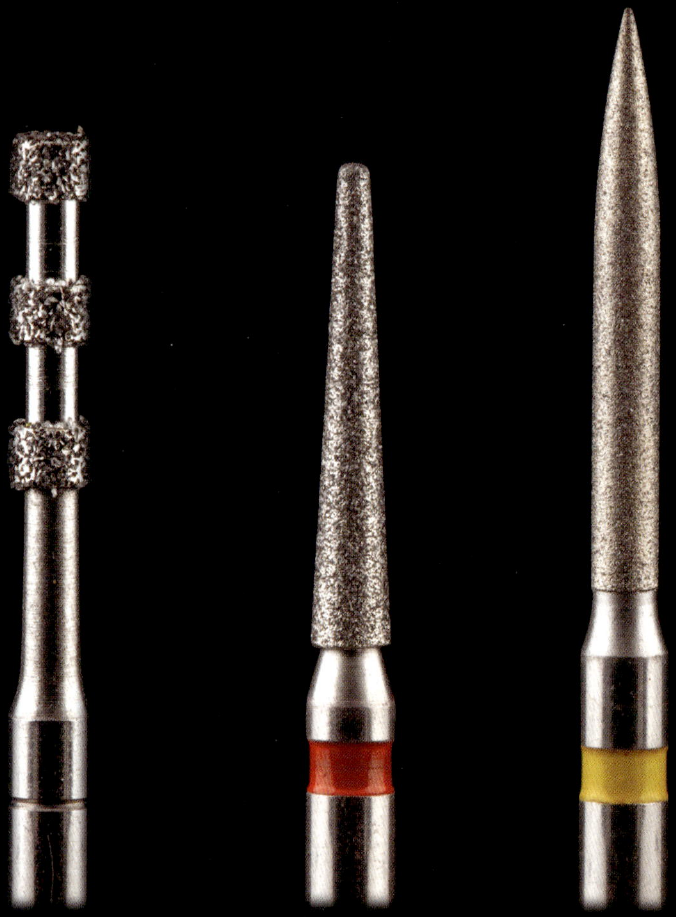

Medium depth cutter 0.3 mm

Fine round-end taper 016

Extra-fine flame 012

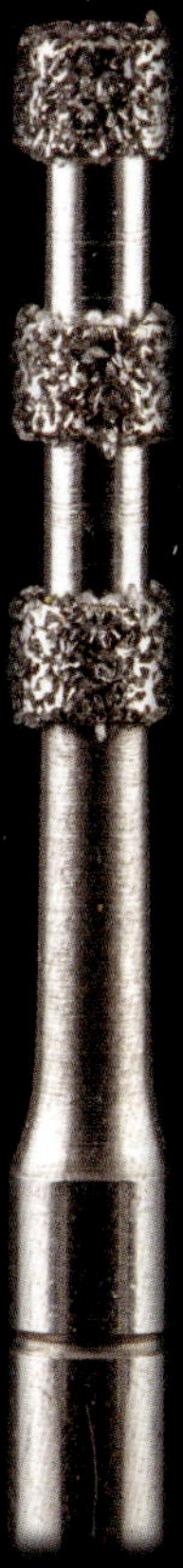
Medium depth cutter
0.3 mm

Depth cutter

Limit the choice to a **0.3-mm** depth cutter as a 0.5-mm one may lead to "overprepping" of the enamel, especially in the cervical areas where the enamel is thin

Round-end taper

This is for pretty much **EVERYTHING**…

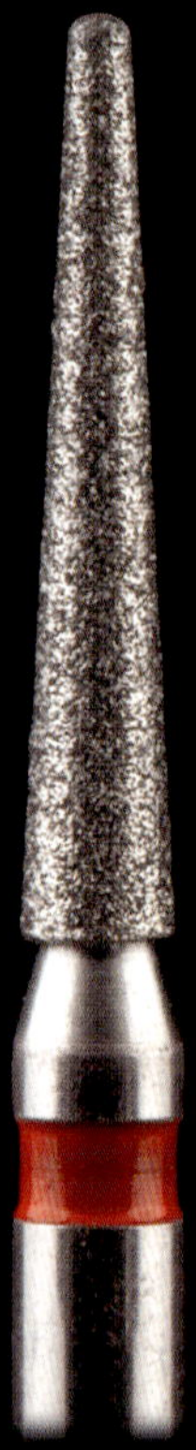

Fine round-end taper
016

NOTE: Do **not** go **beyond the tip** of the bur to avoid a **"lip"**

If a slight "ledge" is created, remove with a hand instrument or end-cutting bur

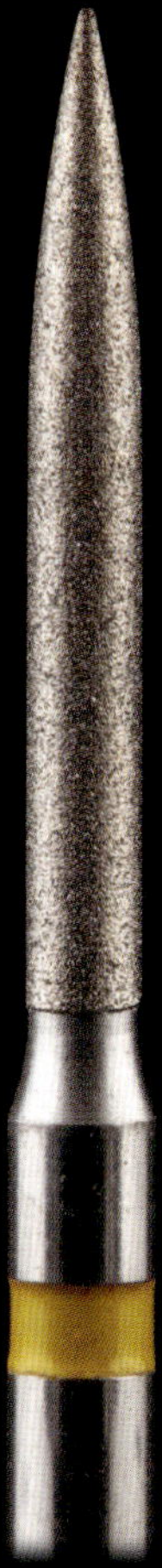

Extra-fine flame
012

Flame

For rounding and **finishing** select areas such as the connection between the incisal and interproximal preparation

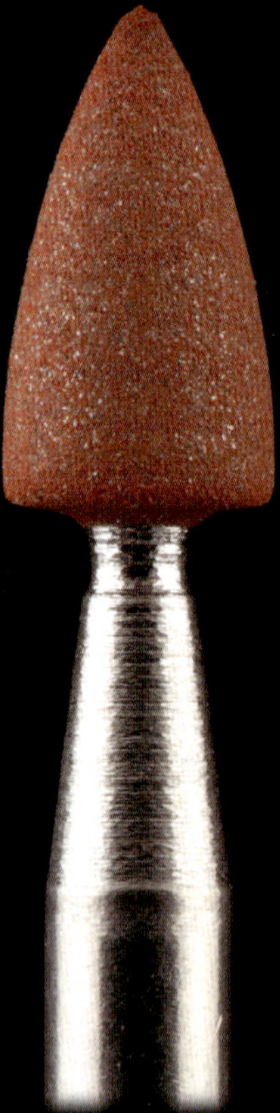

Optional polish

Rounded/smooth preparation leads to **better fit** and higher success rates

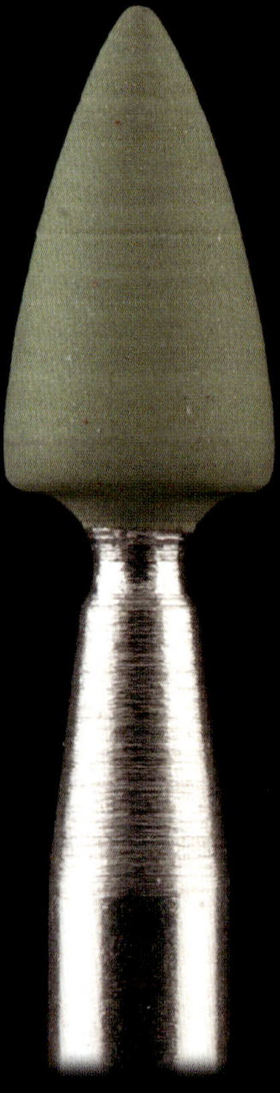

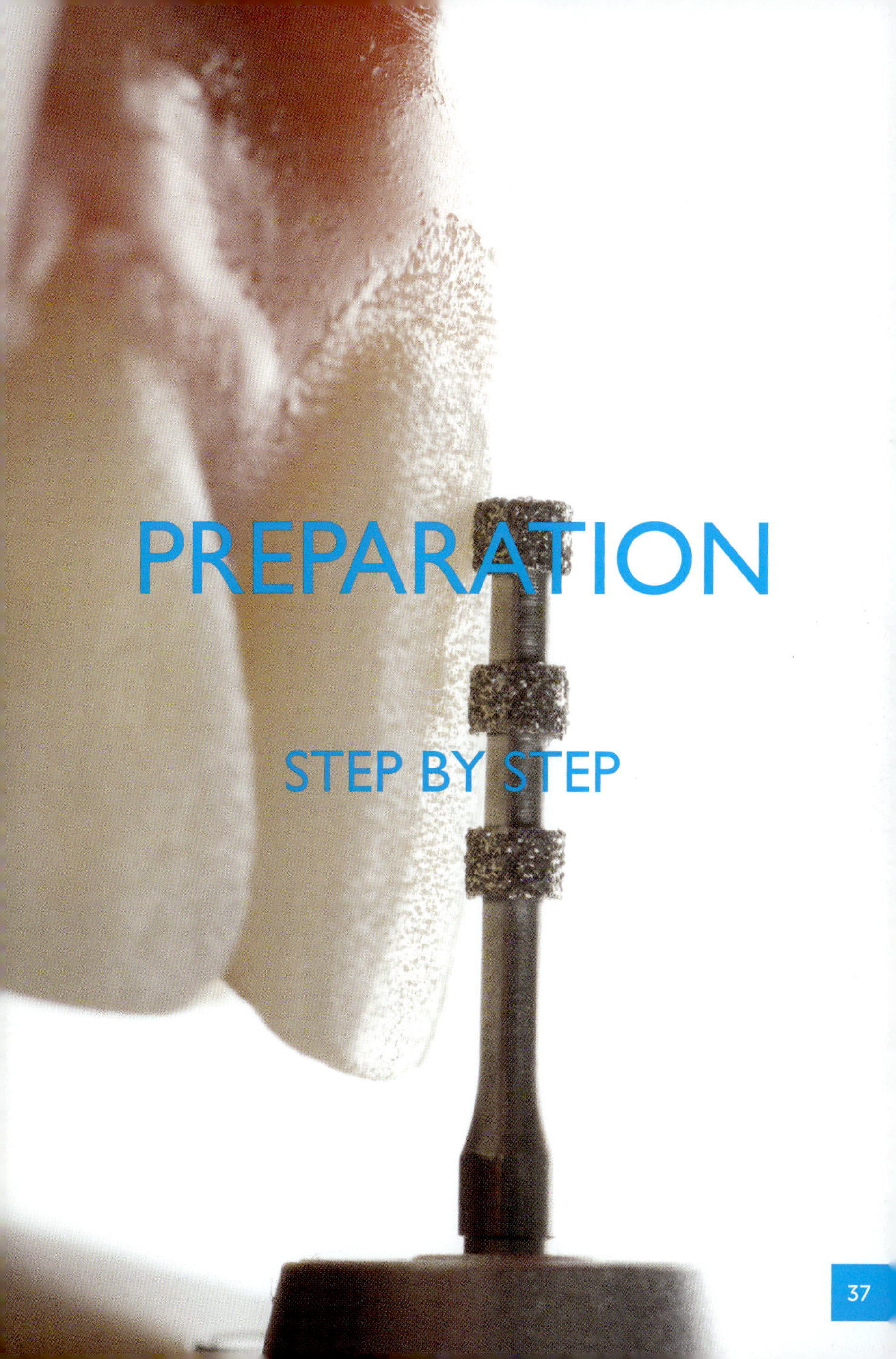

PREPARATION

STEP BY STEP

Make a **mock-up** from the digital/analog wax-up (do not bond to the teeth) 1

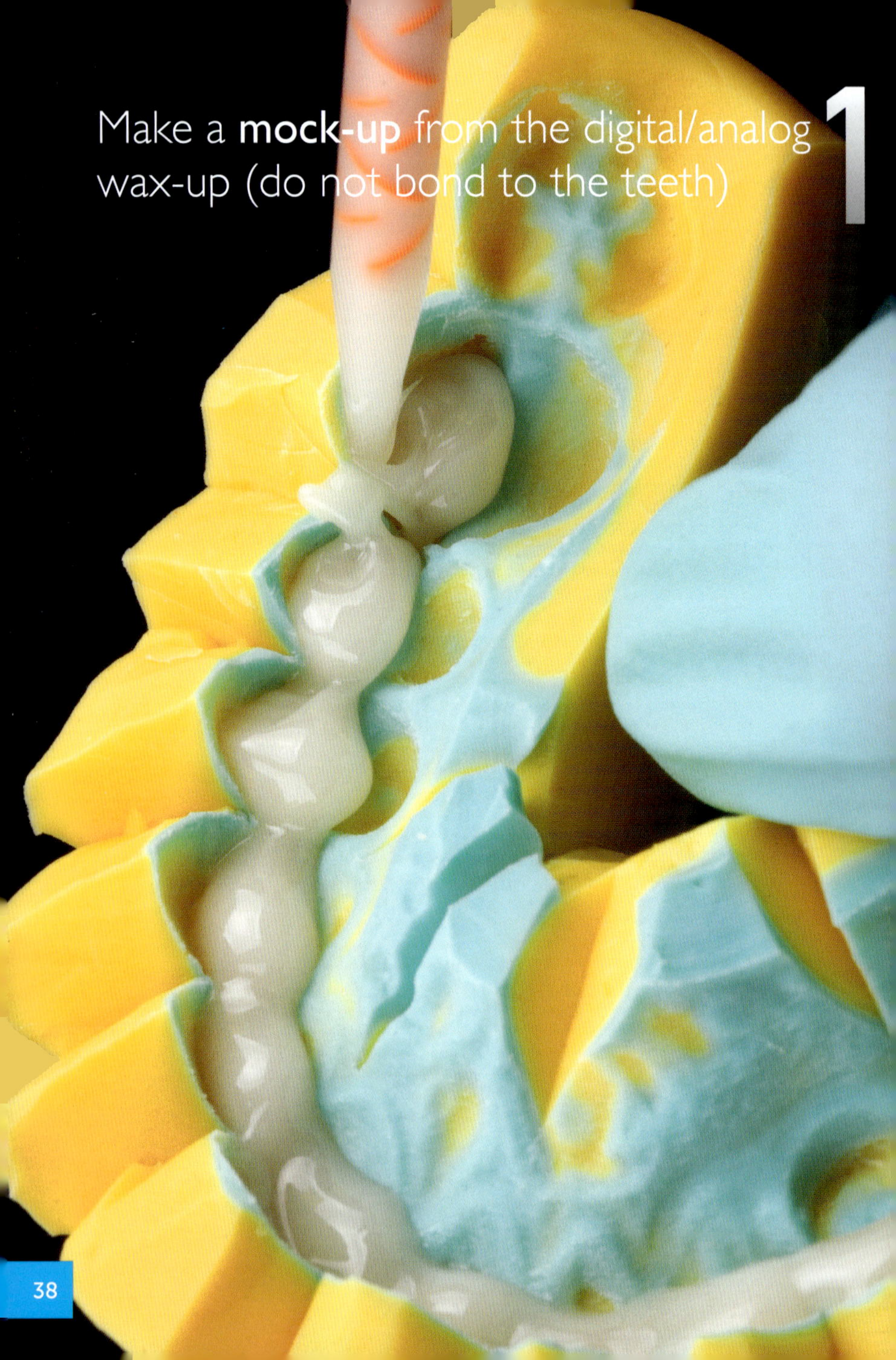

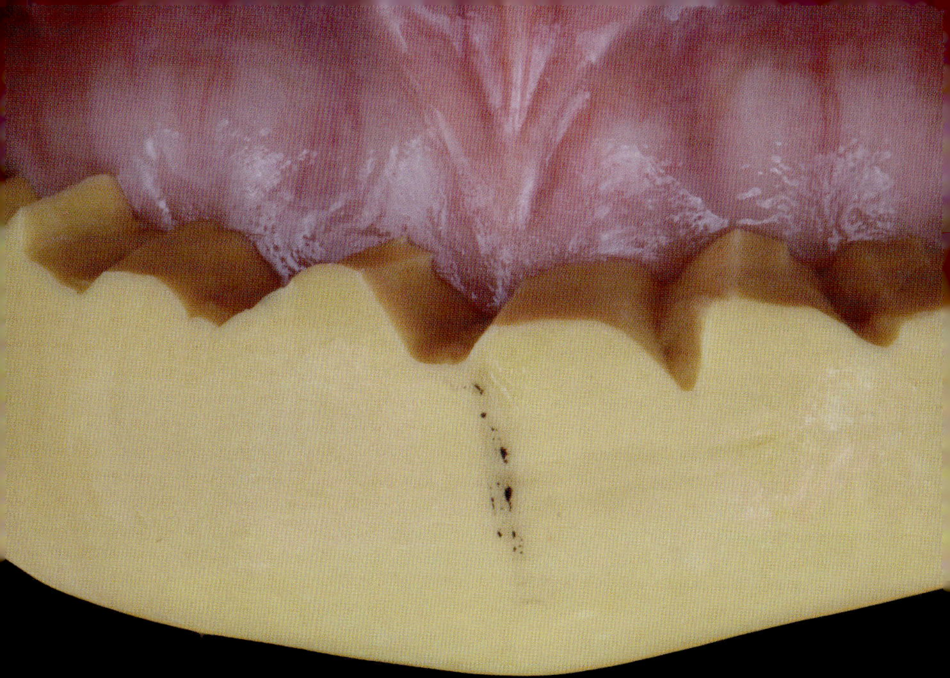

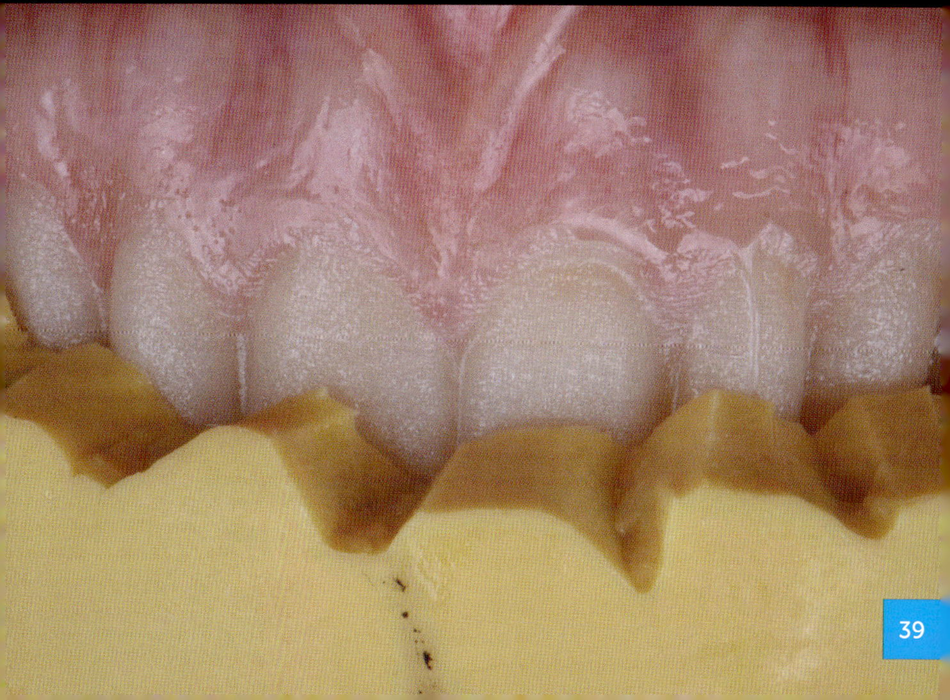

Prepare into the **mock-up** with a 0.3-mm depth cutter

2

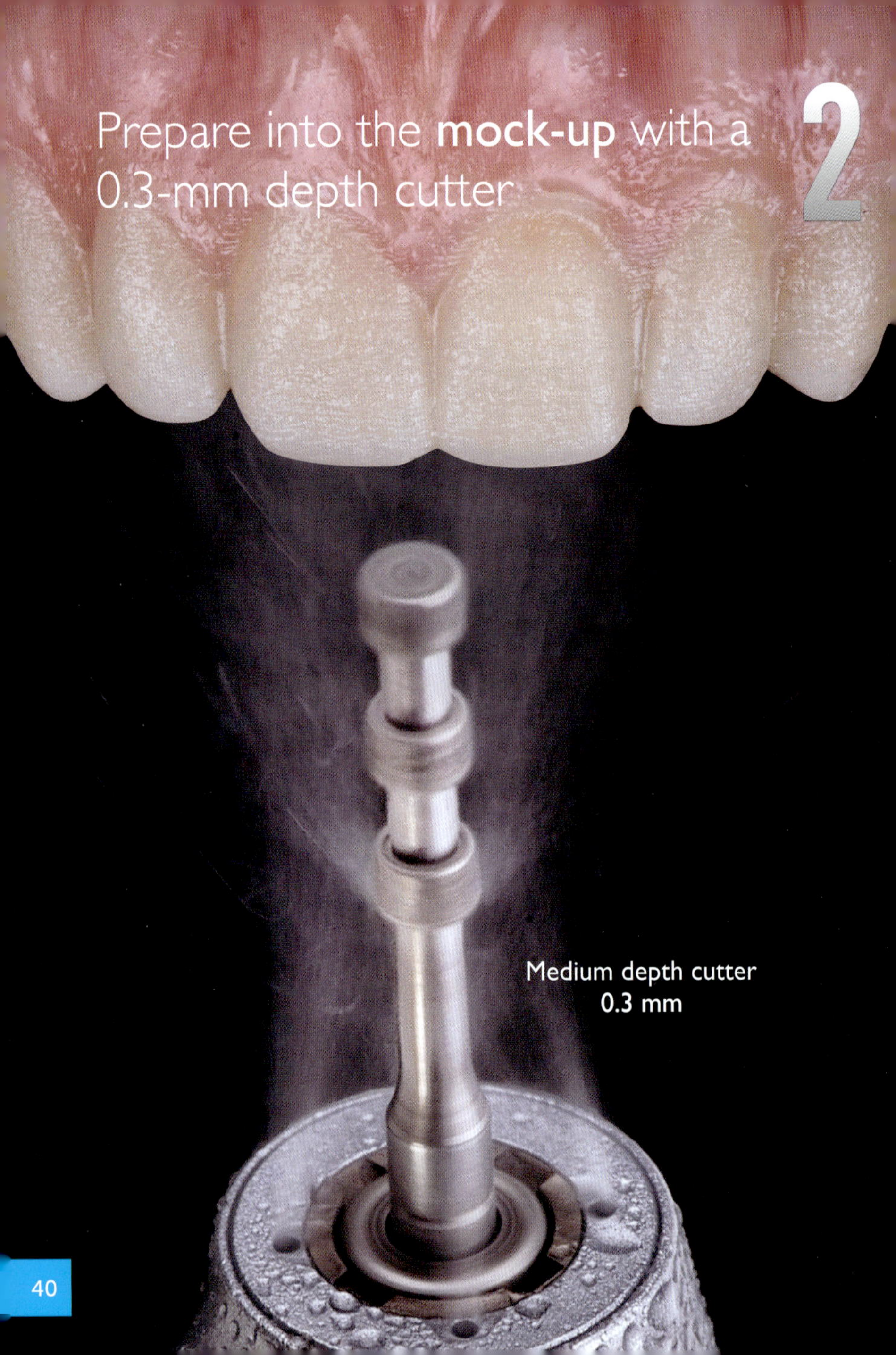

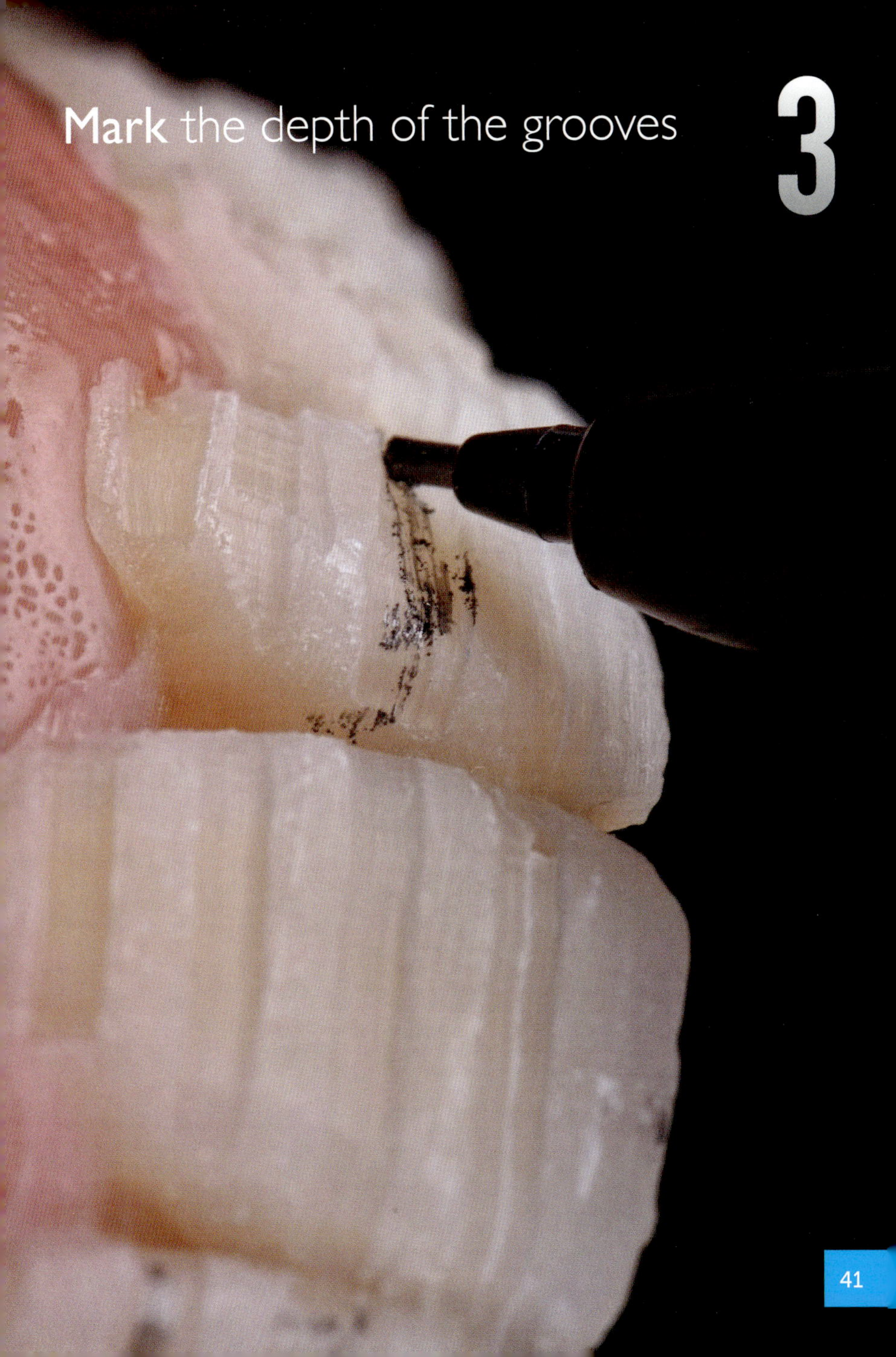

Mark the depth of the grooves

3

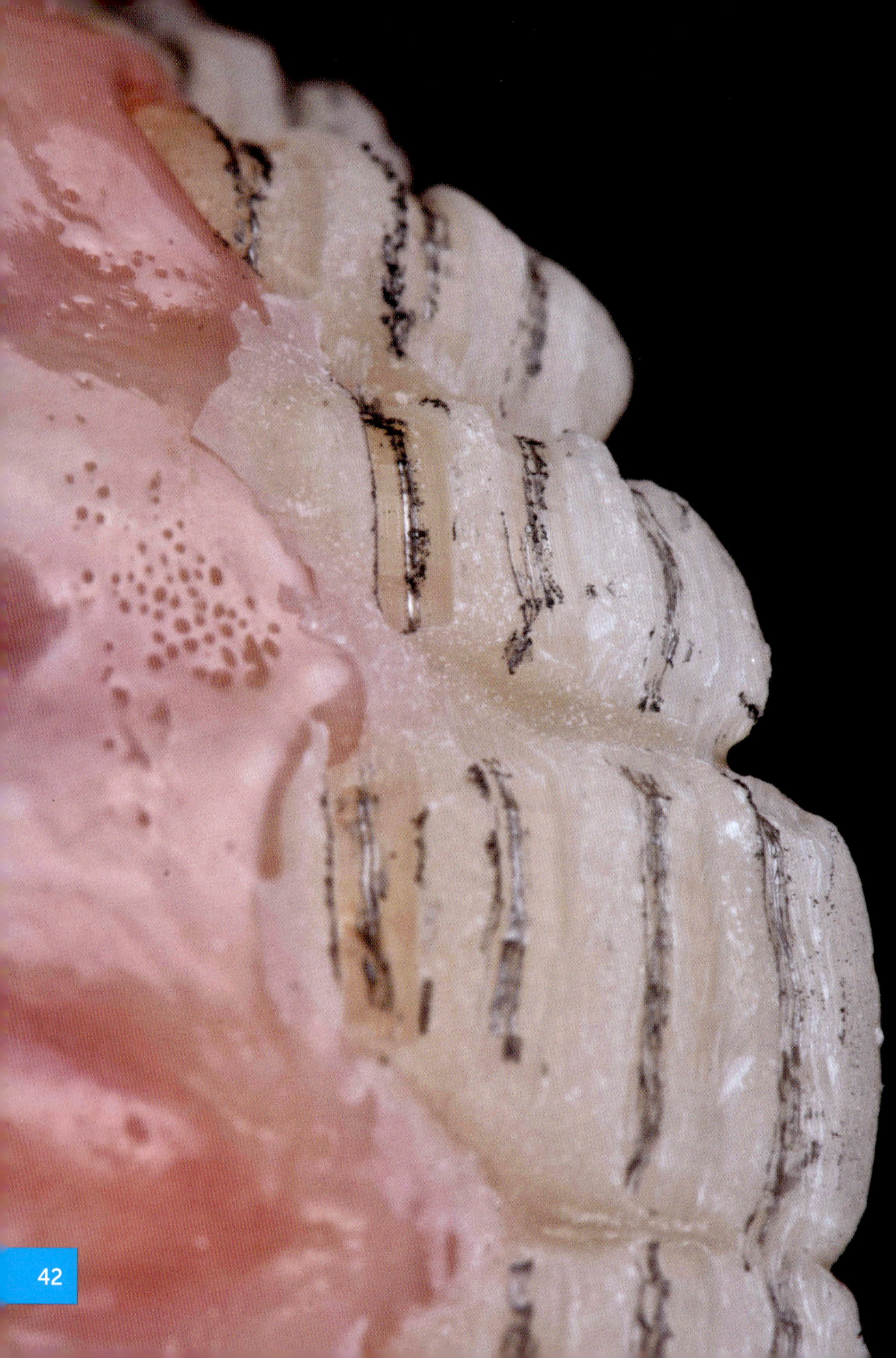

Prepare into the mock-up

4

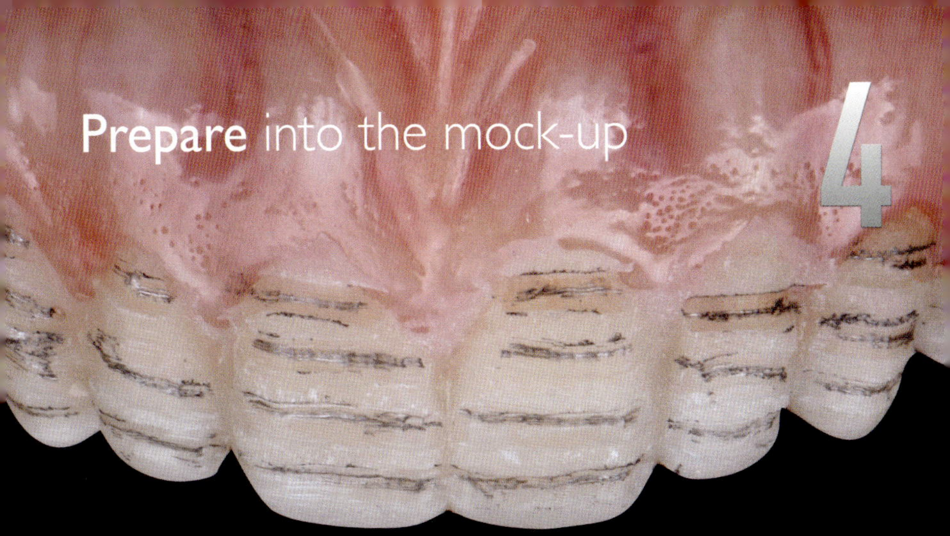

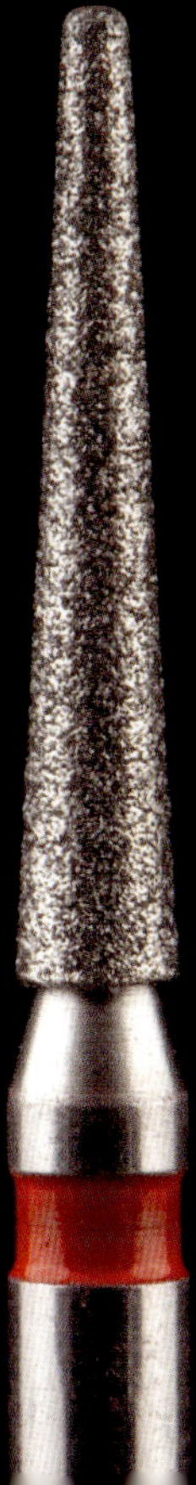

Fine round-end taper
016

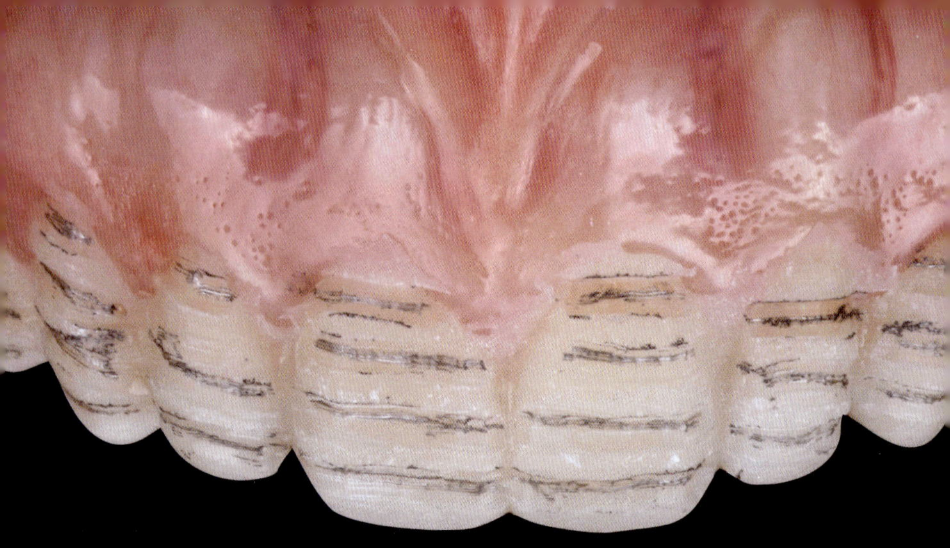

Prepare into the mock-up and level the areas between the grooves with fine round-end diamond burs **up to the marked lines.**

This ensures that you remove tooth structure **only where needed** to provide sufficient space for the ceramic!

FOLLOW TOOTH CURVATURE

Prepare the **cervical finish line**

5

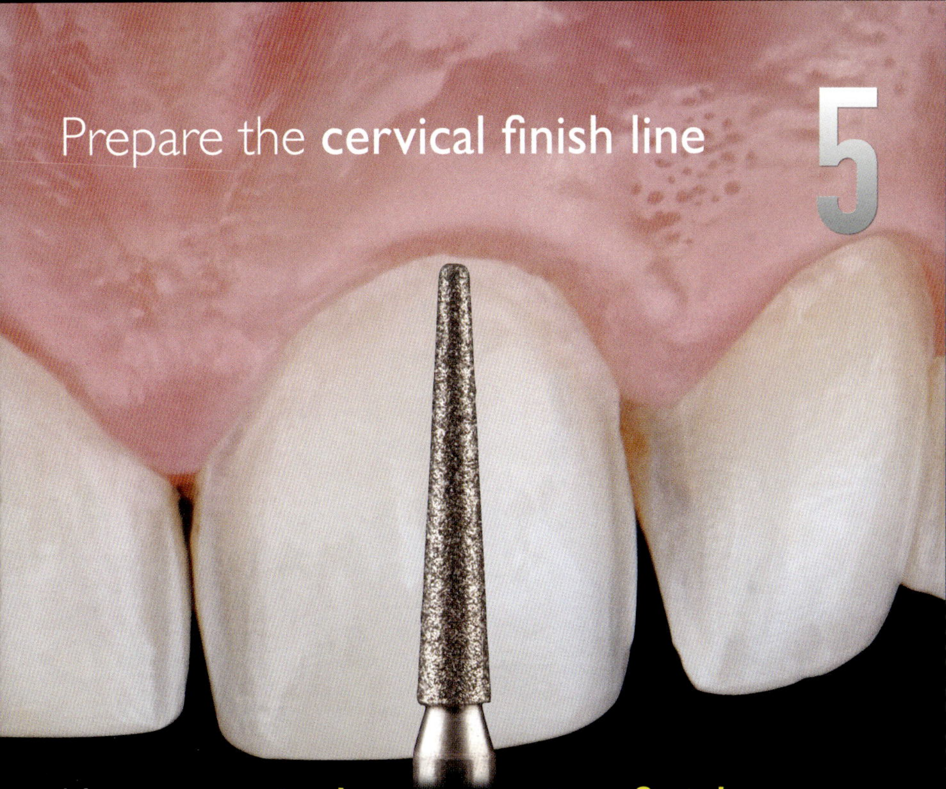

Keep **cervical preparation finish lines** slightly **supragingival**
The "**contact lens effect**" provides optical blending between translucent ceramics and the tooth

For significant **color changes** or opaque ceramics, place the cervical margins **epi-** or **subgingivally**

Prepare the **proximal finish lines** 6

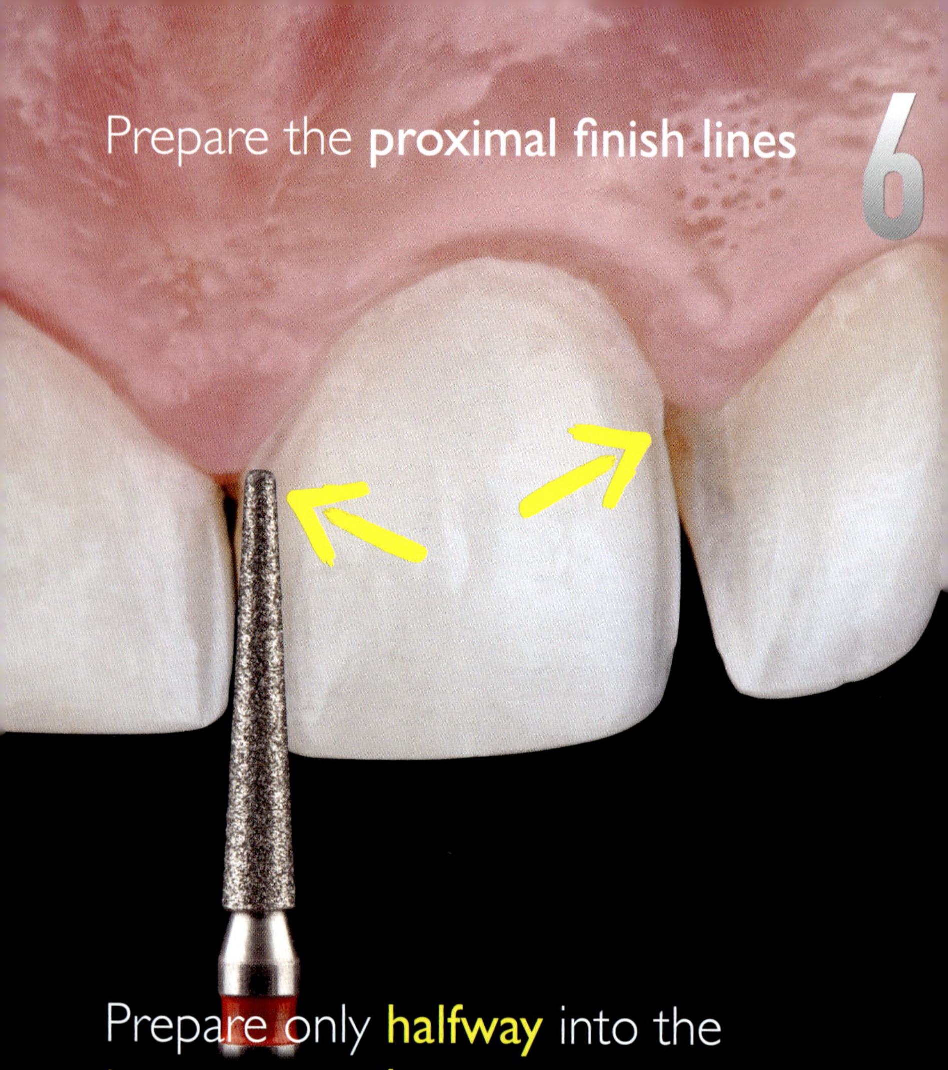

Prepare only **halfway** into the **interproximal contact areas**

Connect to the **cervical margin** with the **"elbow" prep**

Create **incisal space**

7

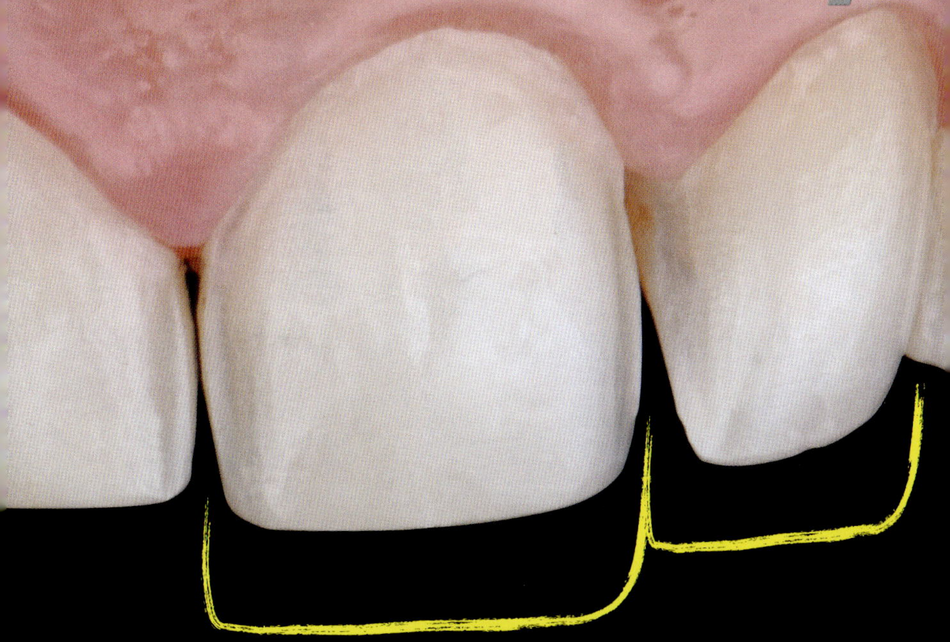

Create **1 to 2 mm incisal space** with reference to the **planned incisal edge**

Create slight interproximal **separation**

8

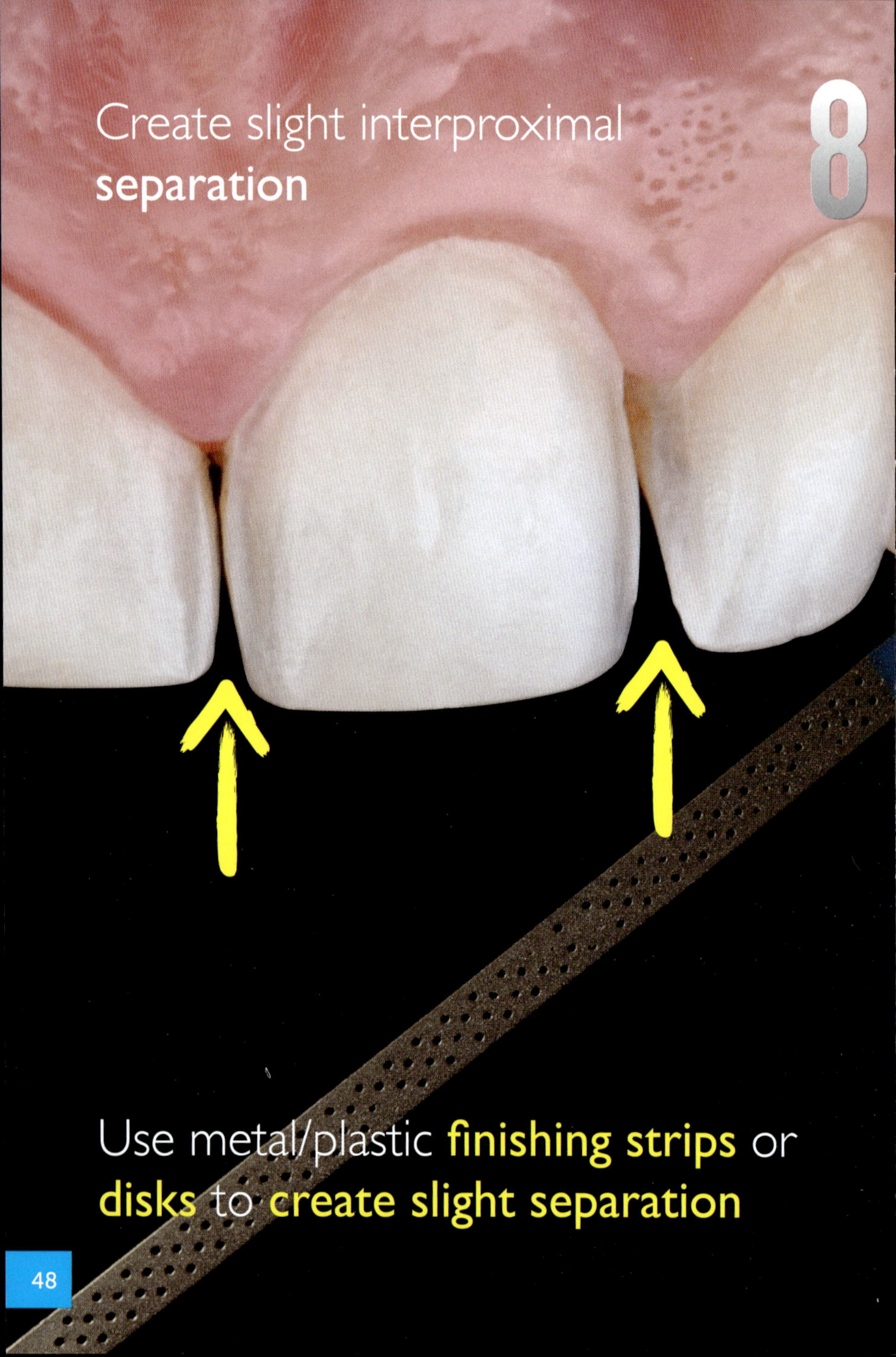

Use metal/plastic **finishing strips** or **disks** to **create slight separation**

Verify uniform reduction with polyvinyl siloxane (PVS) indices

9

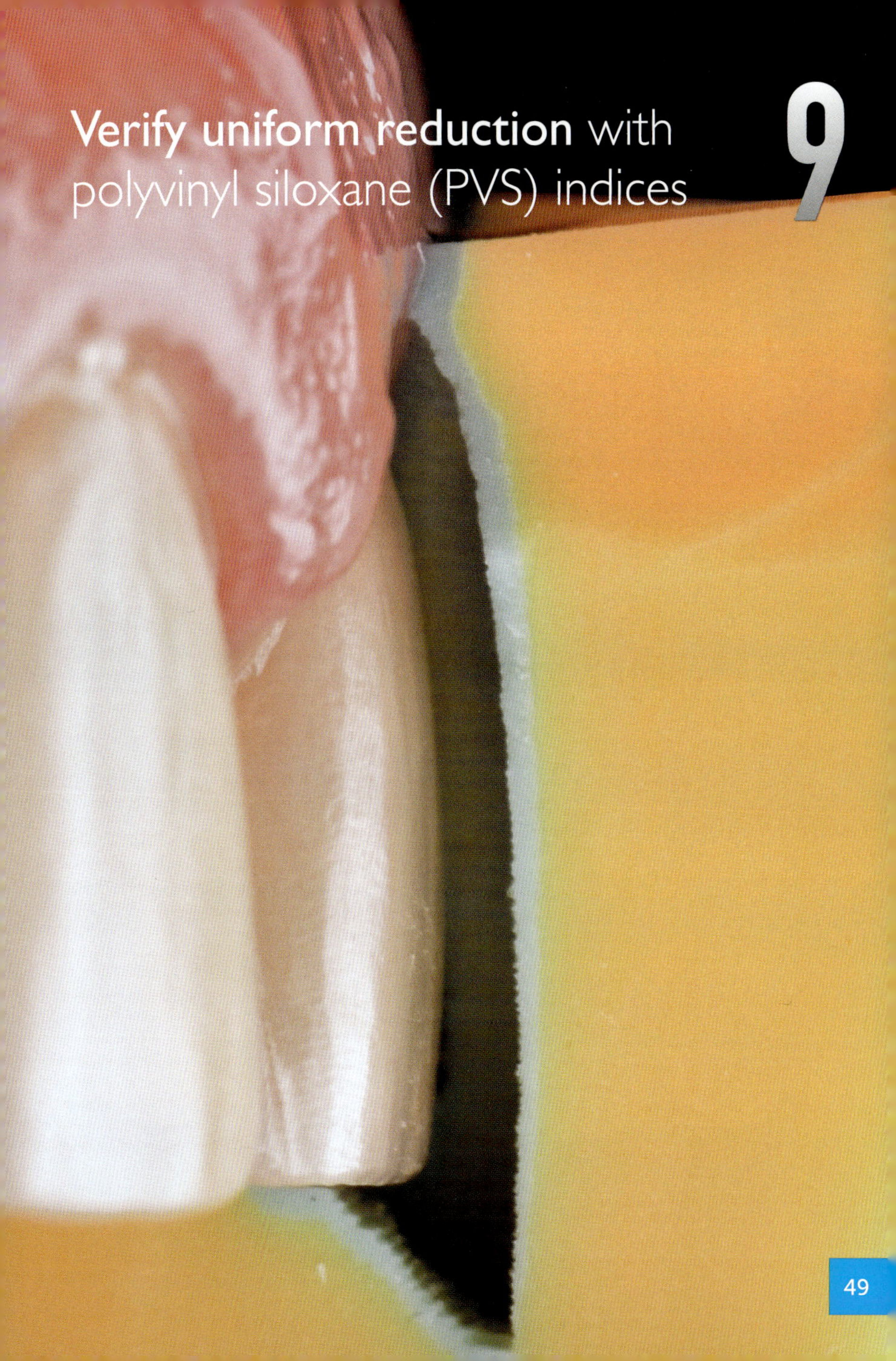

Veneer preparation

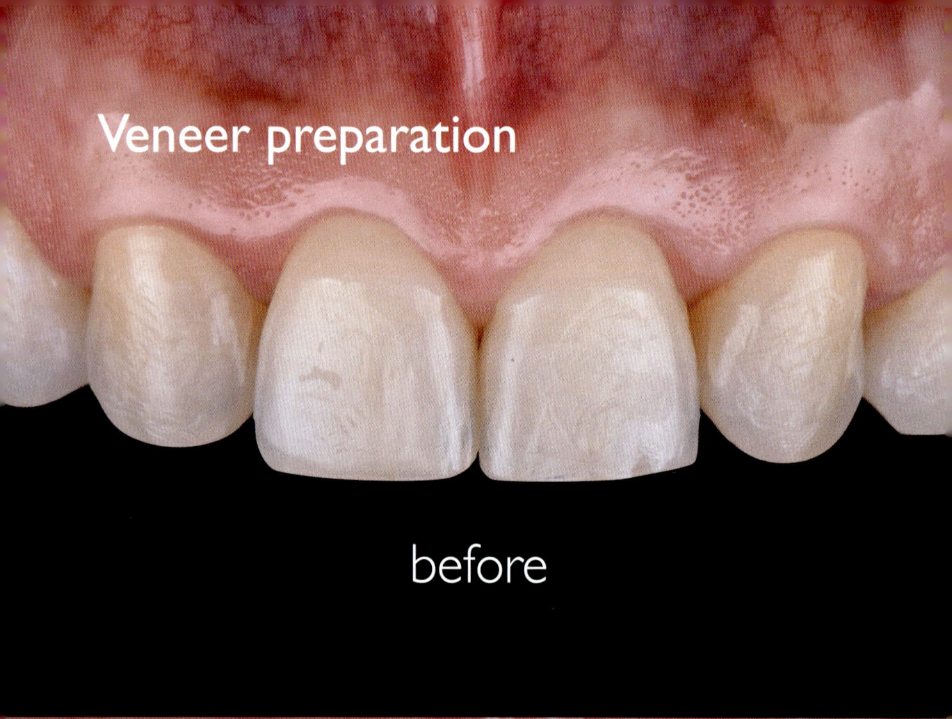

before

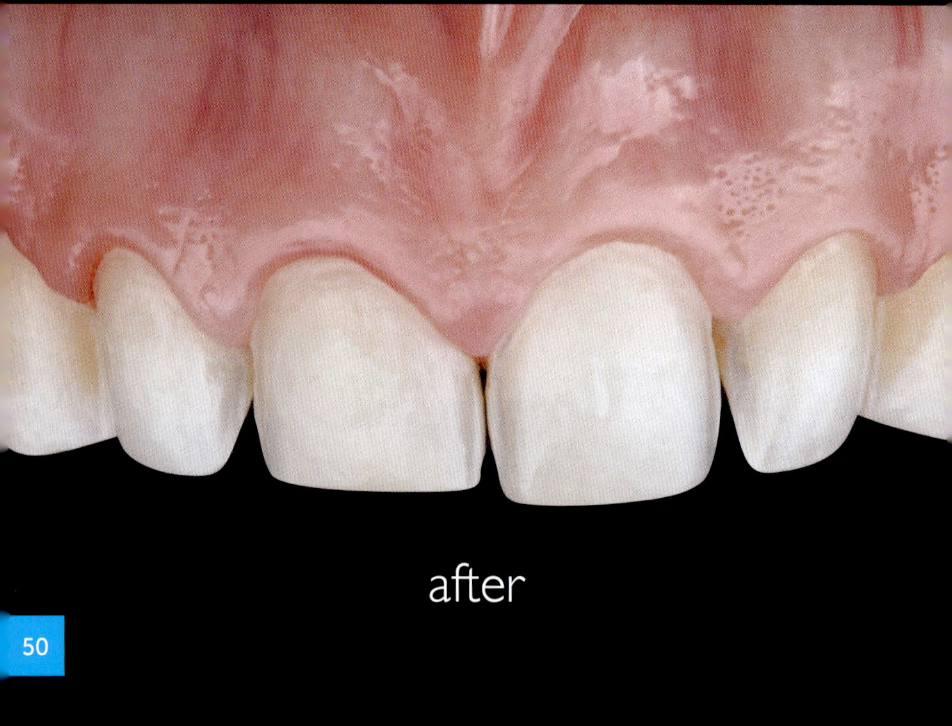

after

PREPARATION

CHEAT SHEET

1. Make a mock-up
2. Prepare into the mock-up with a 0.3-mm depth cutter
3. Mark the depth of the grooves
4. Prepare into the mock-up with a fine round-end taper diamond bur up to the marked lines
5. Prepare the cervical finish line
6. Prepare the proximal finish lines
7. Create incisal space
8. Create slight interproximal separation
9. Verify uniform reduction with PVS indices

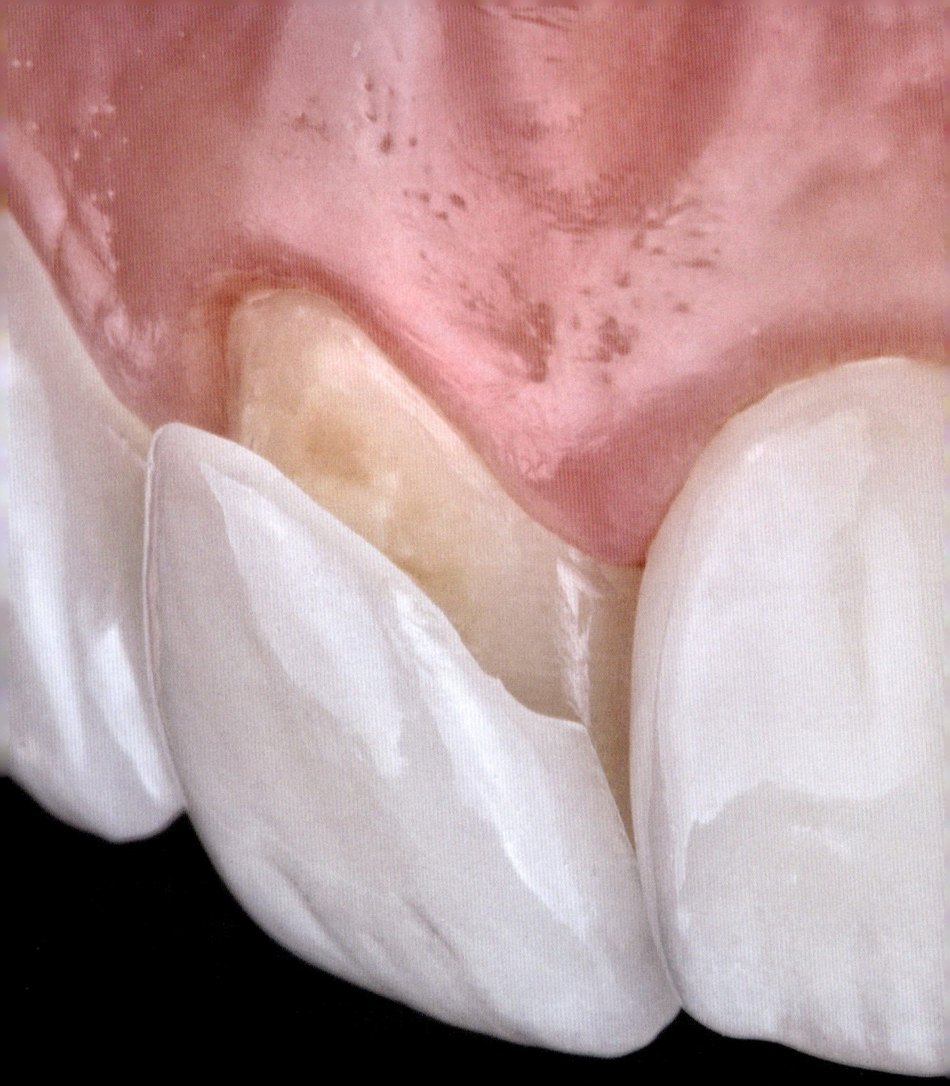

HOW MUCH ENAMEL DO YOU NEED?

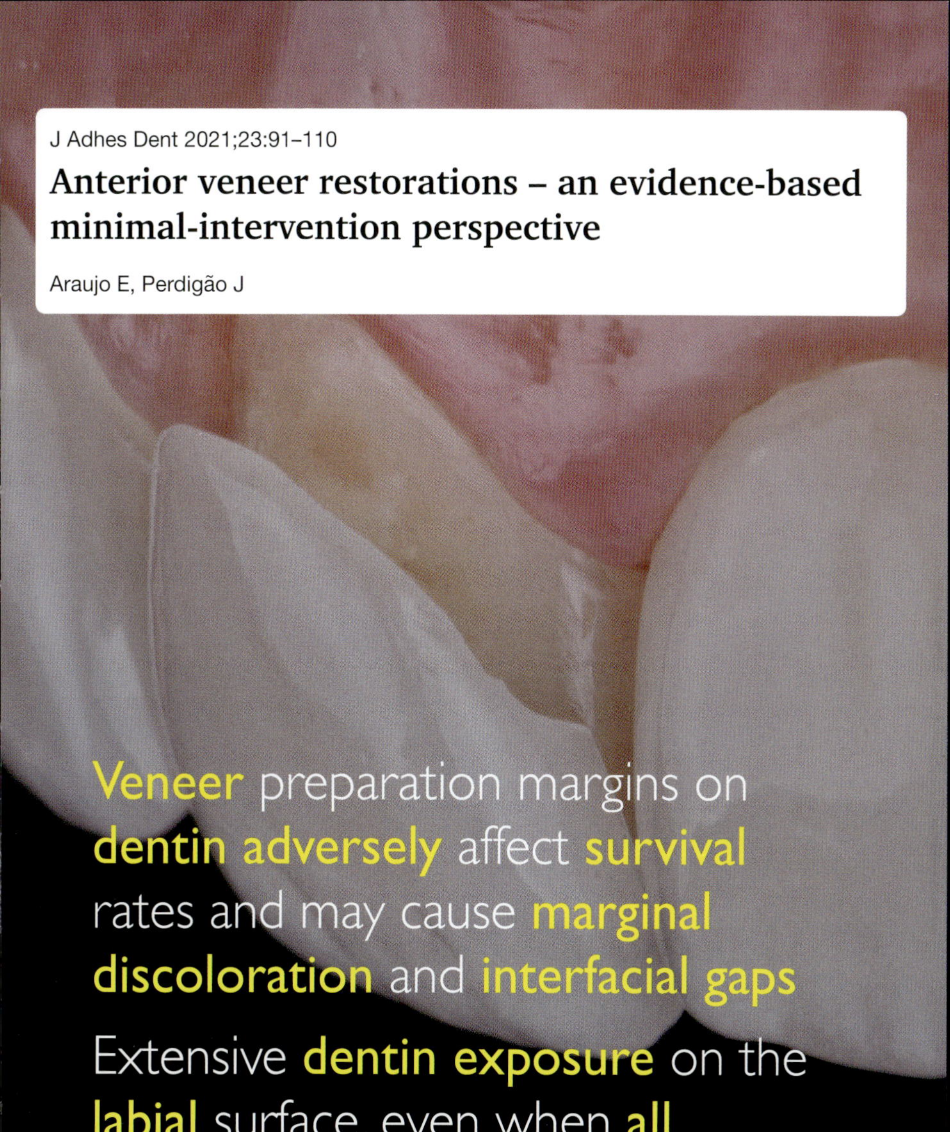

J Adhes Dent 2021;23:91–110

Anterior veneer restorations – an evidence-based minimal-intervention perspective

Araujo E, Perdigão J

Veneer preparation margins on **dentin adversely** affect **survival** rates and may cause **marginal discoloration** and **interfacial gaps**

Extensive **dentin exposure** on the **labial** surface, even when **all margins** are in **enamel**, **reduces** the **survival** rate of laminate veneers

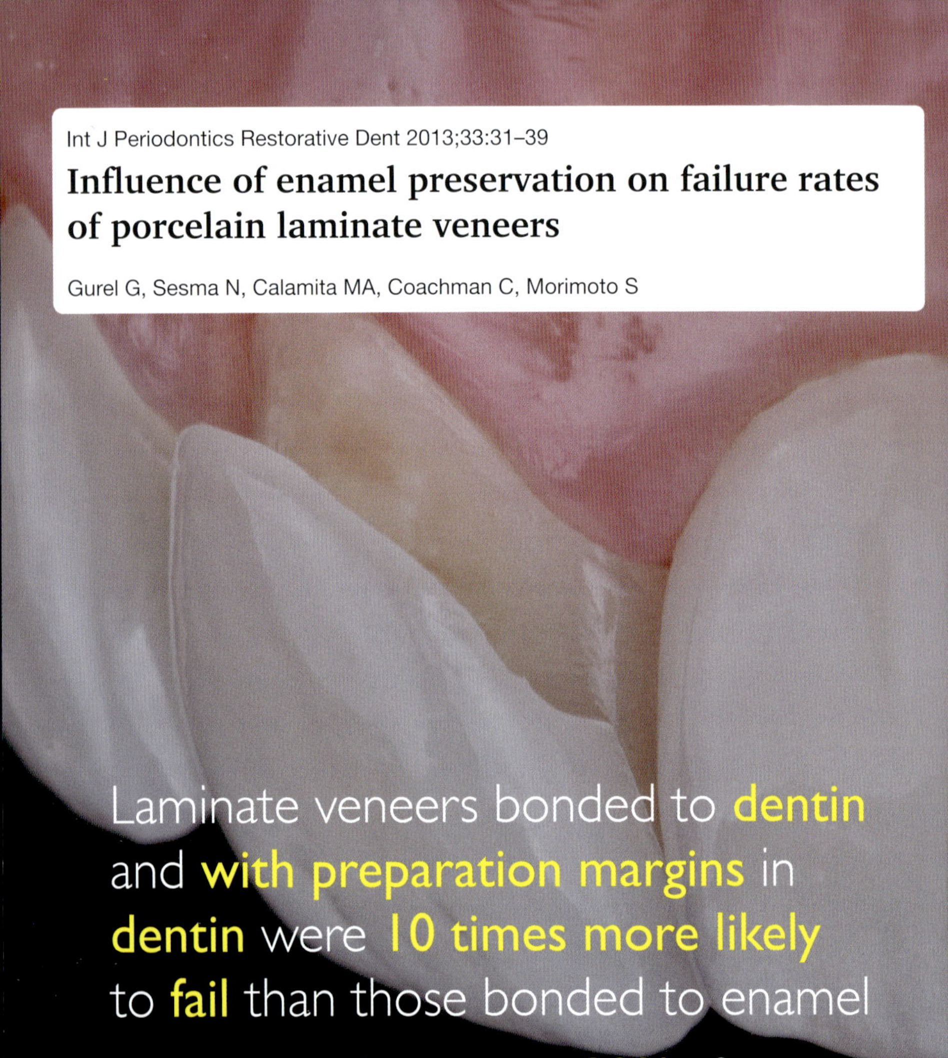

Int J Periodontics Restorative Dent 2013;33:31–39

Influence of enamel preservation on failure rates of porcelain laminate veneers

Gurel G, Sesma N, Calamita MA, Coachman C, Morimoto S

Laminate veneers bonded to **dentin** and **with preparation margins** in **dentin** were **10 times more likely** to **fail** than those bonded to enamel

The **survival** rate was **99%** after 12 years when bonded to **enamel** and **94%** for veneers with **enamel** only at the **margins**

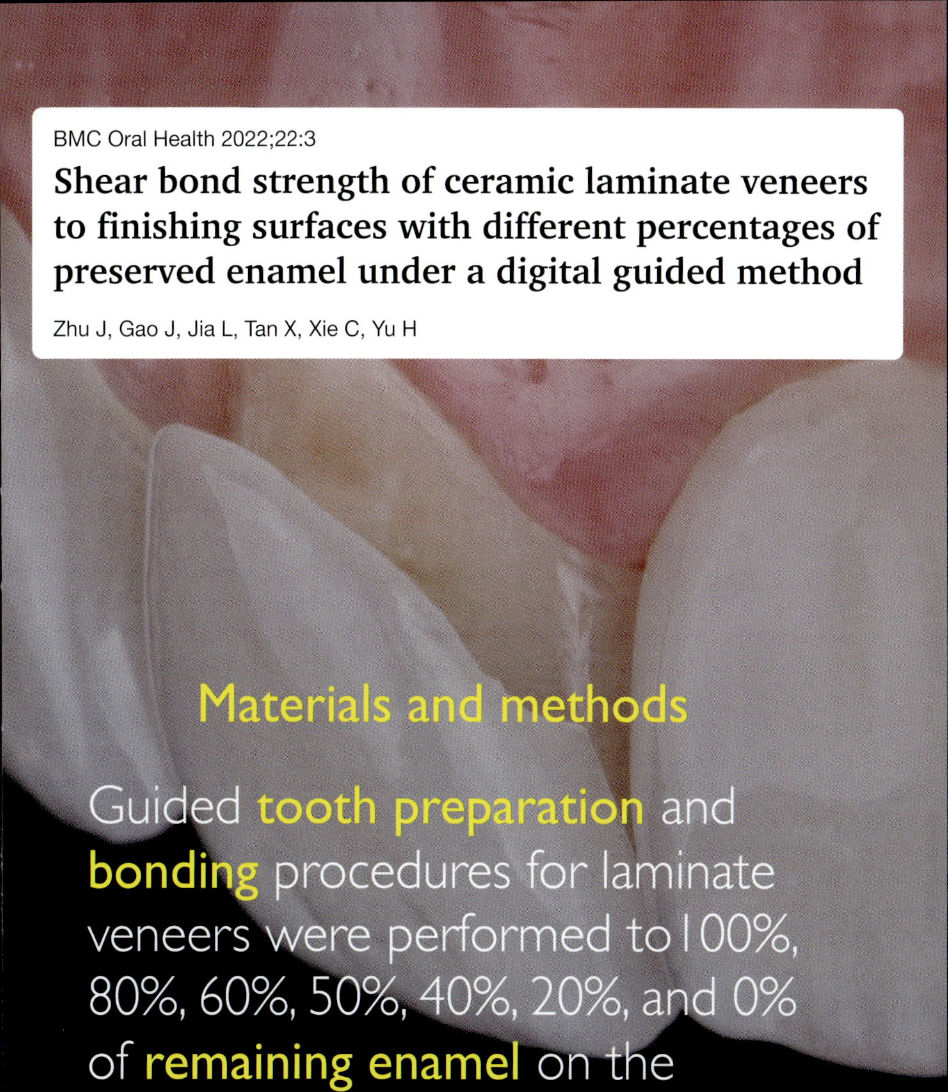

BMC Oral Health 2022;22:3

Shear bond strength of ceramic laminate veneers to finishing surfaces with different percentages of preserved enamel under a digital guided method

Zhu J, Gao J, Jia L, Tan X, Xie C, Yu H

Materials and methods

Guided **tooth preparation** and **bonding** procedures for laminate veneers were performed to 100%, 80%, 60%, 50%, 40%, 20%, and 0% of **remaining enamel** on the bonding surface

Shear bond strength (SBS) was tested

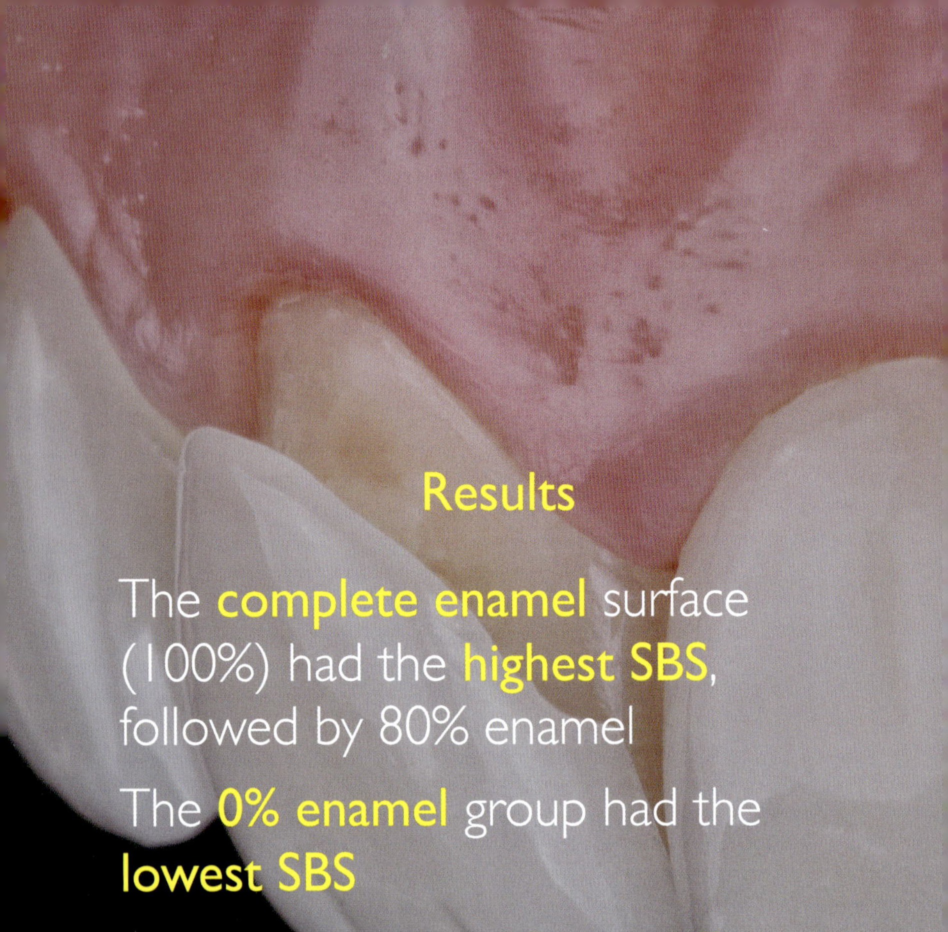

Results

The **complete enamel** surface (100%) had the **highest SBS**, followed by 80% enamel

The **0% enamel** group had the **lowest SBS**

There was no **significant difference** among the **40% to100% enamel groups**, while the **20% or 0% enamel** groups had a significantly **lower** mean **SBS** than the **40% enamel** group

Zhu et al BMC Oral Health 2022;22:3

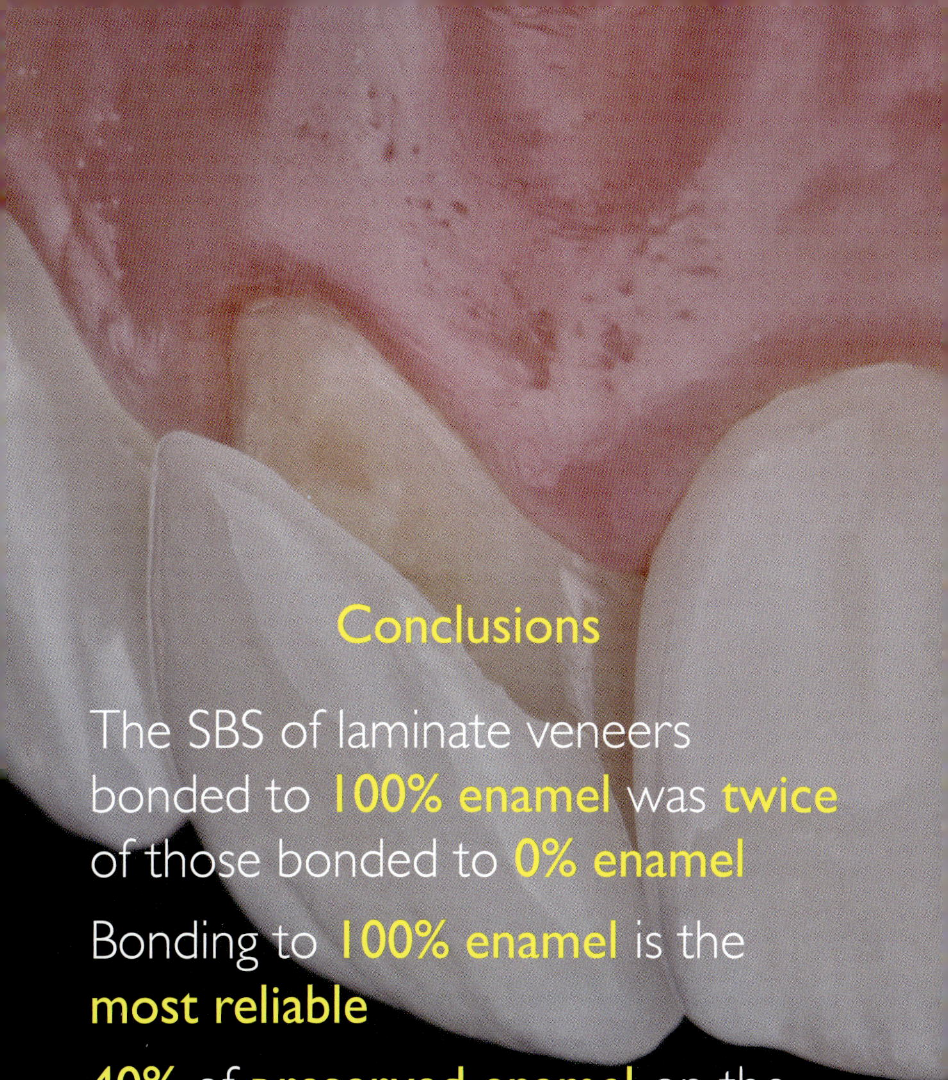

Conclusions

The SBS of laminate veneers bonded to **100% enamel** was **twice** of those bonded to **0% enamel**

Bonding to **100% enamel** is the **most reliable**

40% of **preserved enamel** on the bonding surface was the absolute **minimal acceptable** value in this laboratory study

Zhu et al. BMC Oral Health 2022;22:3

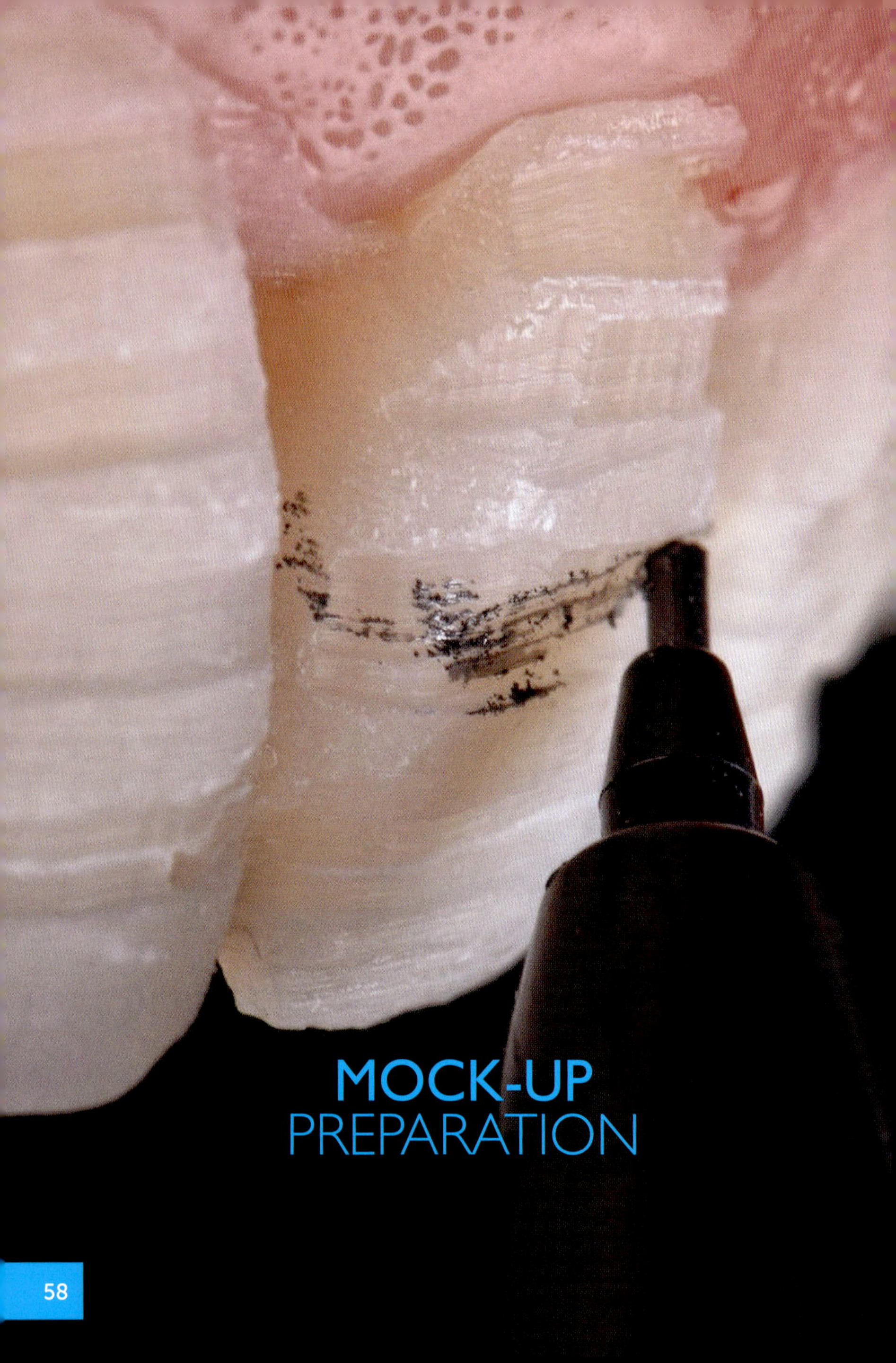

MOCK-UP
PREPARATION

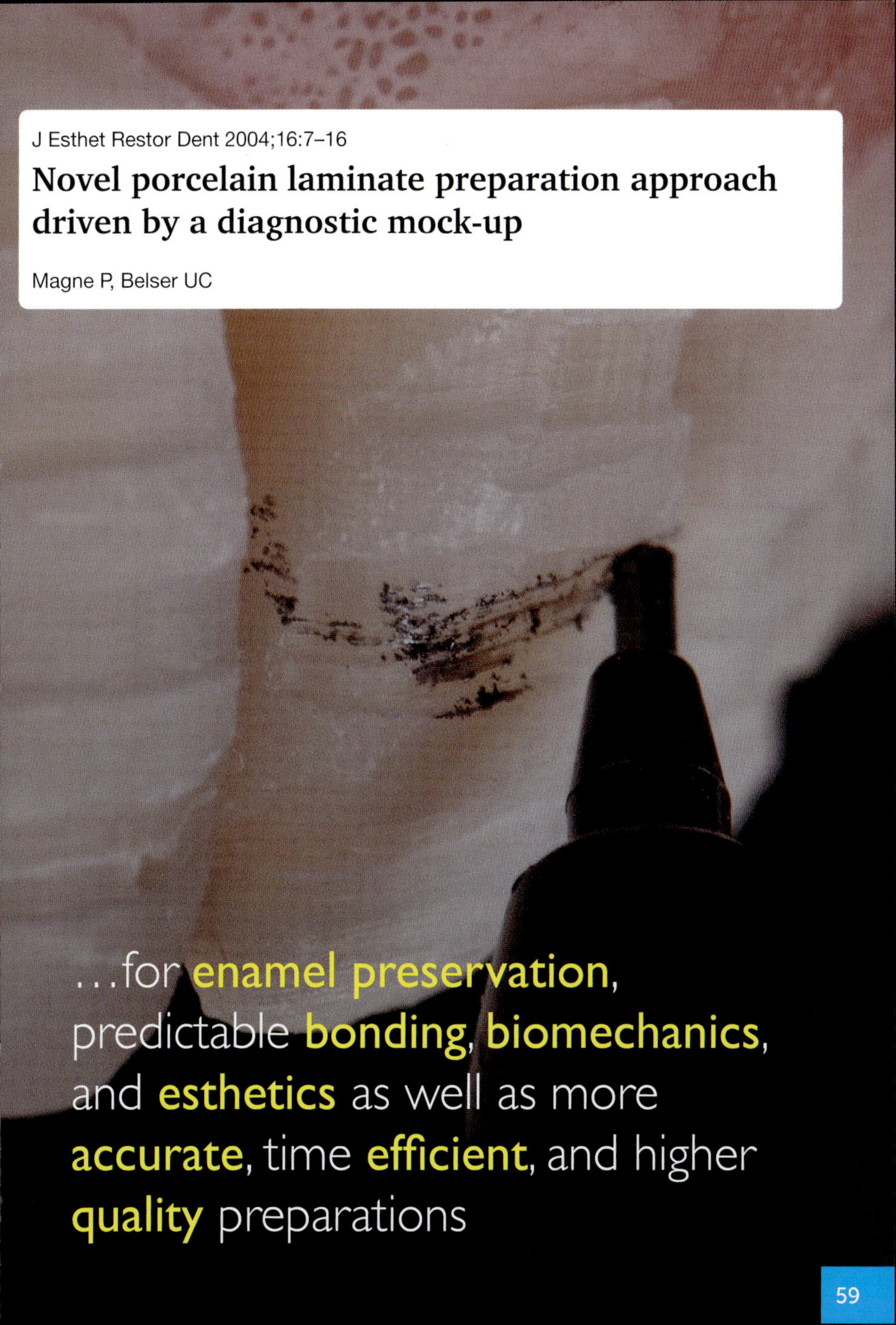

J Esthet Restor Dent 2004;16:7–16

Novel porcelain laminate preparation approach driven by a diagnostic mock-up

Magne P, Belser UC

…for **enamel preservation**, predictable **bonding**, **biomechanics**, and **esthetics** as well as more **accurate**, time **efficient**, and higher **quality** preparations

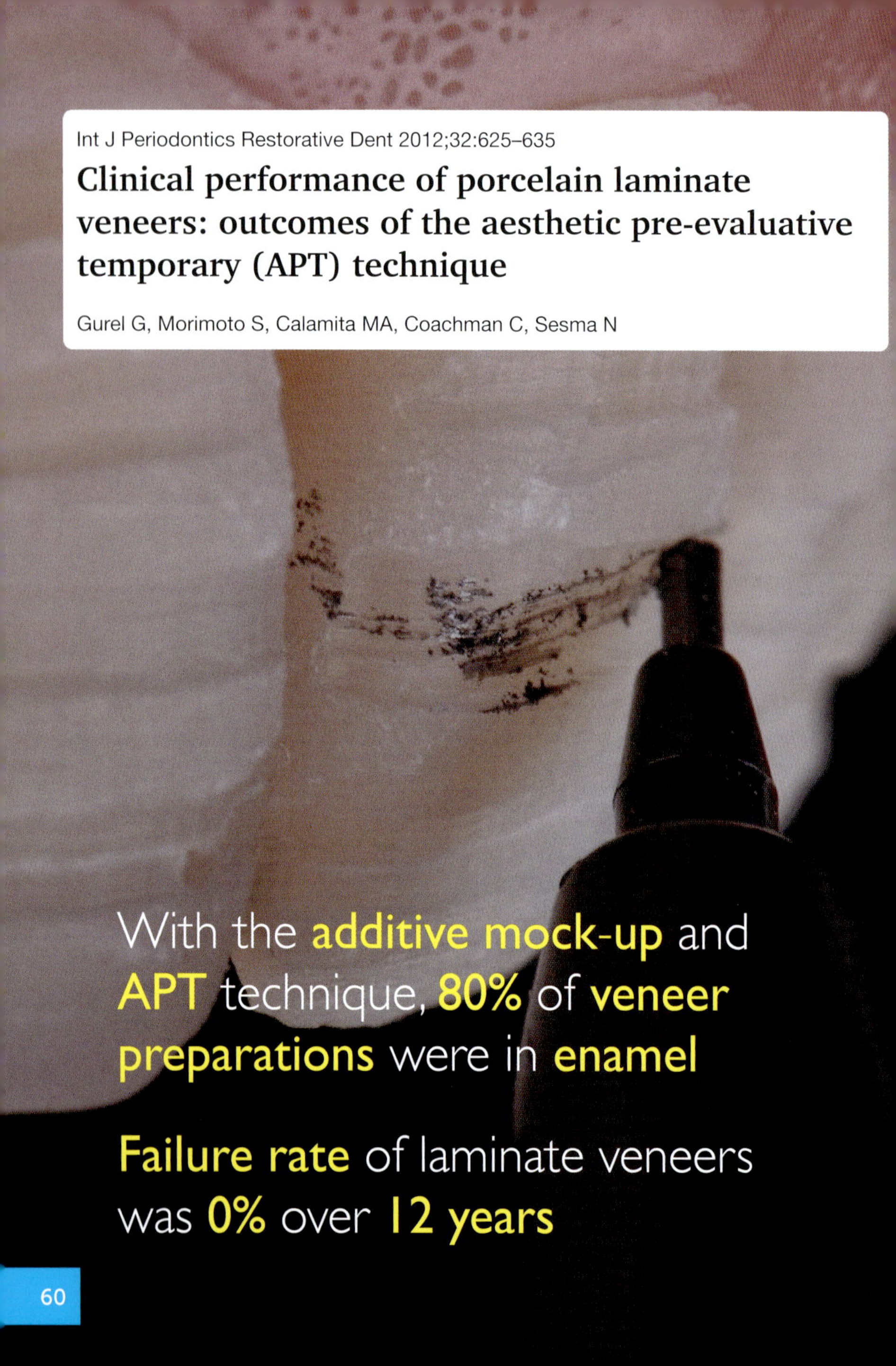

Int J Periodontics Restorative Dent 2012;32:625–635

Clinical performance of porcelain laminate veneers: outcomes of the aesthetic pre-evaluative temporary (APT) technique

Gurel G, Morimoto S, Calamita MA, Coachman C, Sesma N

With the **additive mock-up** and **APT** technique, **80%** of **veneer preparations** were in **enamel**

Failure rate of laminate veneers was **0%** over **12 years**

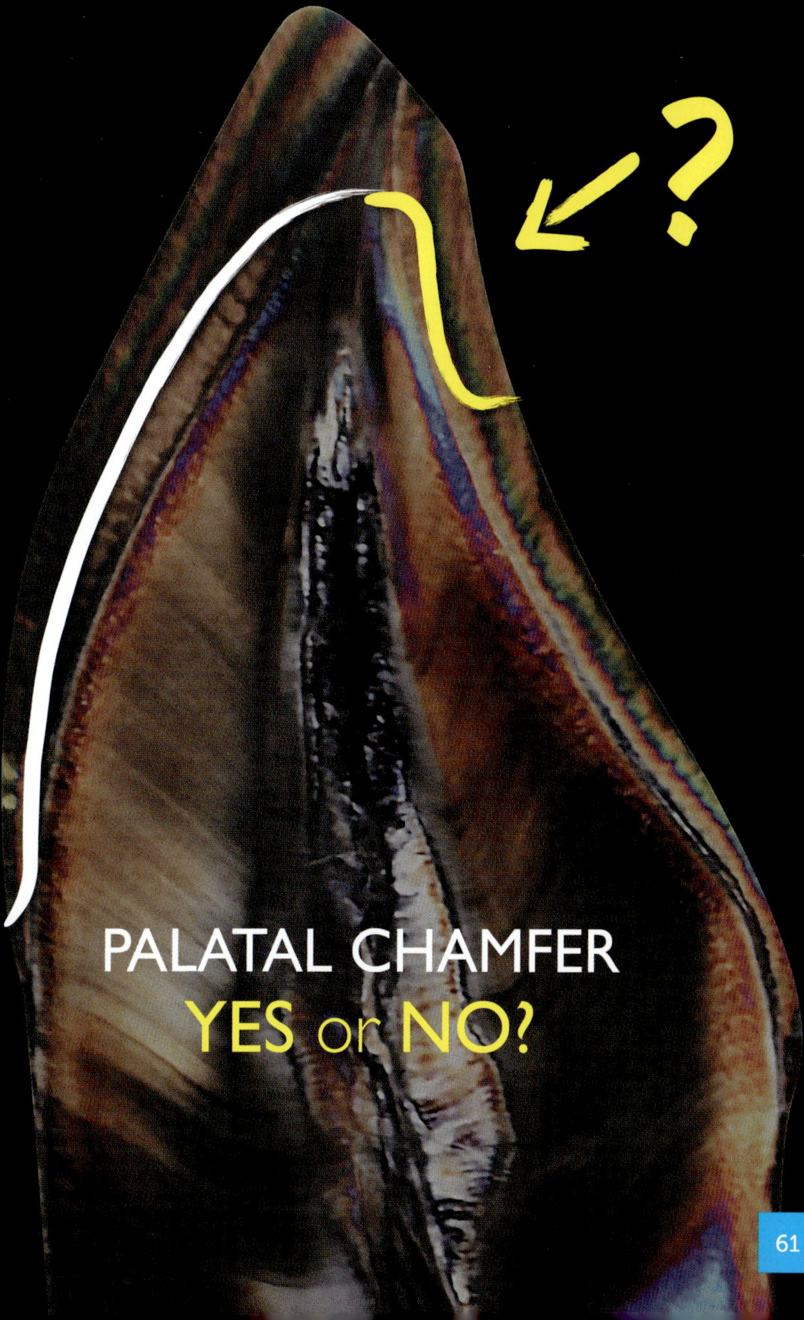

PALATAL CHAMFER
YES or NO?

J Am Dent Assoc 2018;149:25–37

Incisal preparation design for ceramic veneers: A critical review

Chai SY, Bennani V, Aarts JM, Lyons K

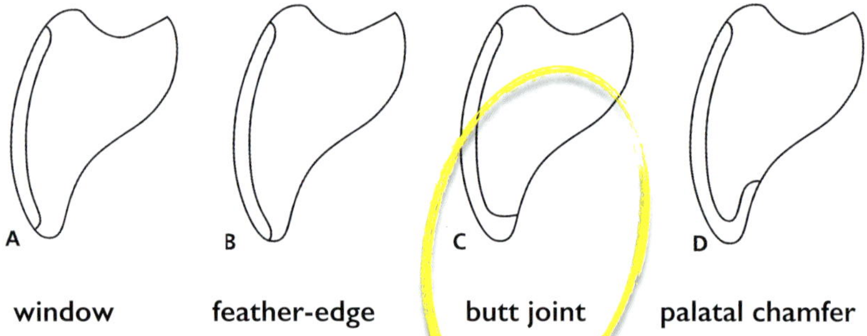

Evidence supports **butt joint** over **palatal chamfer** and other incisal preparation designs

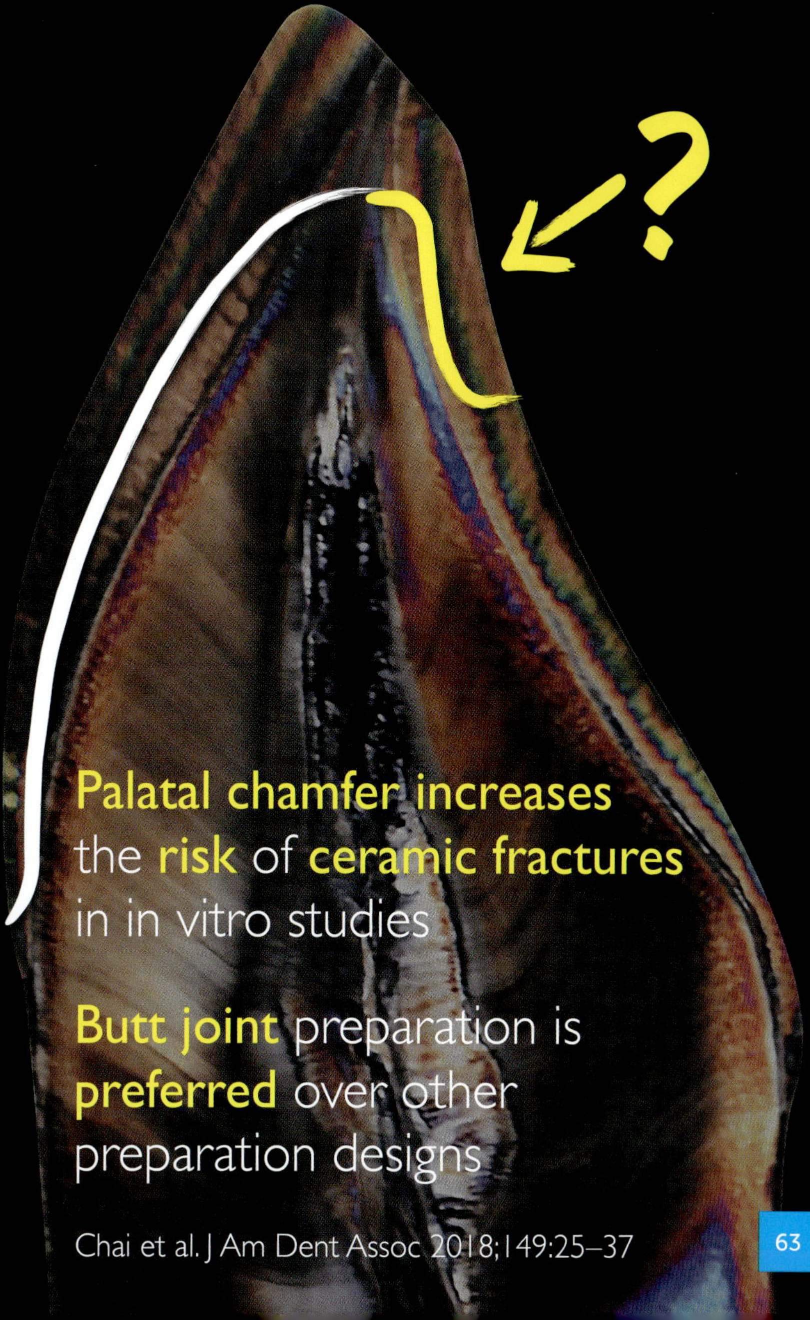

Palatal chamfer increases the **risk** of **ceramic fractures** in in vitro studies

Butt joint preparation is **preferred** over other preparation designs

Chai et al. J Am Dent Assoc 2018;149:25–37

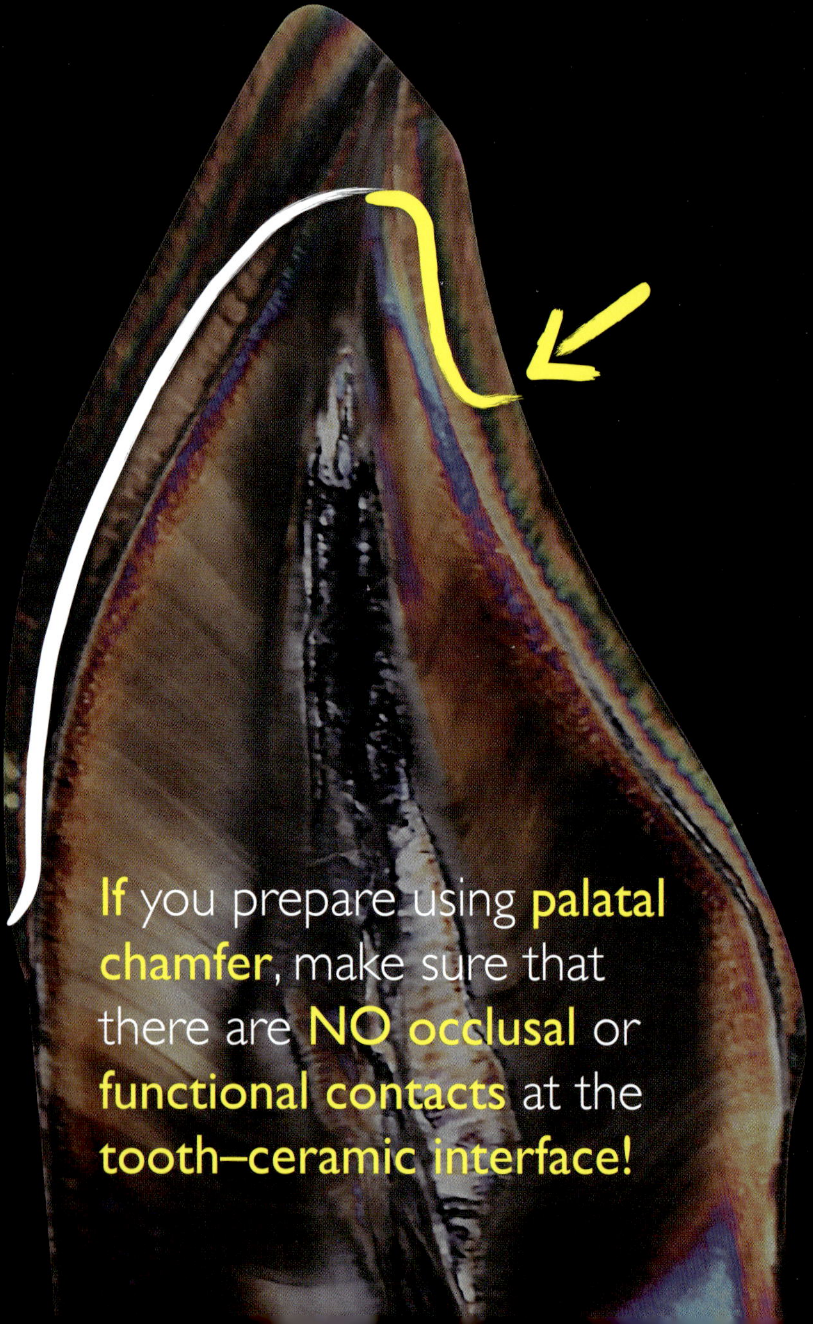

If you prepare using palatal chamfer, make sure that there are NO occlusal or functional contacts at the tooth–ceramic interface!

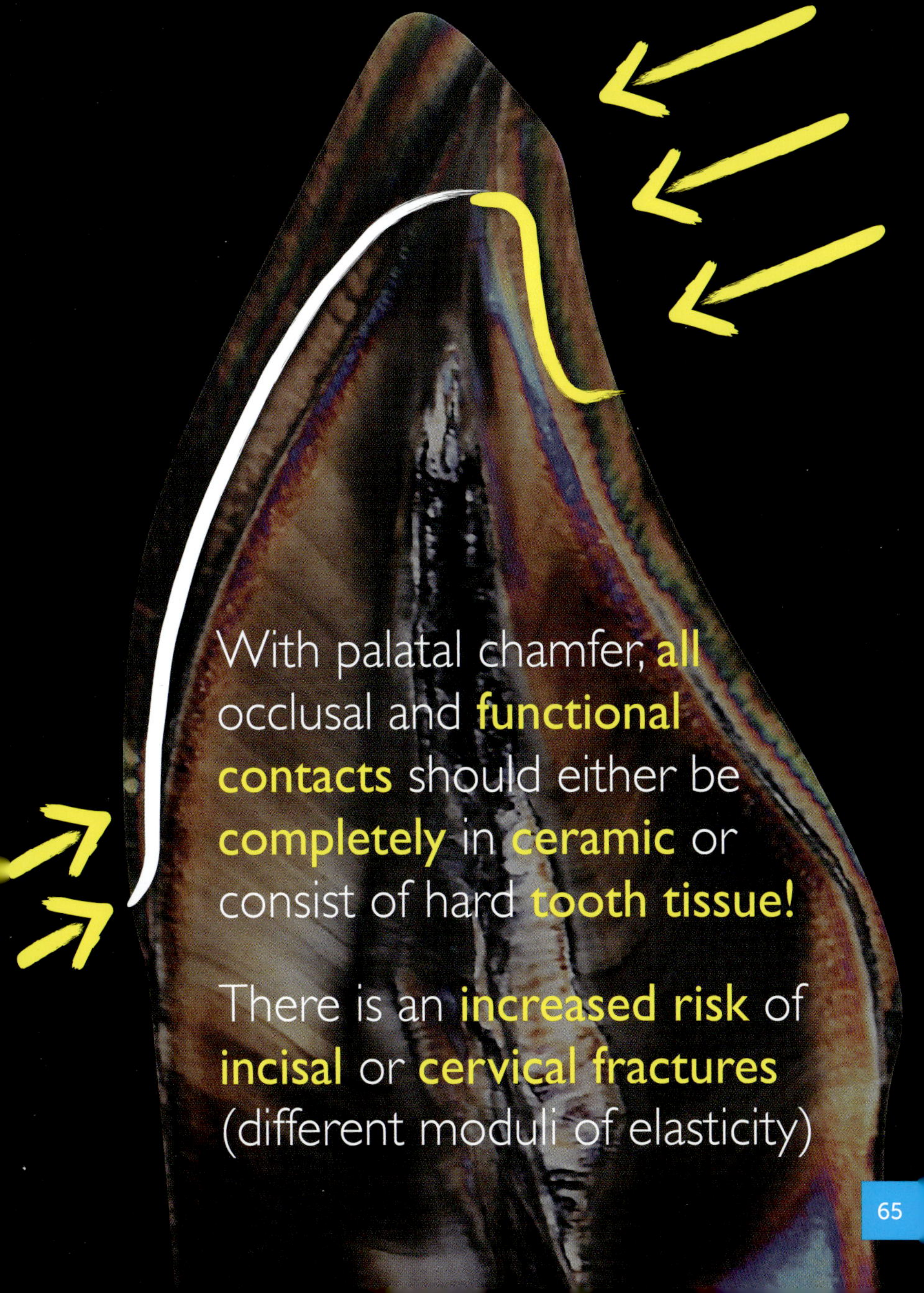

With palatal chamfer, **all** occlusal and **functional contacts** should either be **completely** in **ceramic** or consist of hard **tooth tissue!**

There is an **increased risk** of **incisal** or **cervical fractures** (different moduli of elasticity)

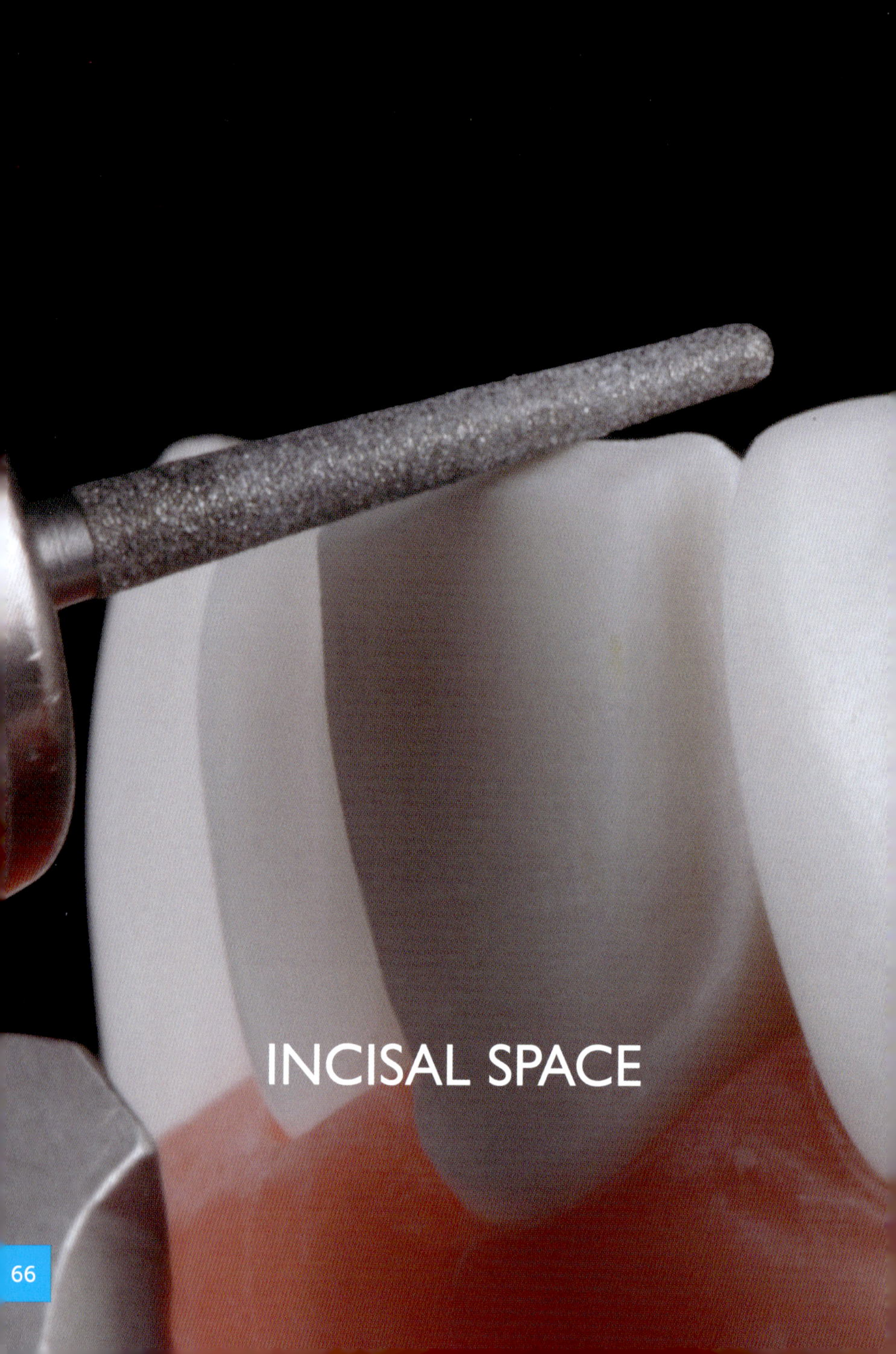

INCISAL SPACE

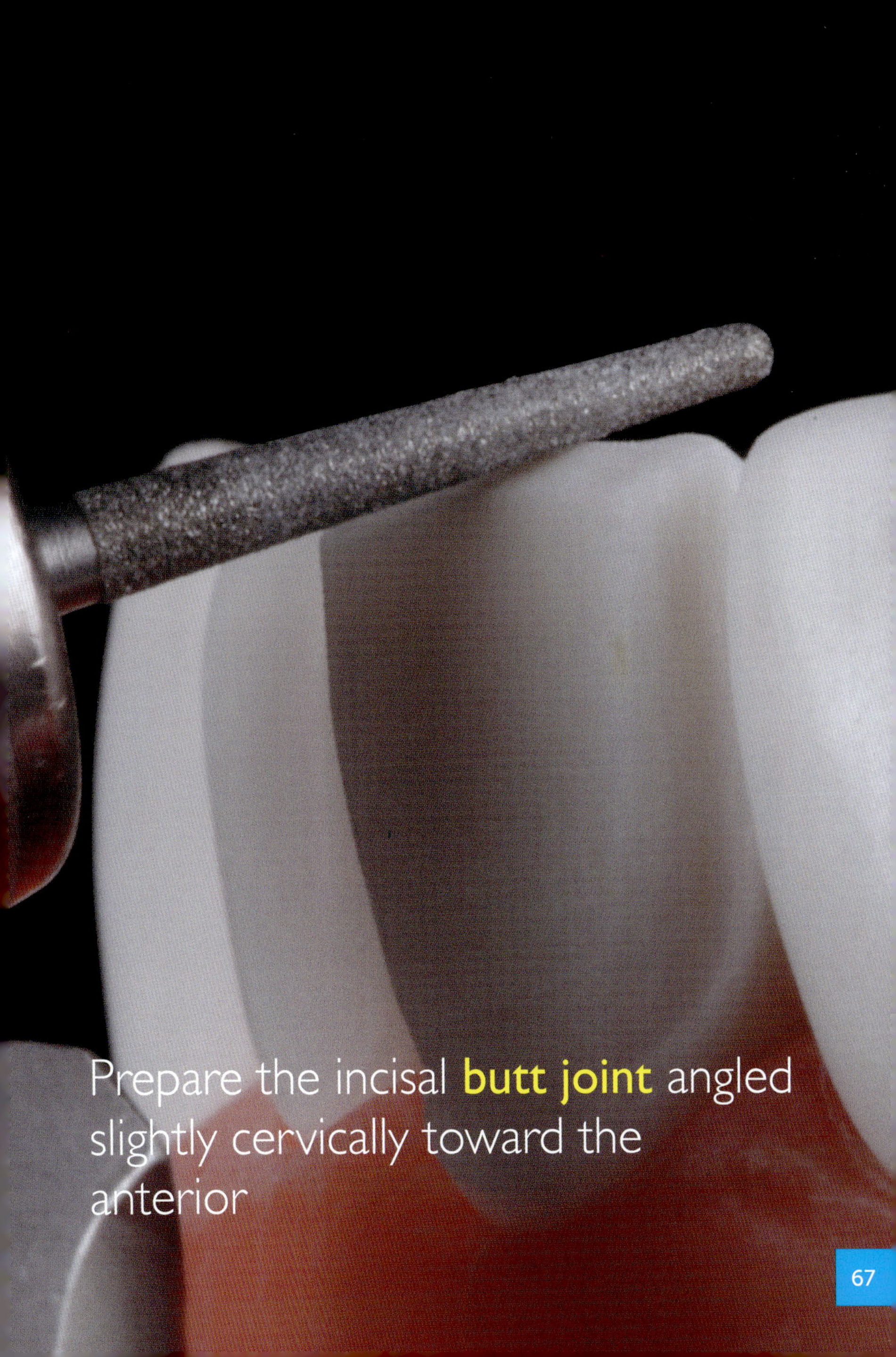

Prepare the incisal **butt joint** angled slightly cervically toward the anterior

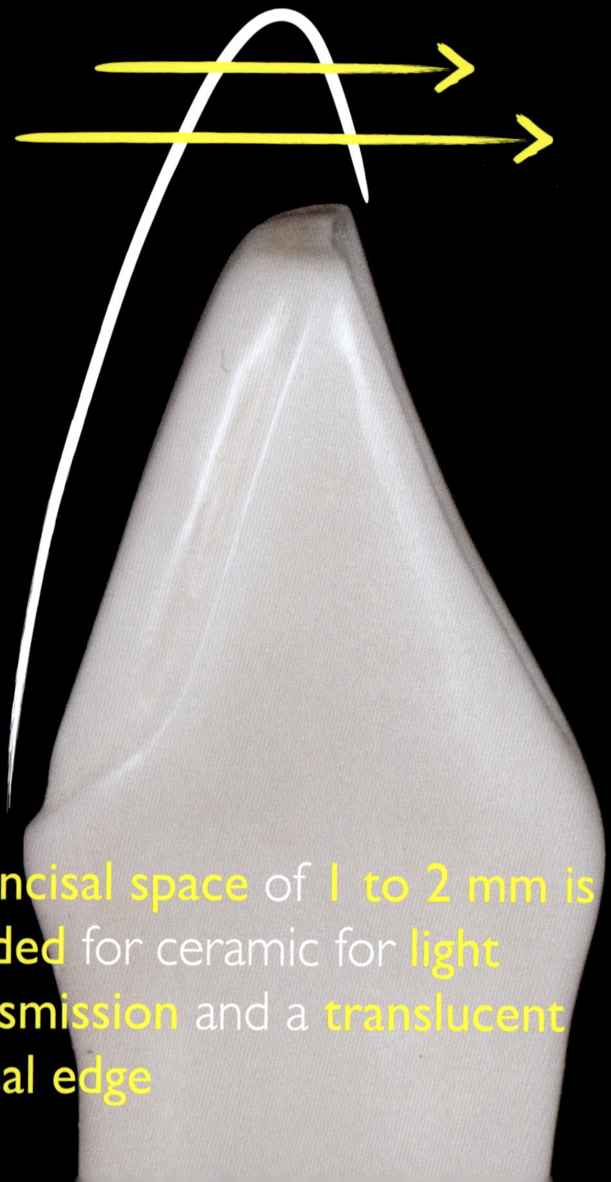

An incisal space of 1 to 2 mm is needed for ceramic for light transmission and a translucent incisal edge

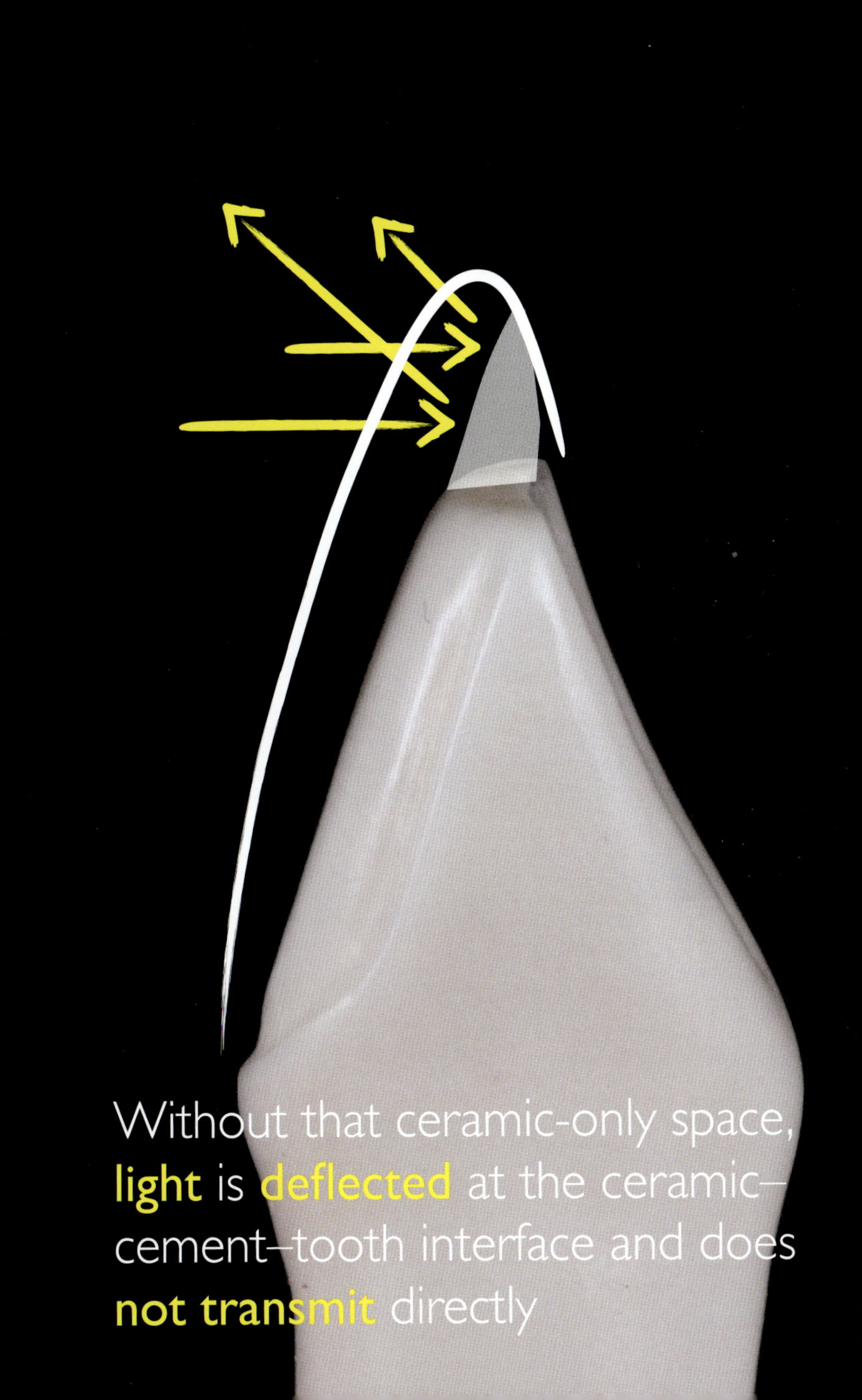

Without that ceramic-only space, **light** is **deflected** at the ceramic–cement–tooth interface and does **not transmit** directly

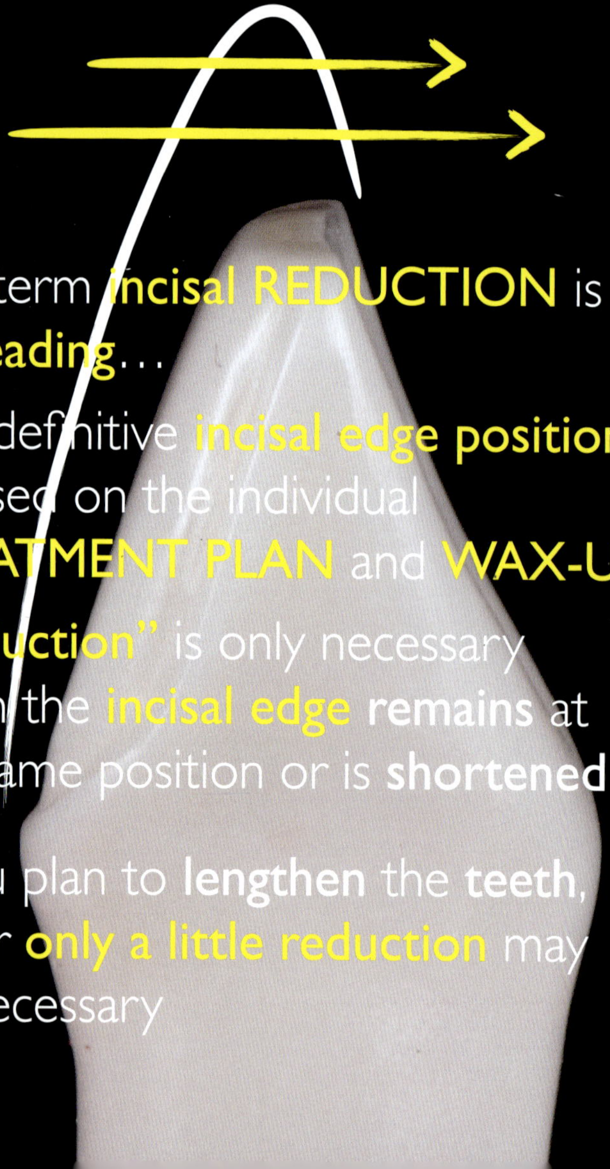

The term incisal REDUCTION is misleading…

The definitive incisal edge position is based on the individual TREATMENT PLAN and WAX-UP

"Reduction" is only necessary when the incisal edge **remains** at the same position or is **shortened**

If you plan to **lengthen** the **teeth**, no or only a little reduction may be necessary

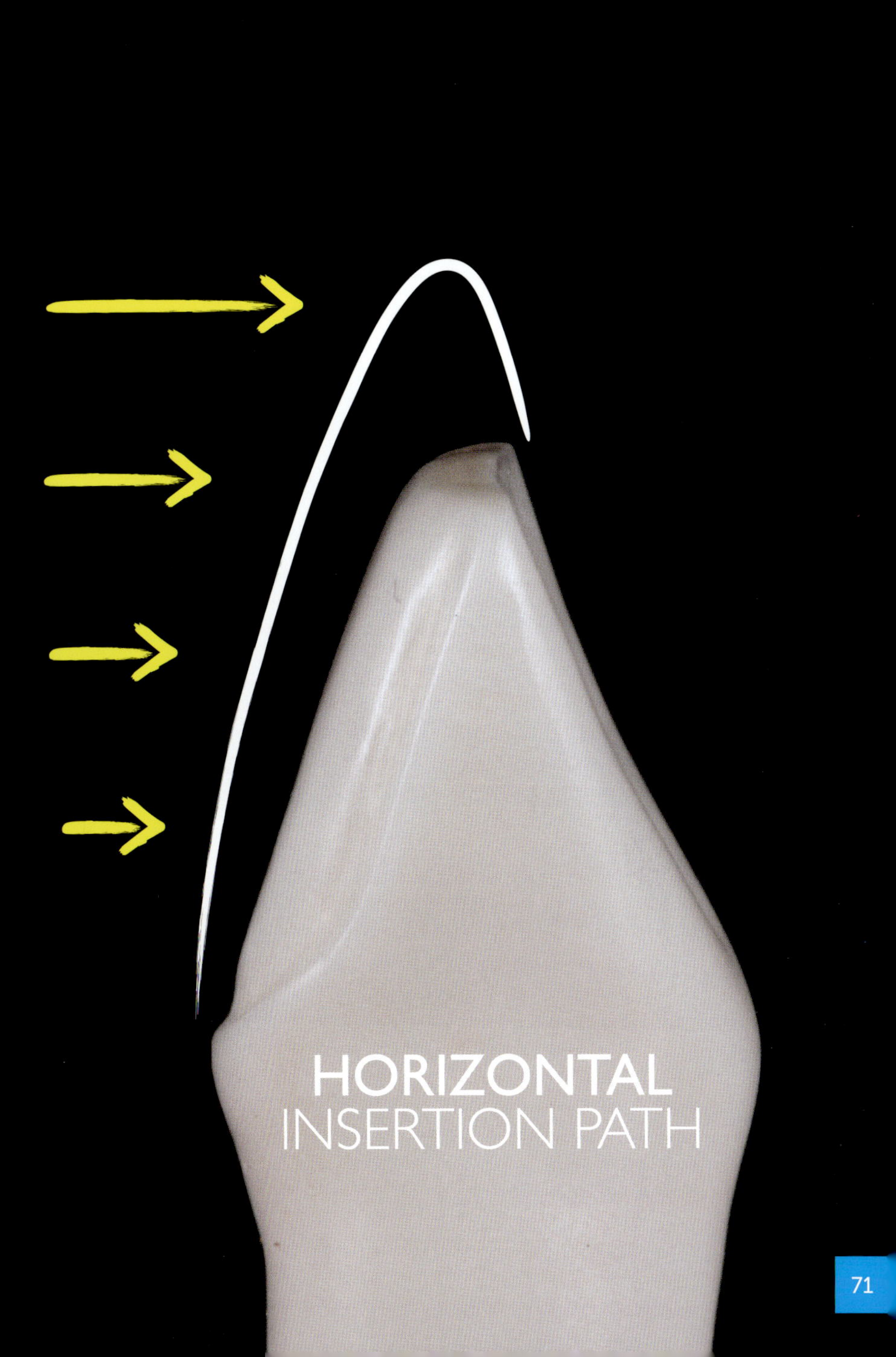

HORIZONTAL
INSERTION PATH

Quint Dent Technol 2016;39:7–25

Novel guidelines for bonded ceramic veneers: Part 1. Is tooth preparation truly necessary?

Clavijo V, Sartori N, Phark JH, Duarte S

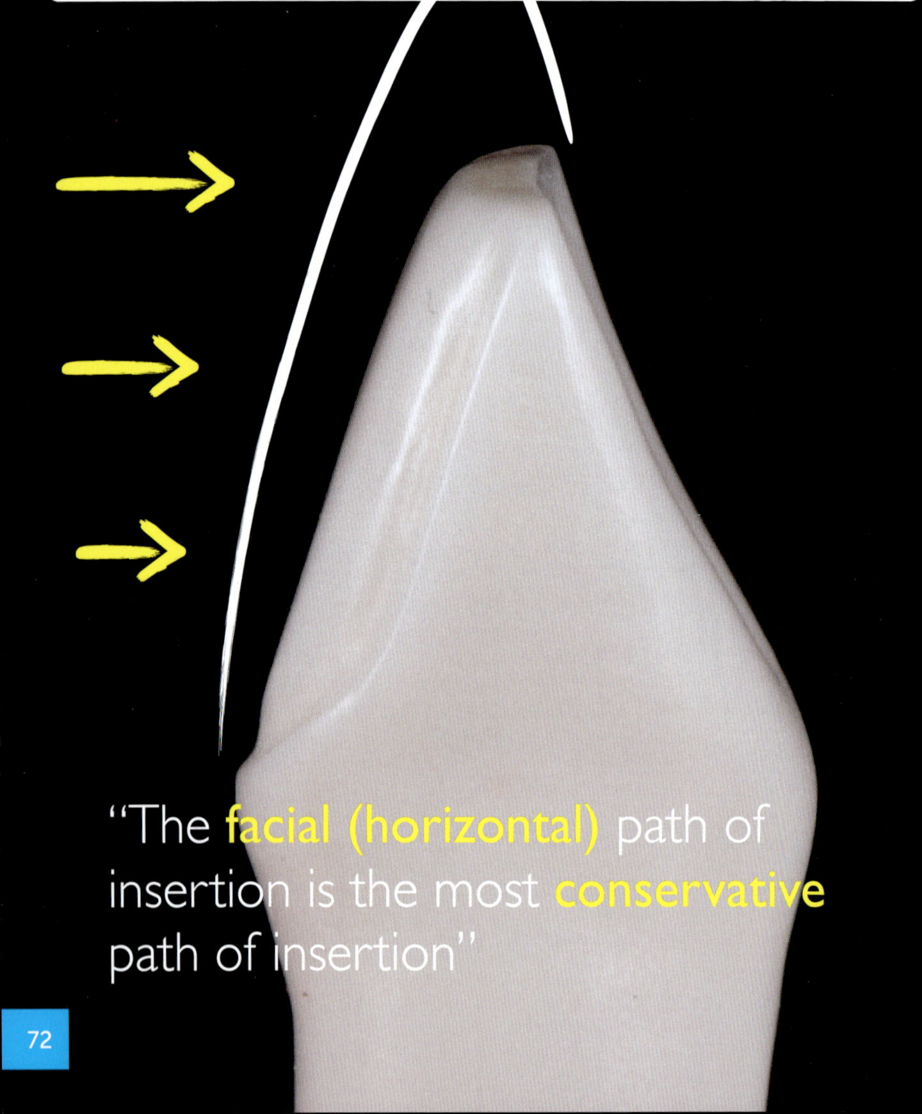

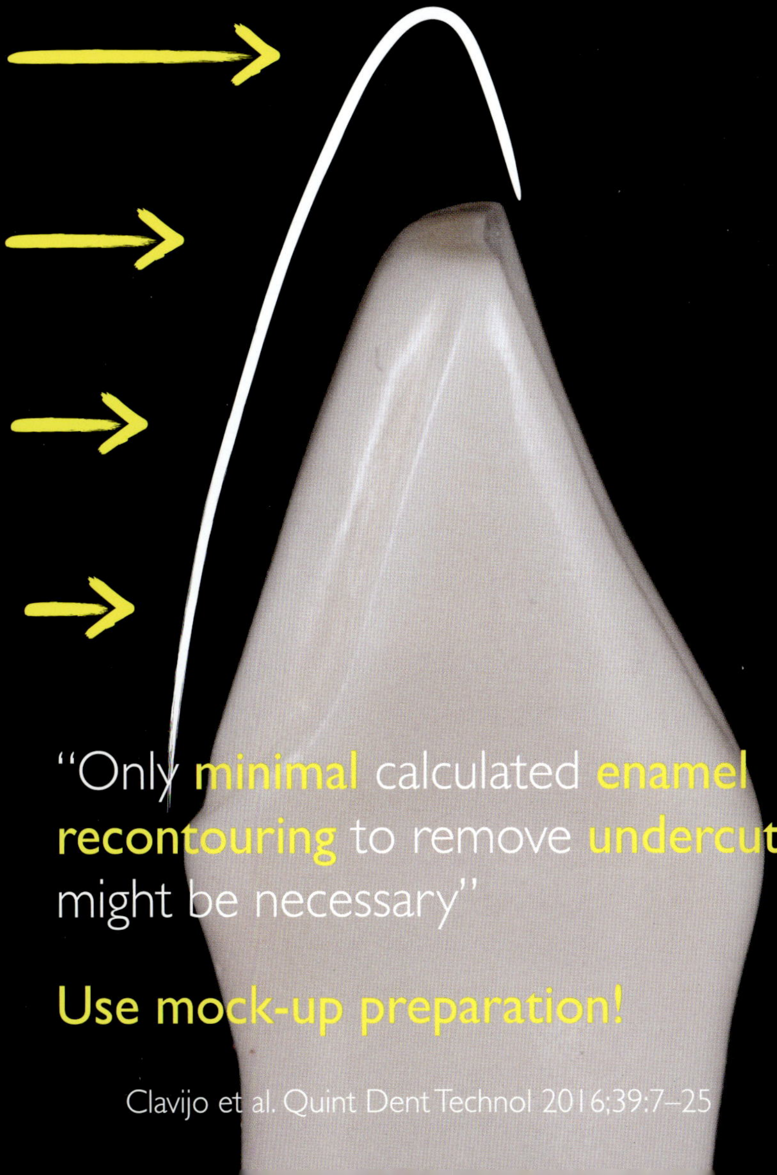

"Only **minimal** calculated **enamel recontouring** to remove **undercuts** might be necessary"

Use mock-up preparation!

Clavijo et al. Quint Dent Technol 2016;39:7–25

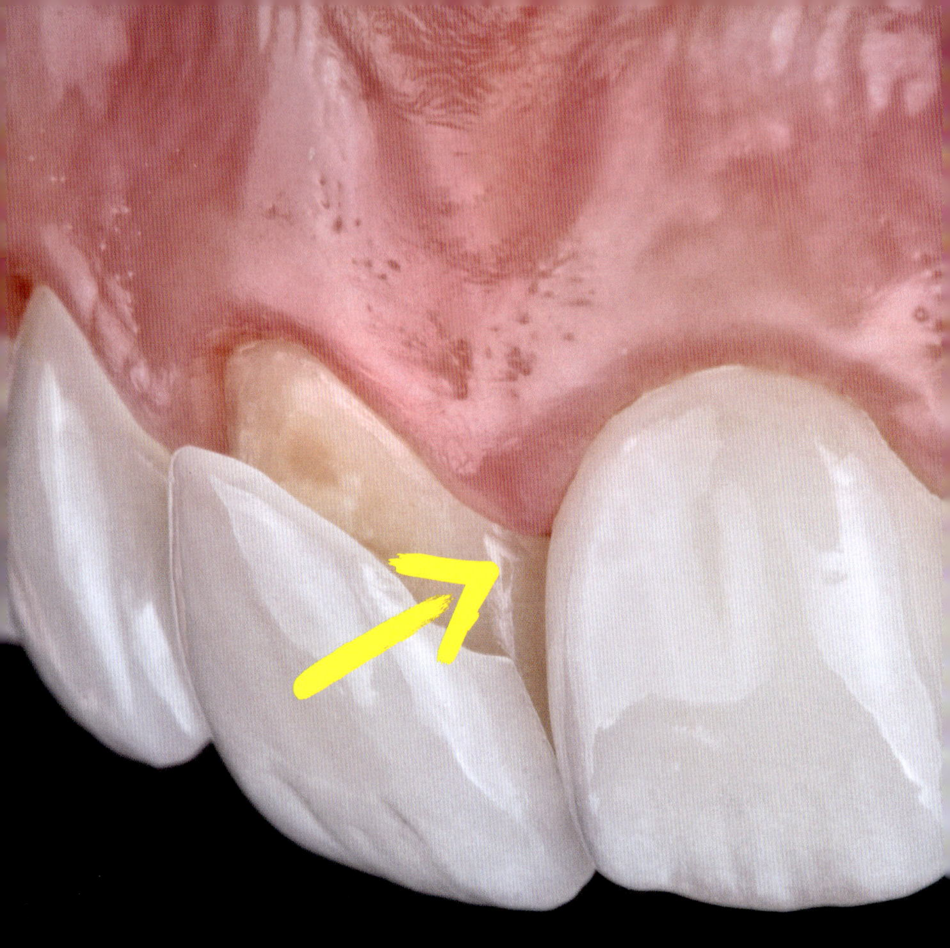

THE "ELBOW" PREP

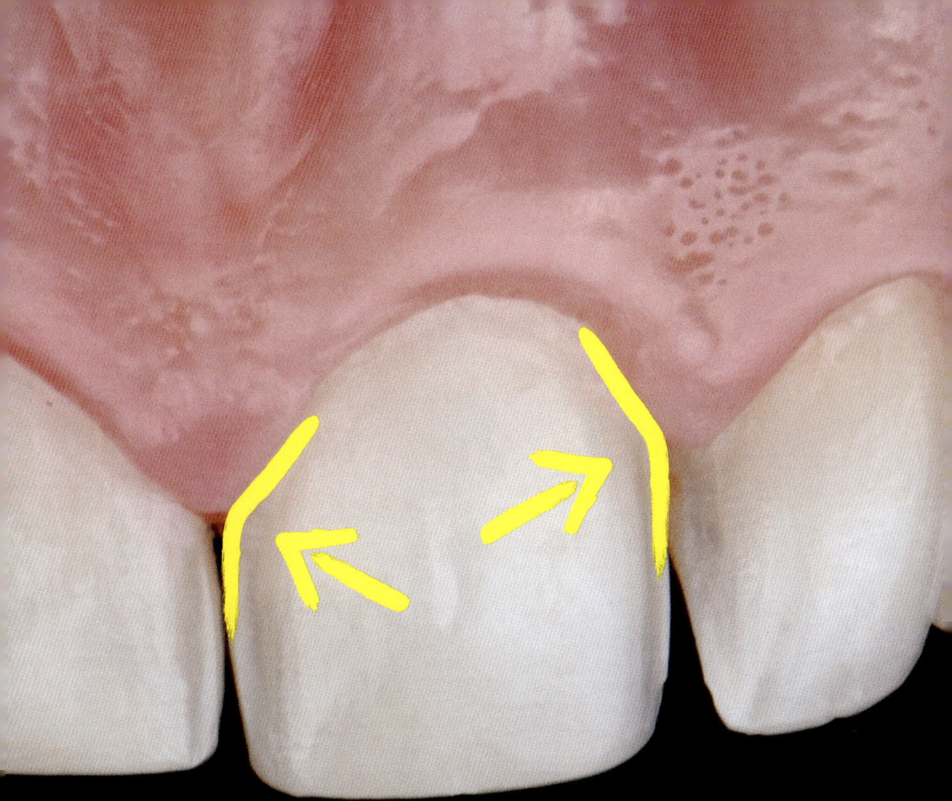

One of the MOST COMMON MISTAKES:

TRIANGLES of remaining cervico-interproximal TOOTH structure are visible from the lateral/profile

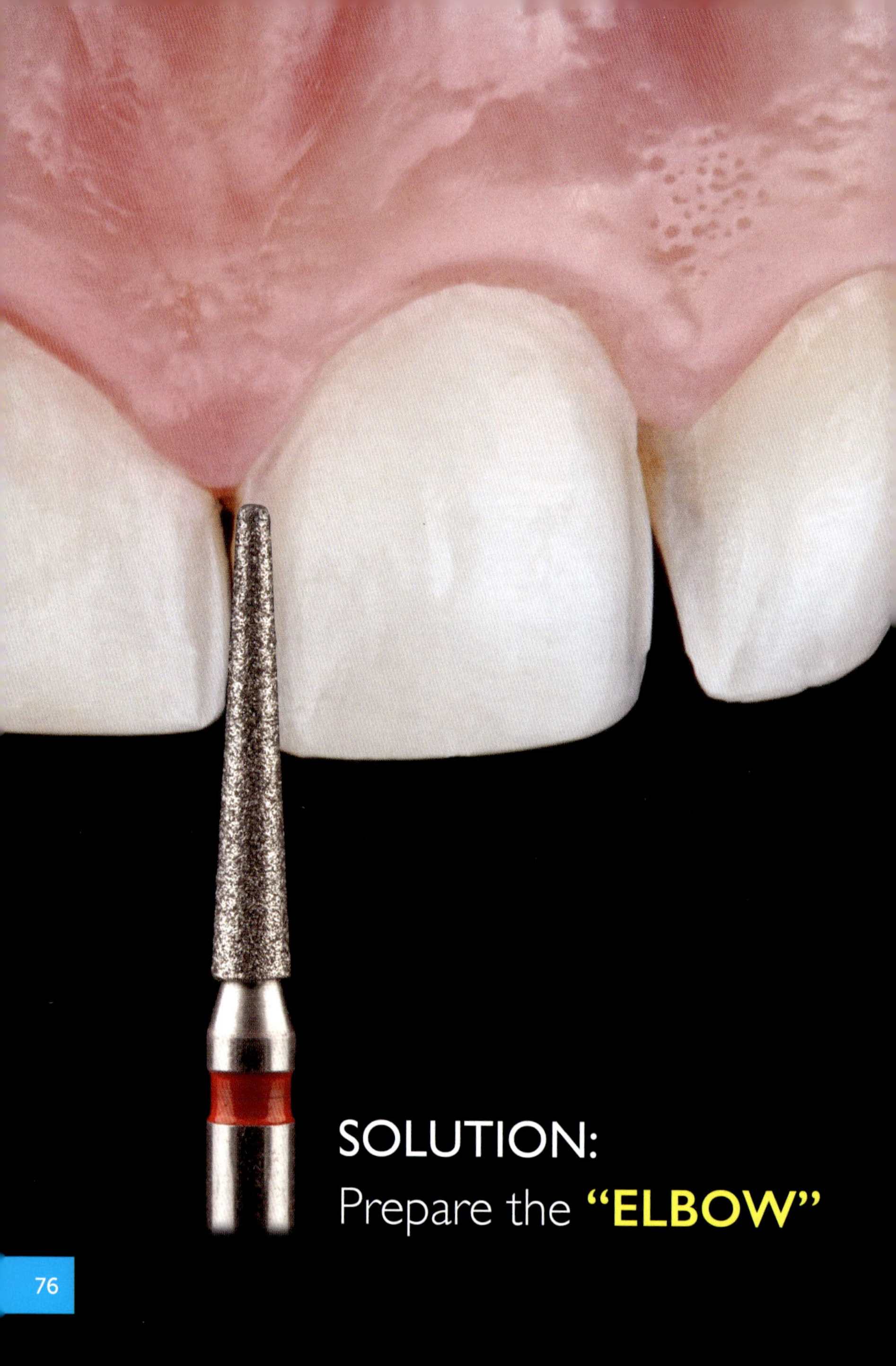

SOLUTION:
Prepare the **"ELBOW"**

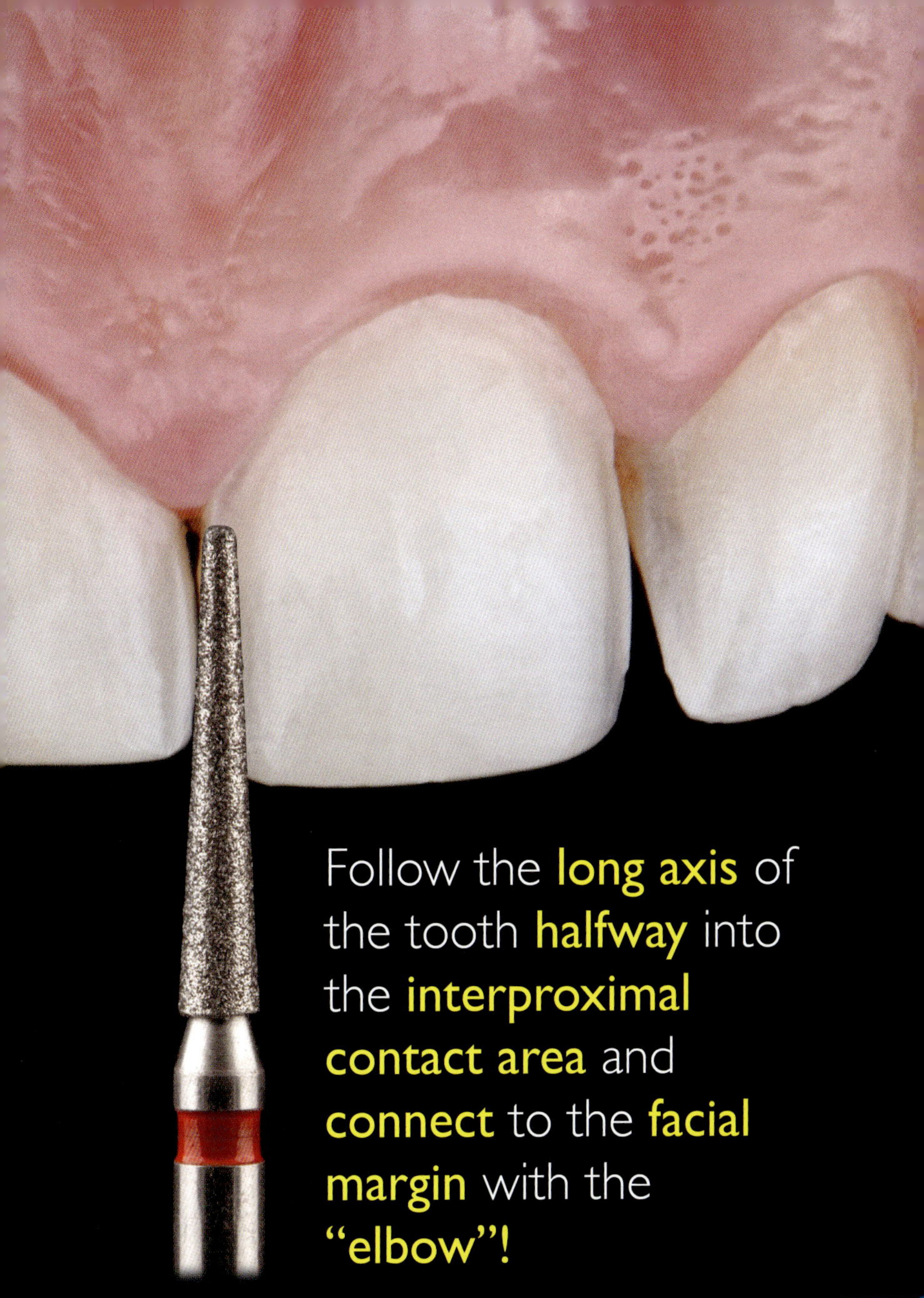

Follow the **long axis** of the tooth **halfway** into the **interproximal contact area** and **connect** to the **facial margin** with the **"elbow"**!

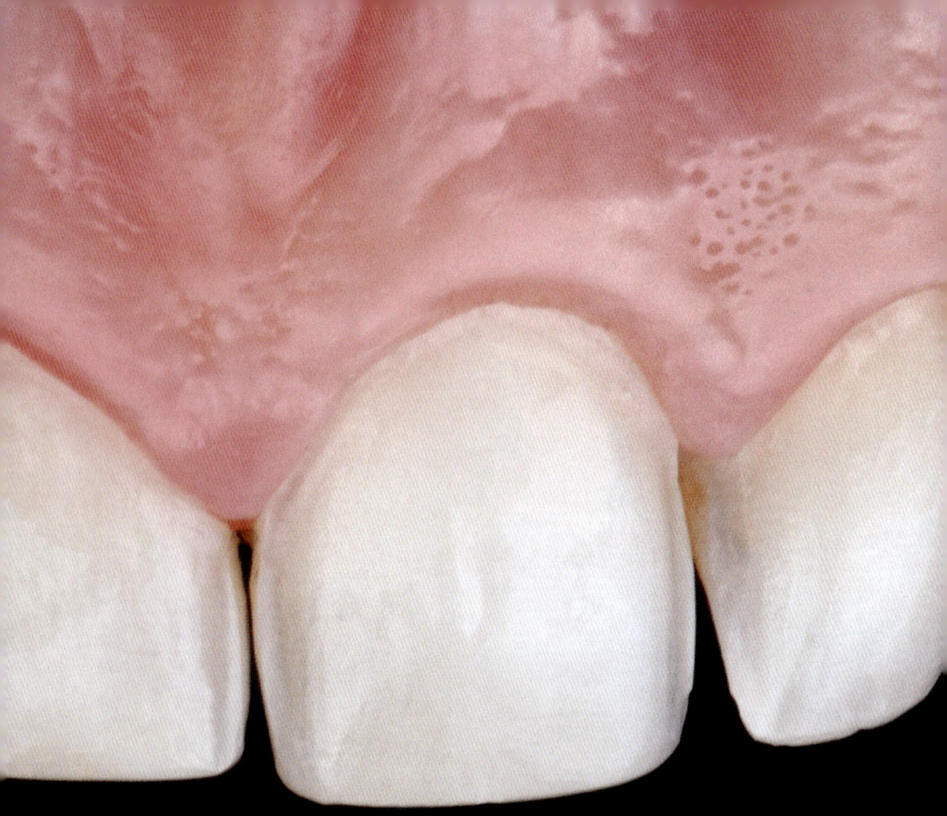

Always **visually check** from **ALL ANGLES** and **ASPECTS** during preparation – **NOT only** from the **frontal view!**

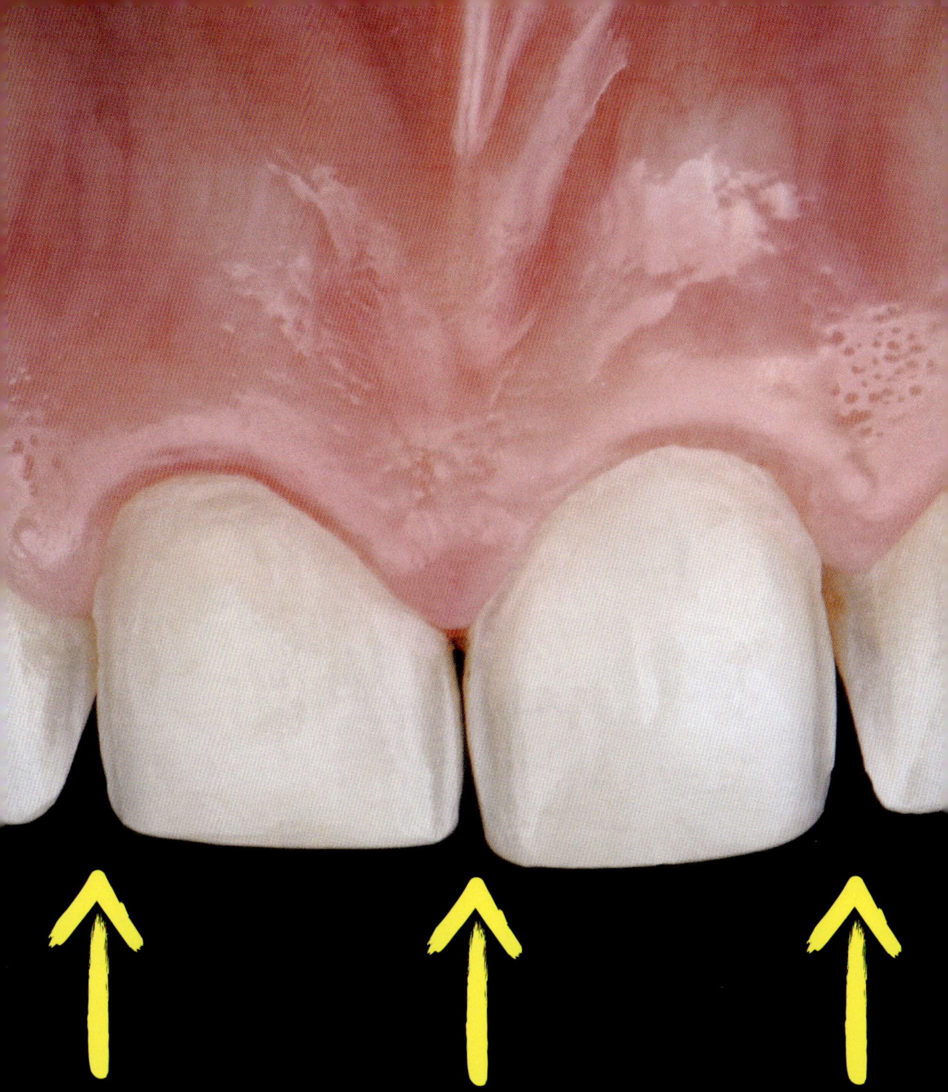

BREAK CONTACT
YES or NO?

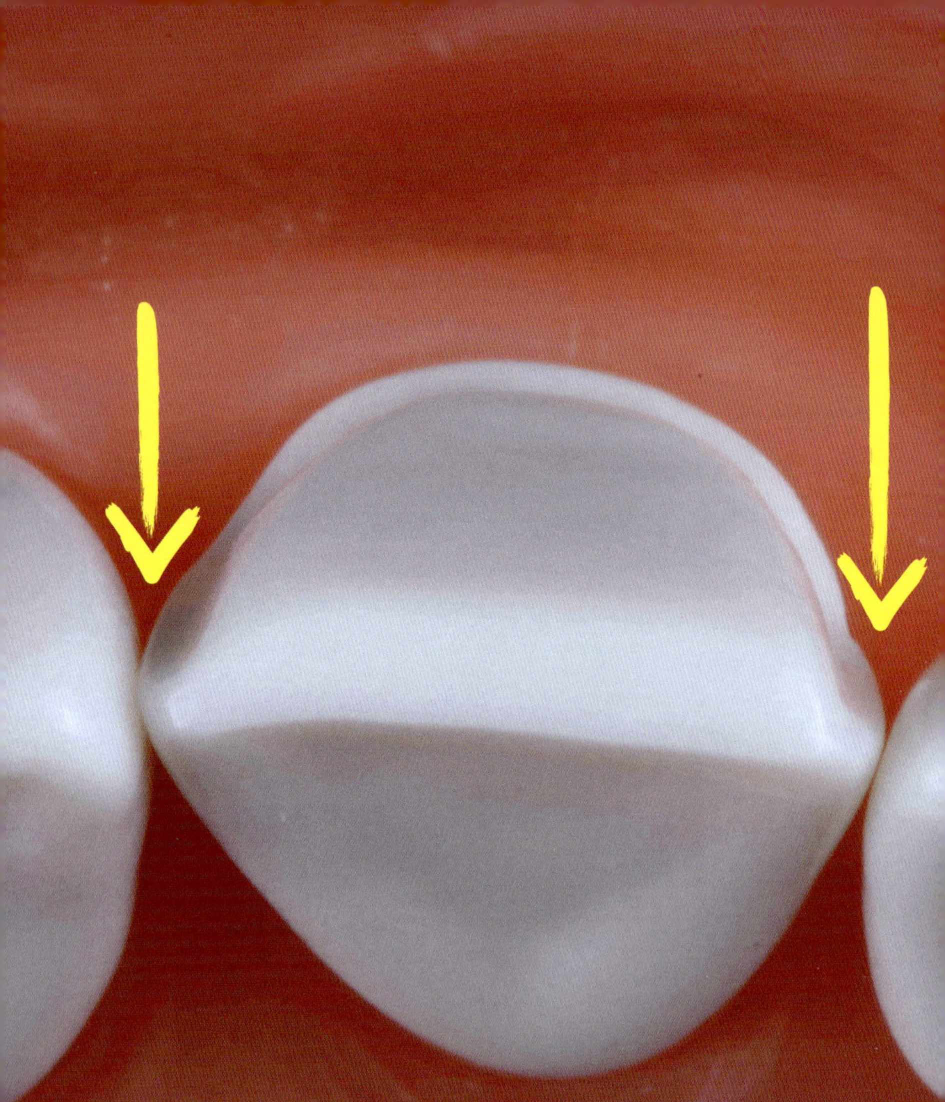

STANDARD PREPARATION:

Prepare only **HALFWAY** into the interproximal contact areas

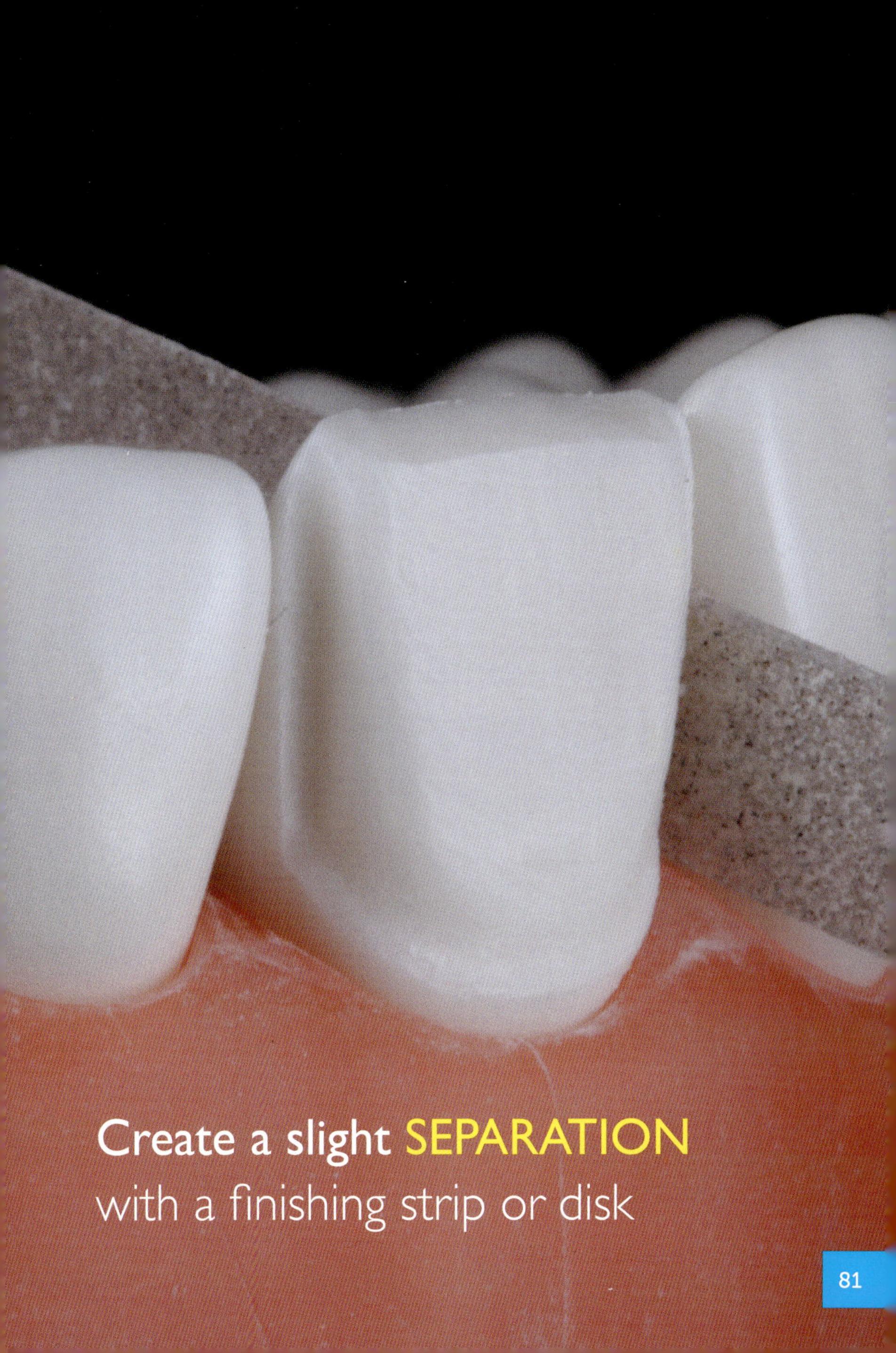

Create a slight SEPARATION
with a finishing strip or disk

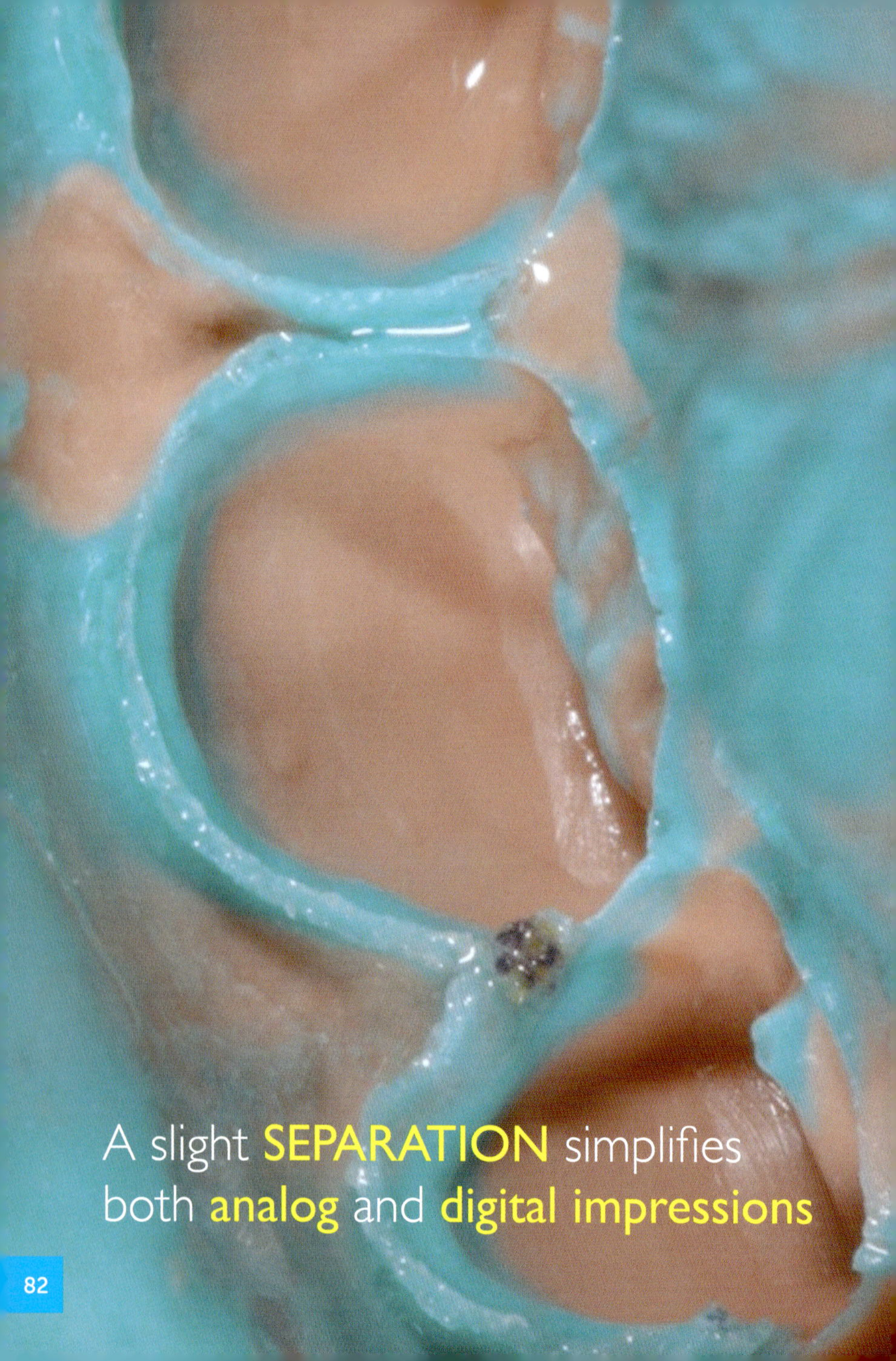

A slight **SEPARATION** simplifies both **analog** and **digital impressions**

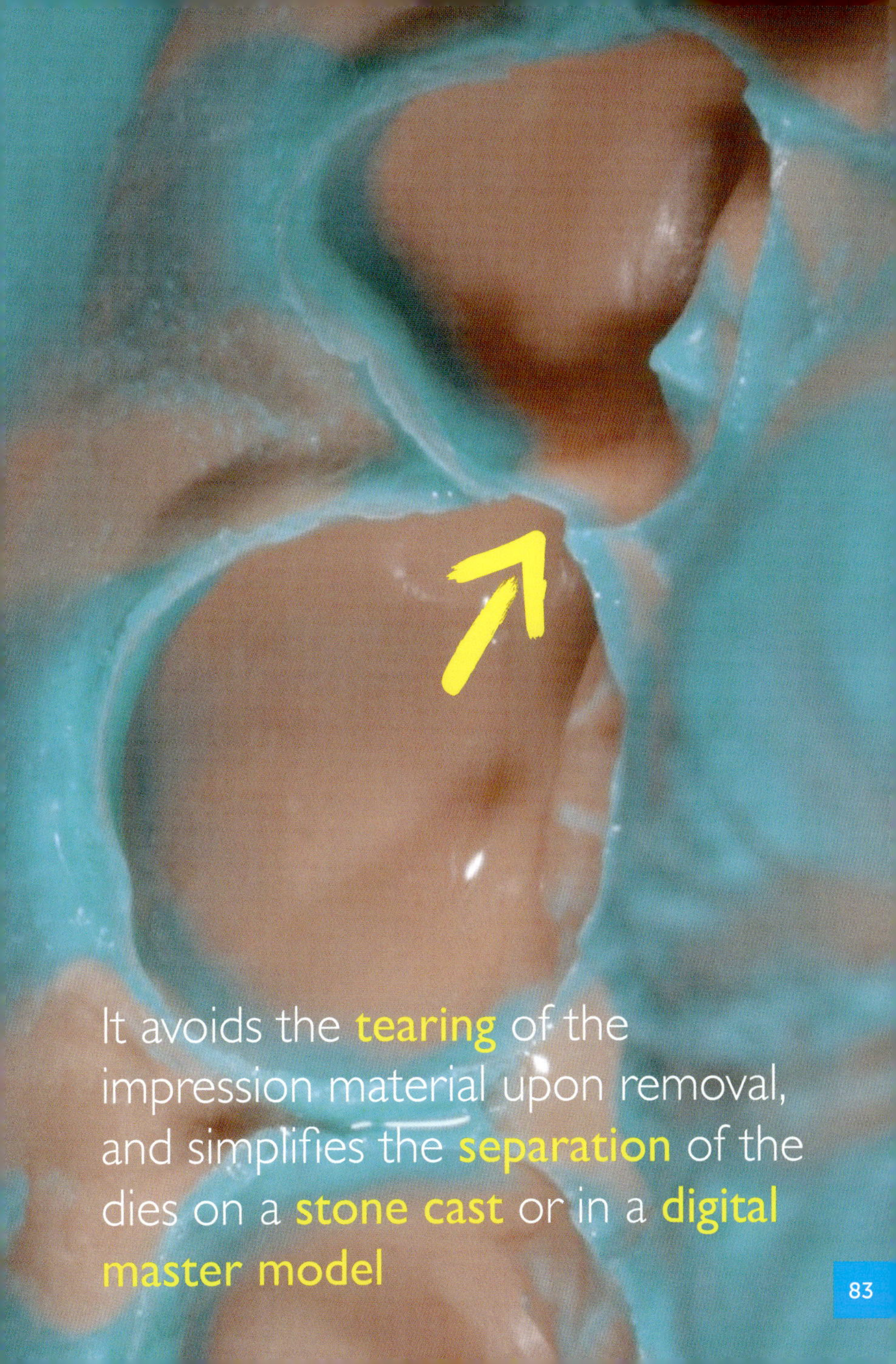

It avoids the **tearing** of the impression material upon removal, and simplifies the **separation** of the dies on a **stone cast** or in a **digital master model**

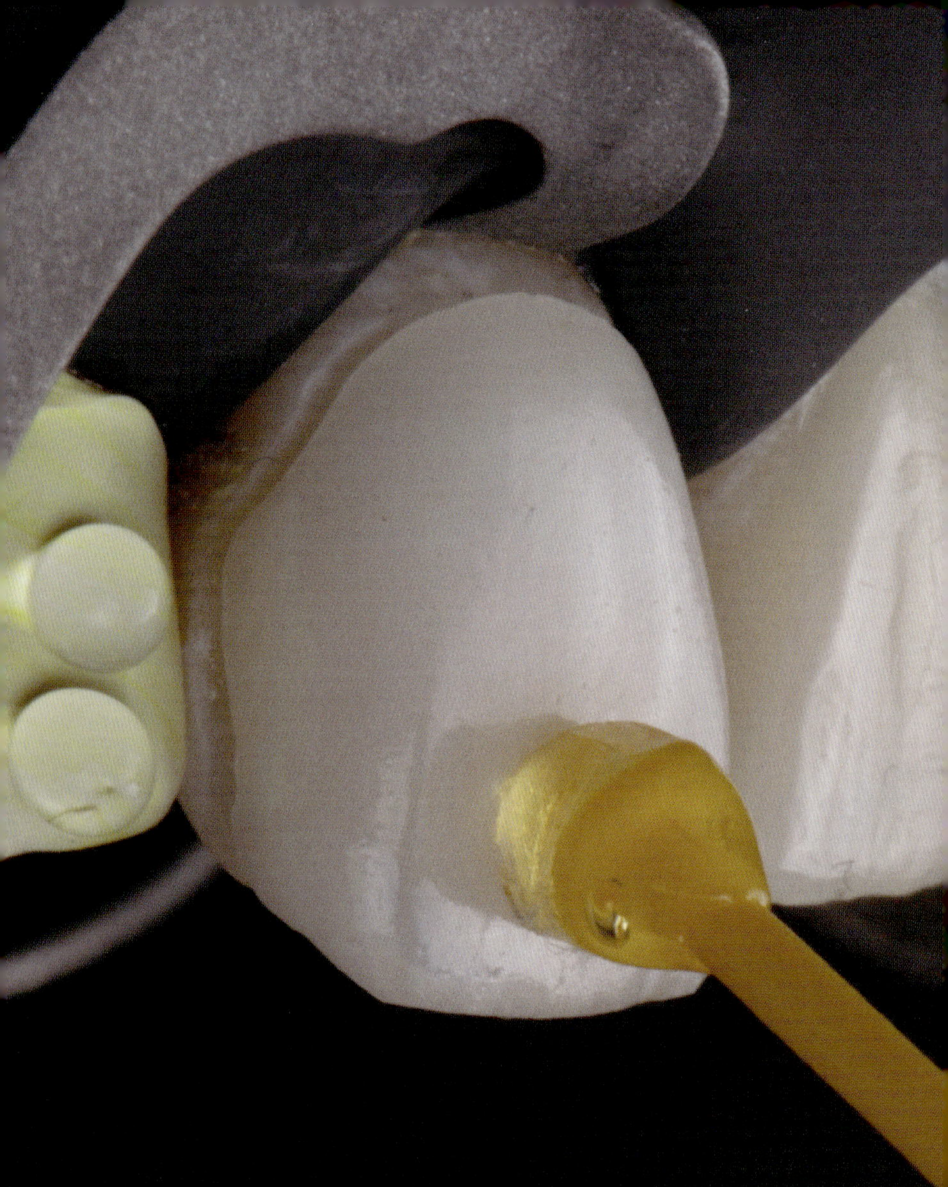

Slight **separation** also makes veneer **bonding easier**

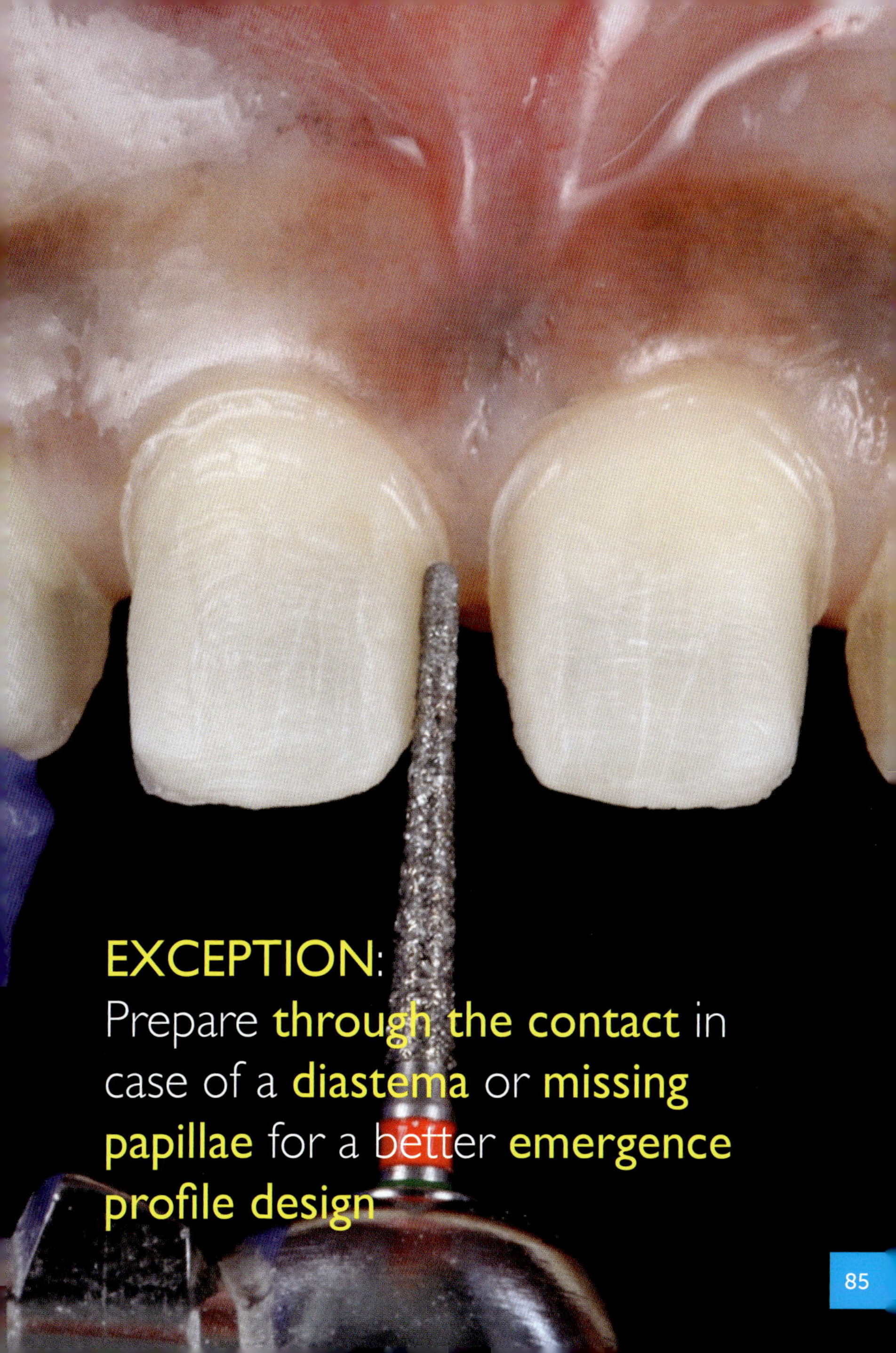

EXCEPTION:

Prepare **through the contact** in case of a **diastema** or **missing papillae** for a better **emergence profile design**

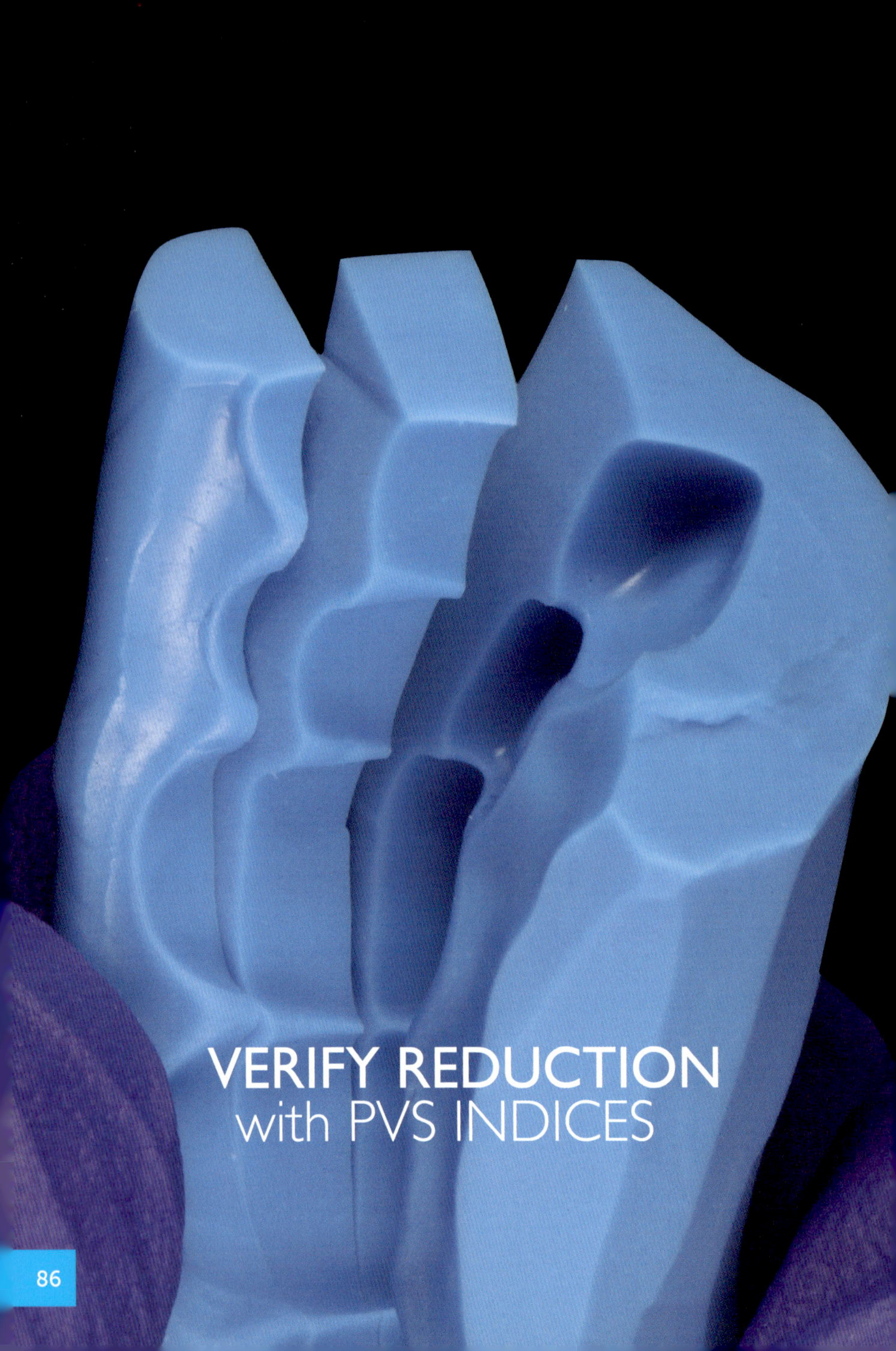

VERIFY REDUCTION with PVS INDICES

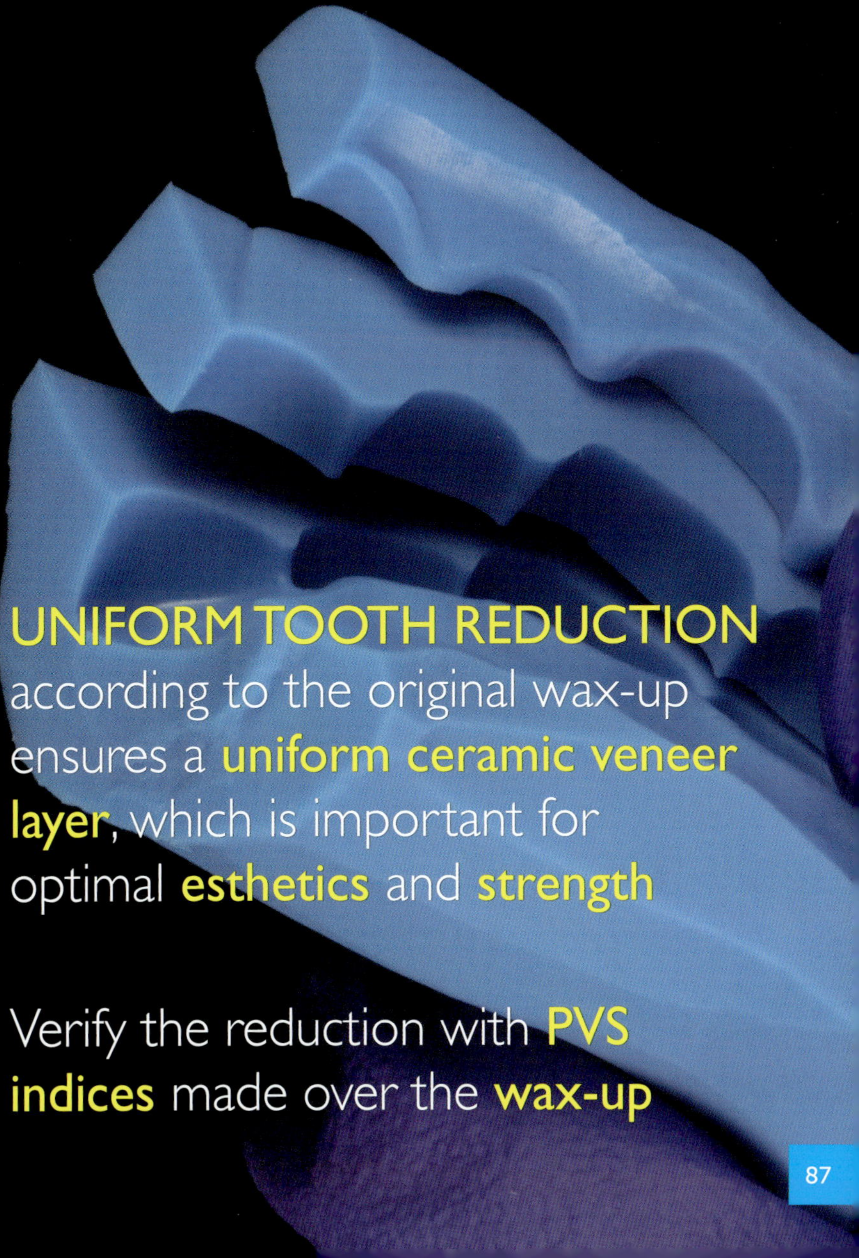

UNIFORM TOOTH REDUCTION

according to the original wax-up ensures a **uniform ceramic veneer layer**, which is important for optimal **esthetics** and **strength**

Verify the reduction with **PVS indices** made over the **wax-up**

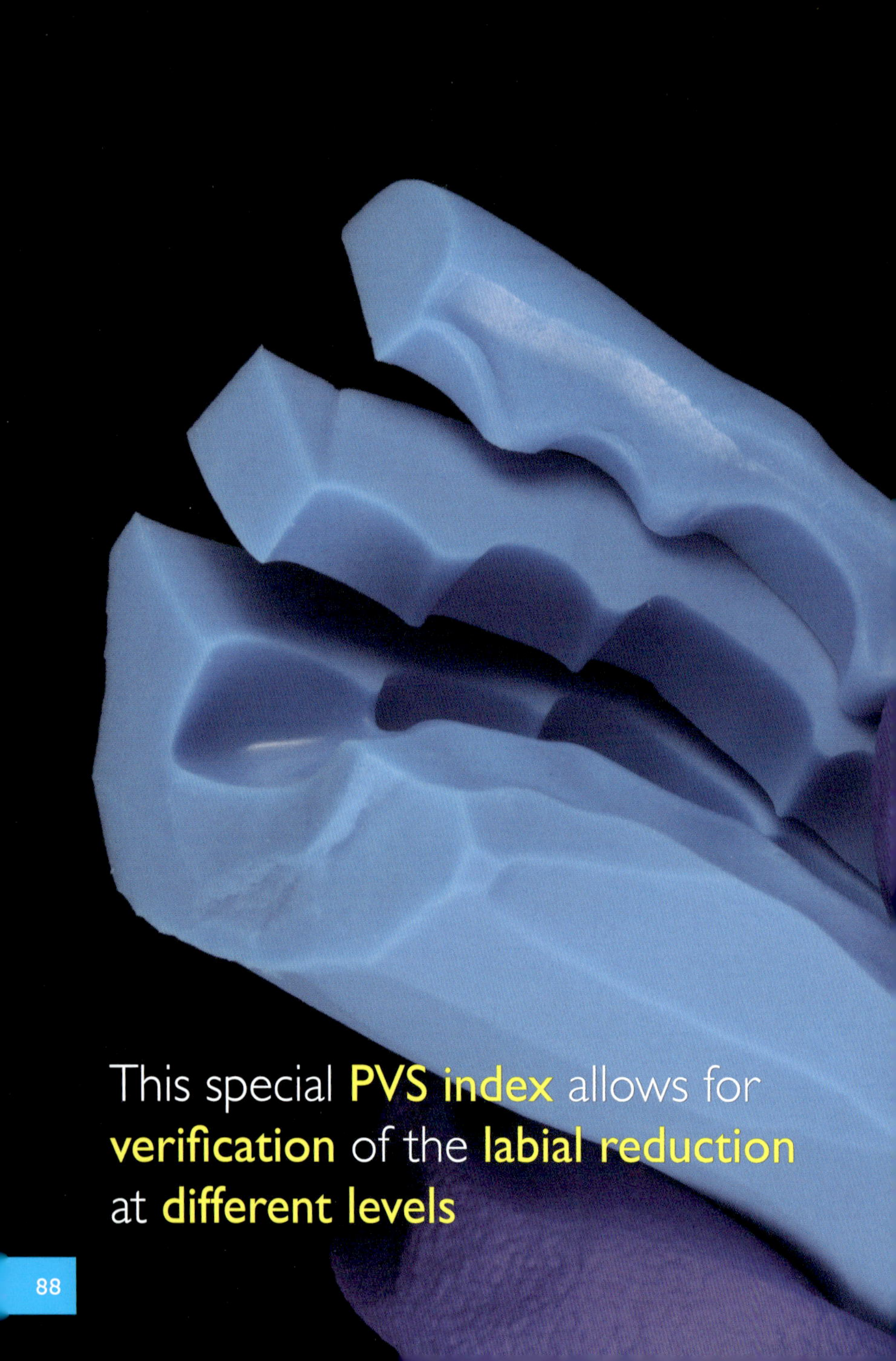

This special **PVS index** allows for **verification** of the **labial reduction** at **different levels**

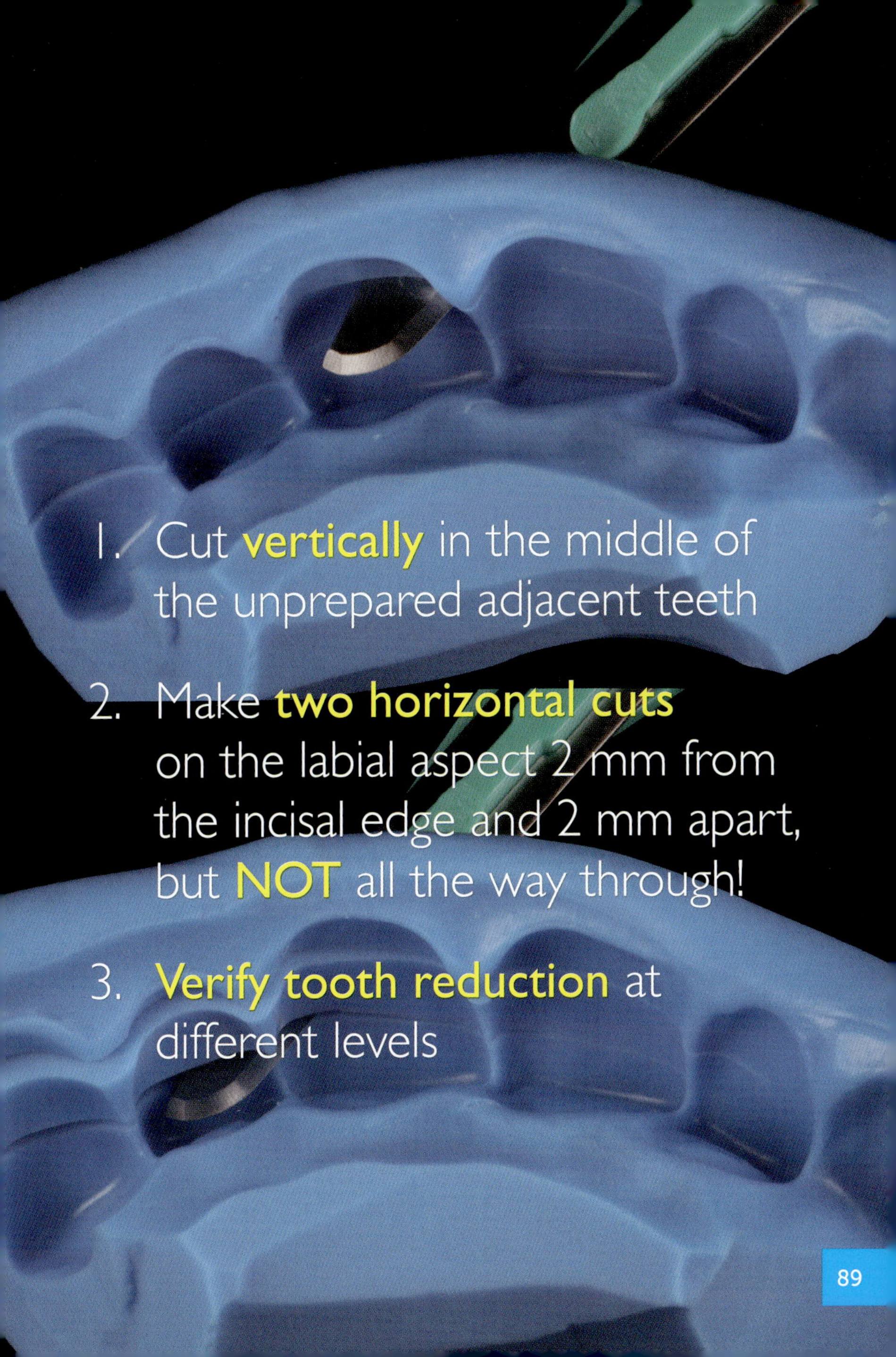

1. Cut **vertically** in the middle of the unprepared adjacent teeth
2. Make **two horizontal cuts** on the labial aspect 2 mm from the incisal edge and 2 mm apart, but **NOT** all the way through!
3. **Verify tooth reduction** at different levels

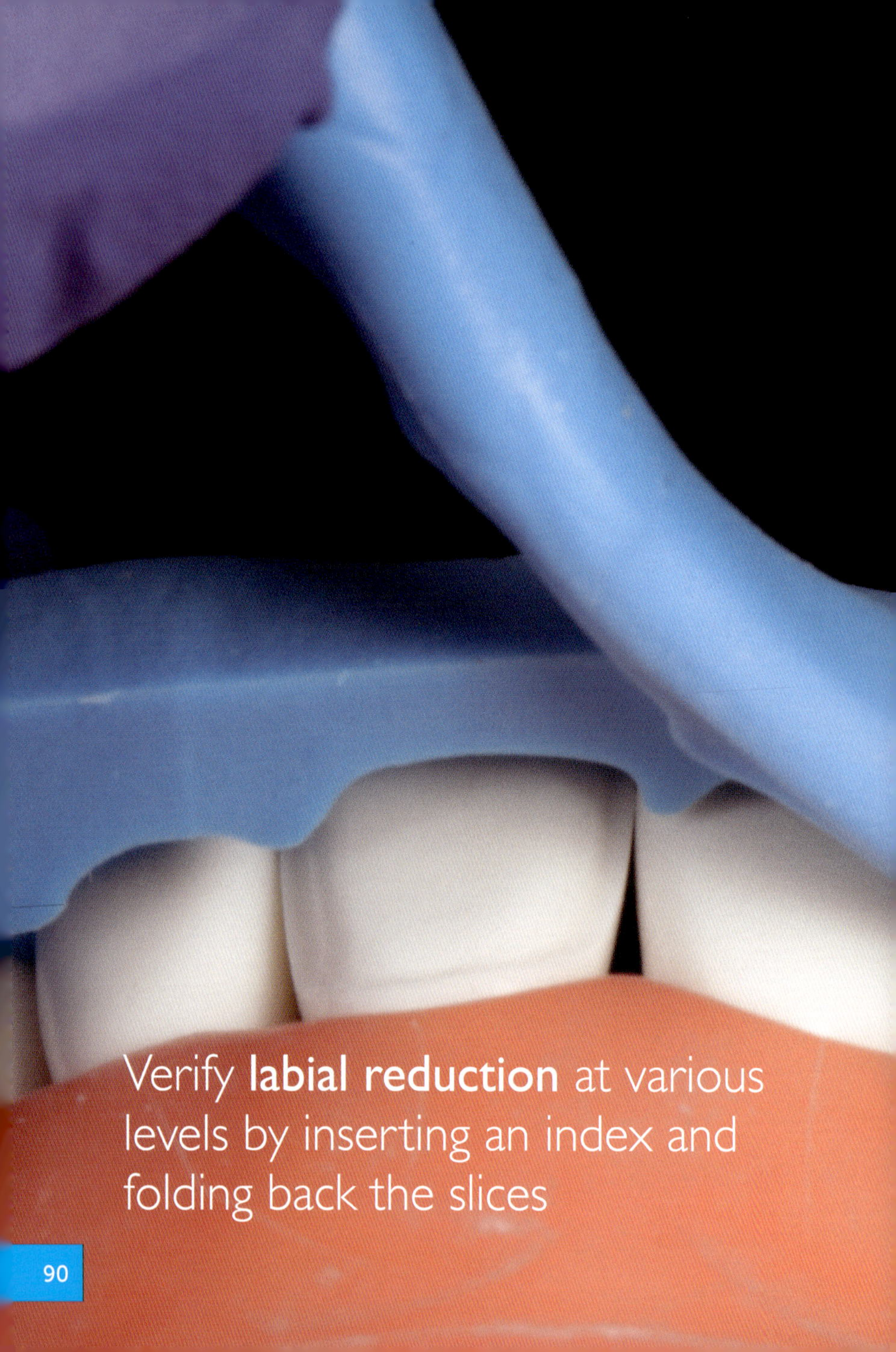

Verify **labial reduction** at various levels by inserting an index and folding back the slices

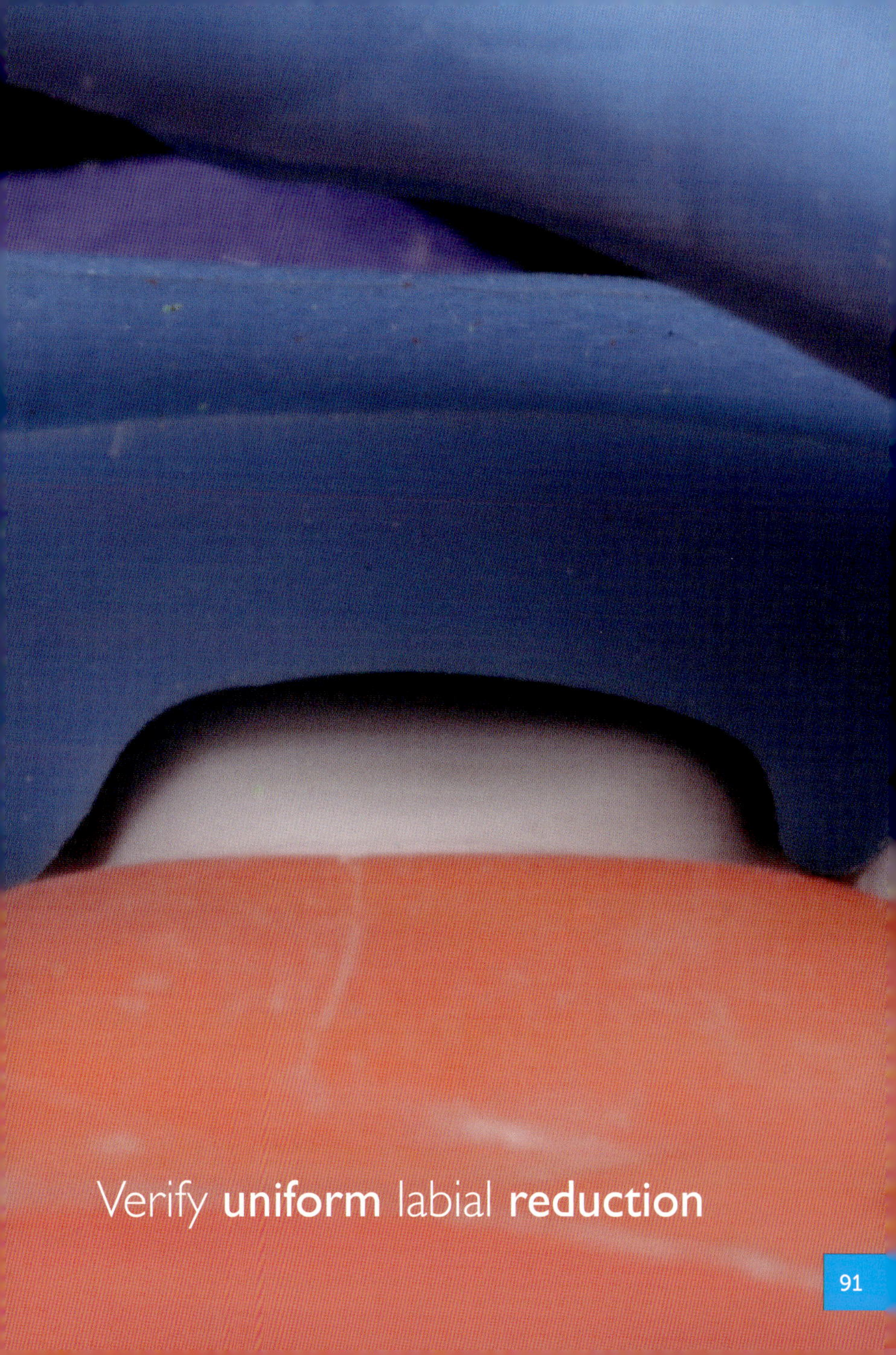

Verify **uniform** labial **reduction**

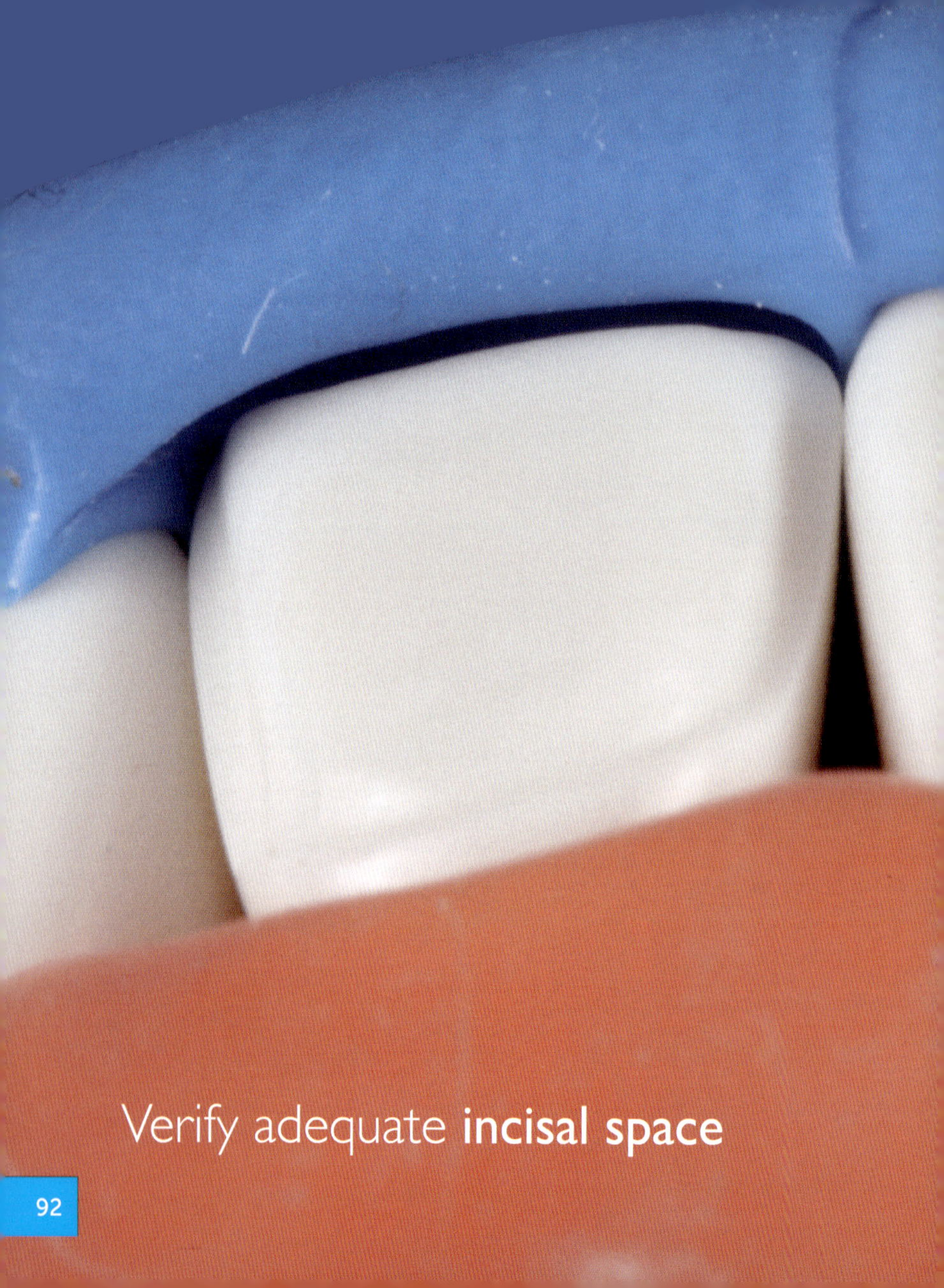

Verify adequate **incisal space**

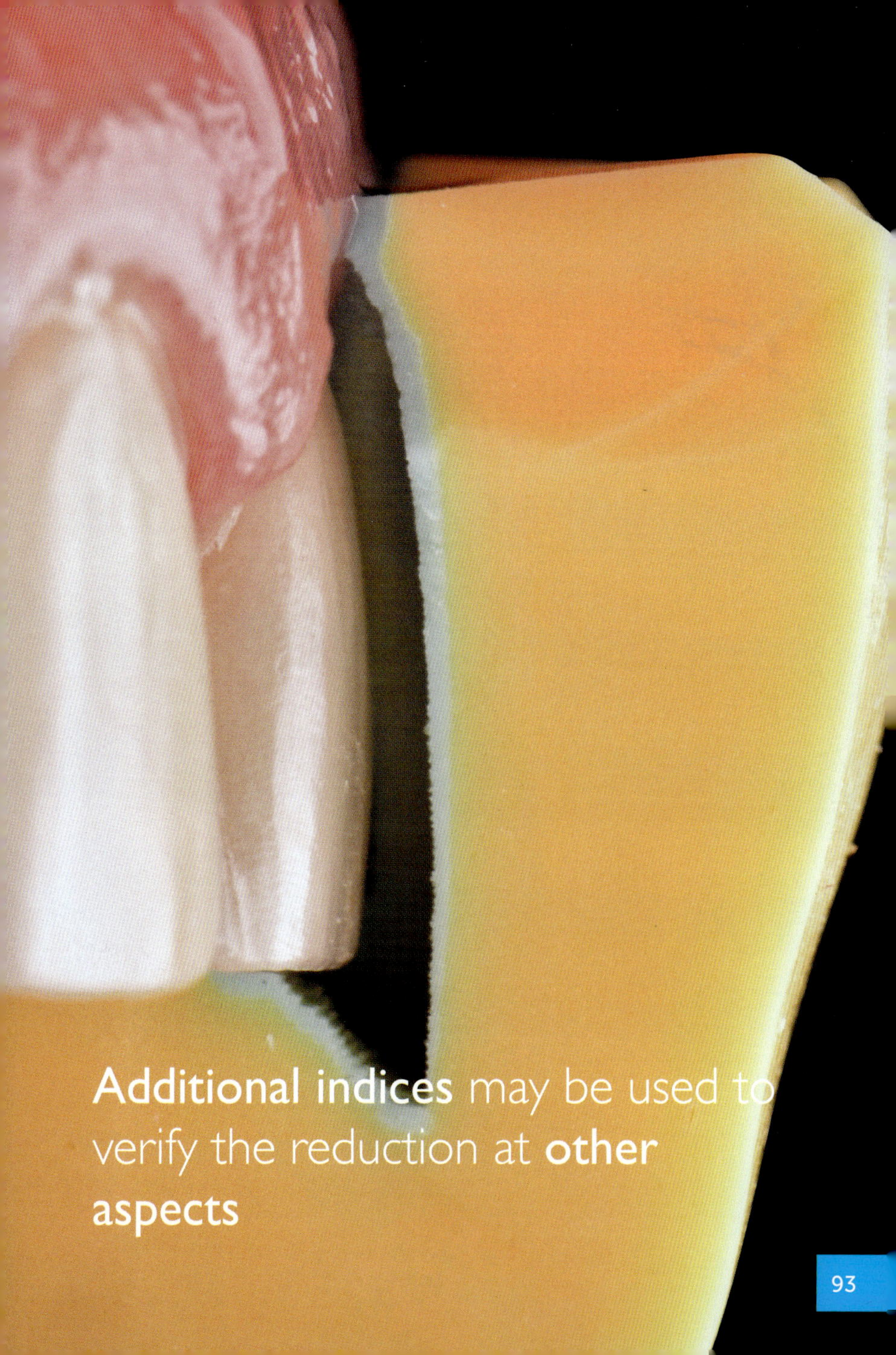

Additional indices may be used to verify the reduction at **other aspects**

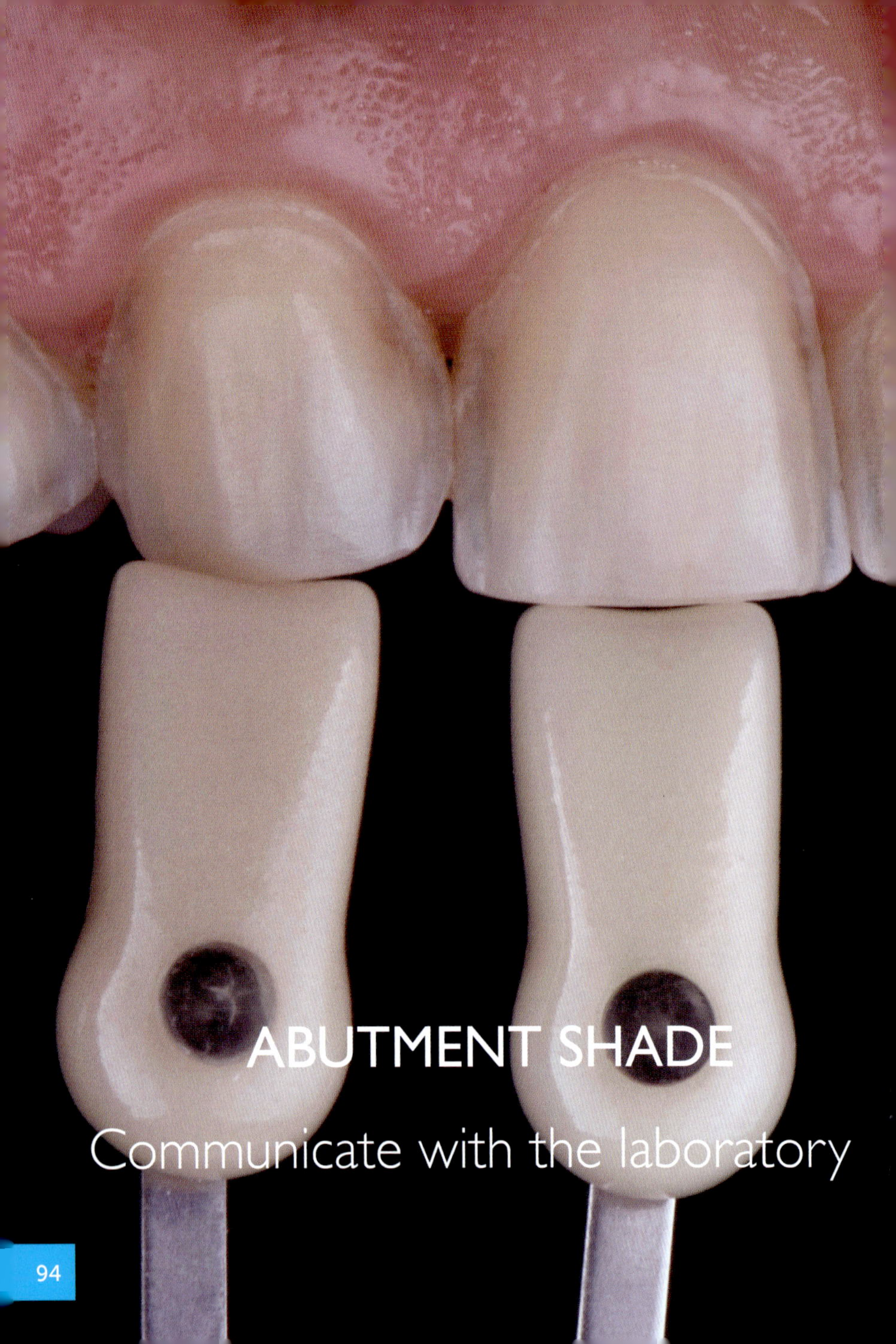

ABUTMENT SHADE

Communicate with the laboratory

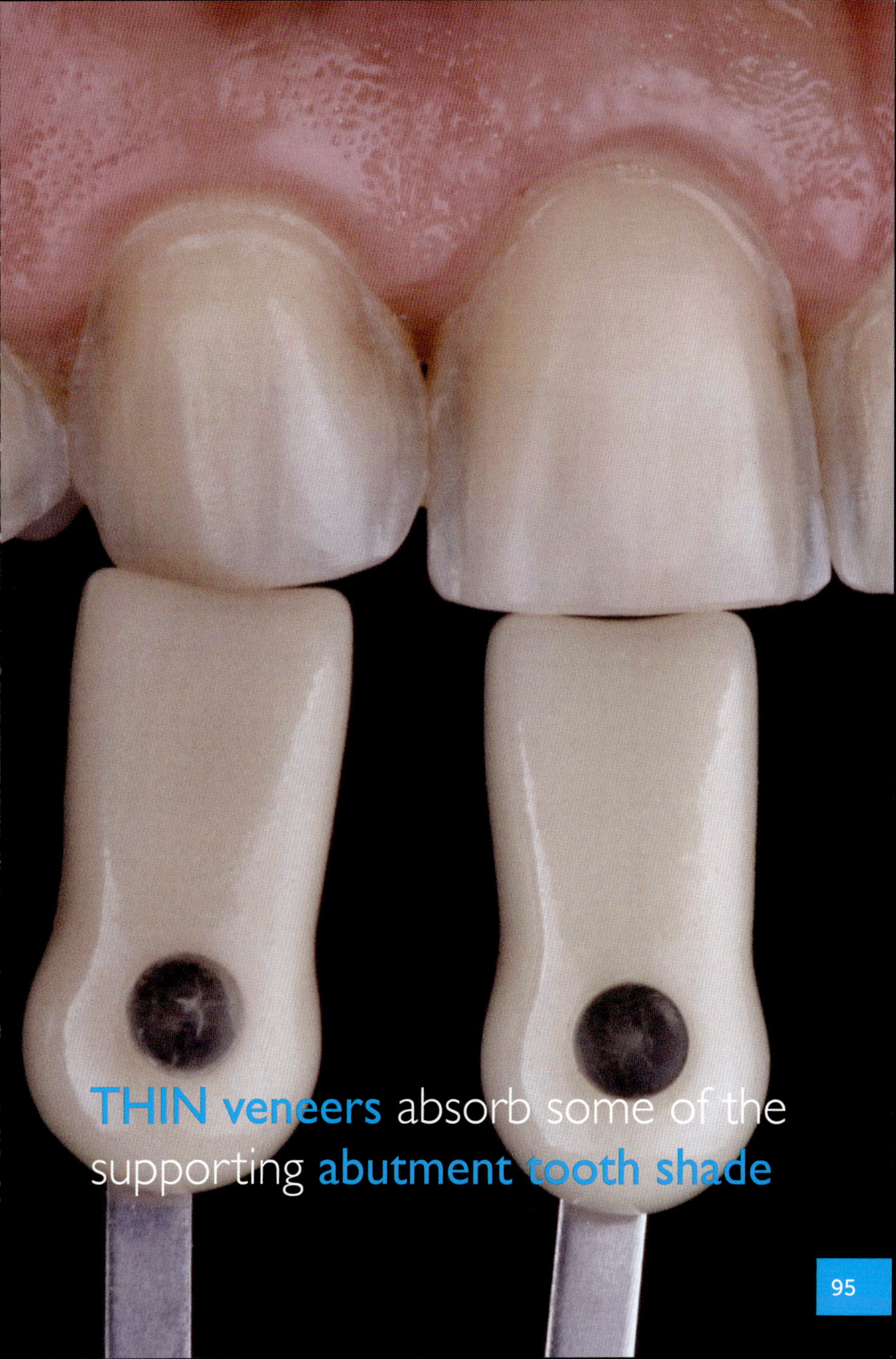

THIN veneers absorb some of the supporting abutment tooth shade

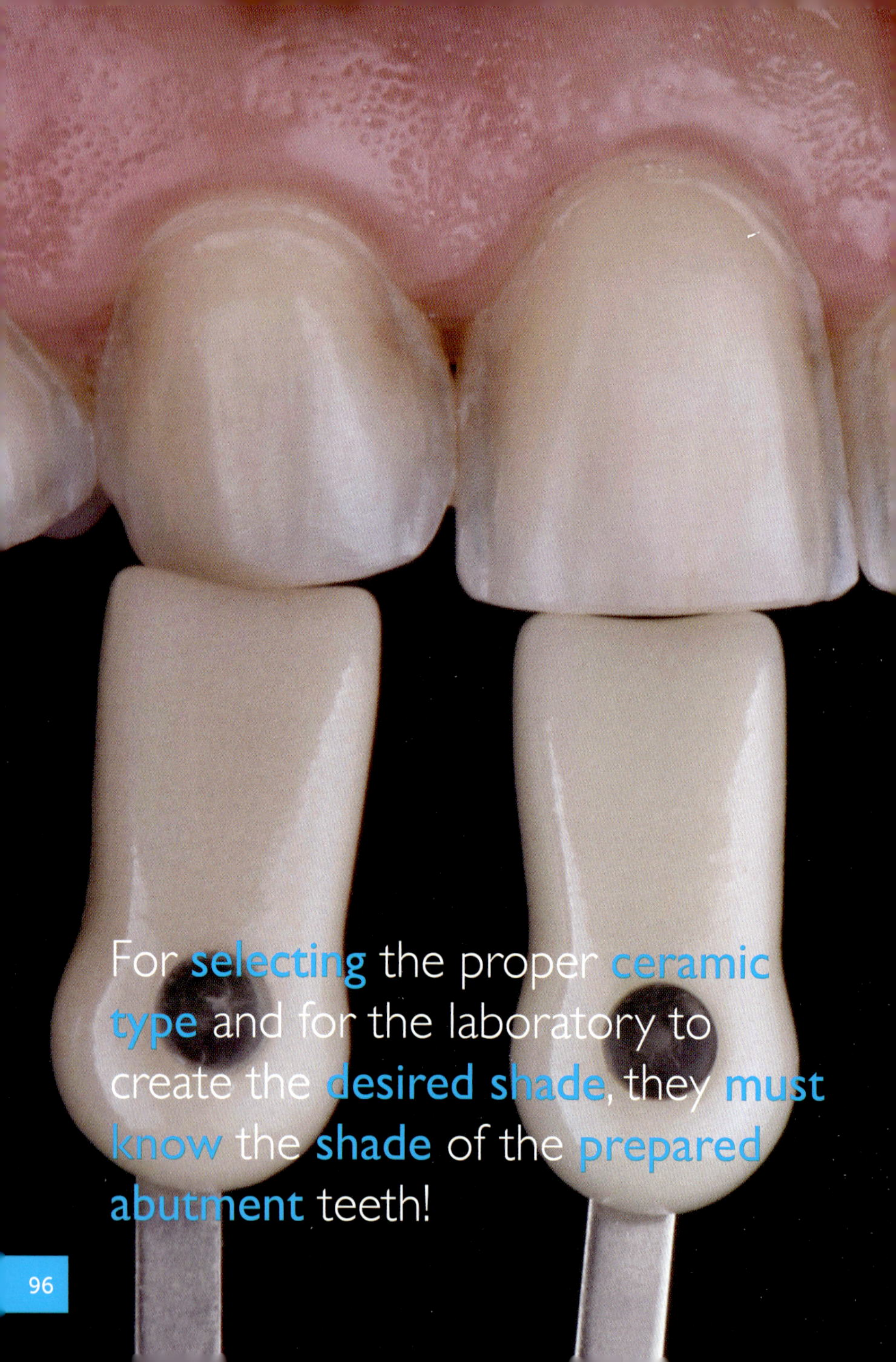

For selecting the proper ceramic type and for the laboratory to create the desired shade, they must know the shade of the prepared abutment teeth!

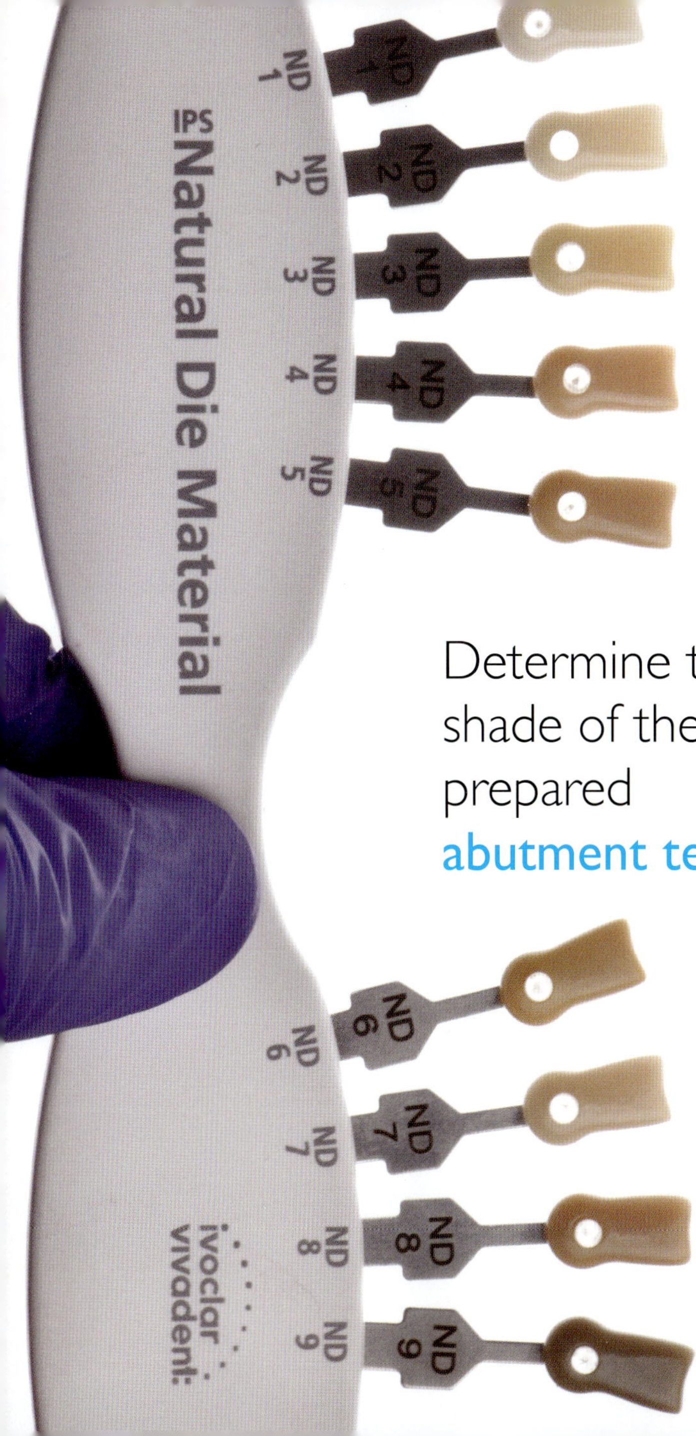

Determine the shade of the prepared **abutment teeth**

The laboratory can make custom dies with the shade of the prepared **abutment teeth**

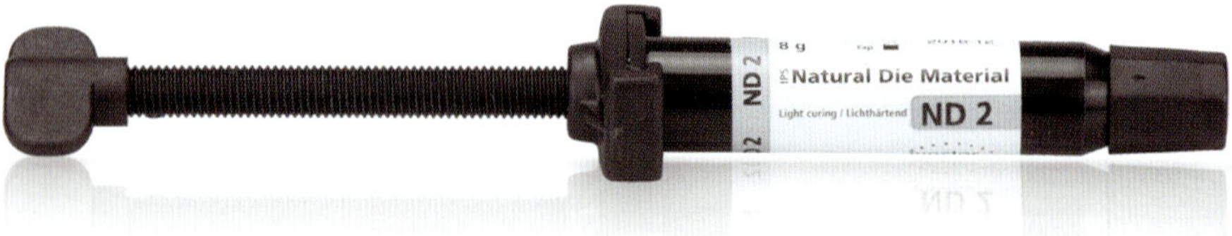

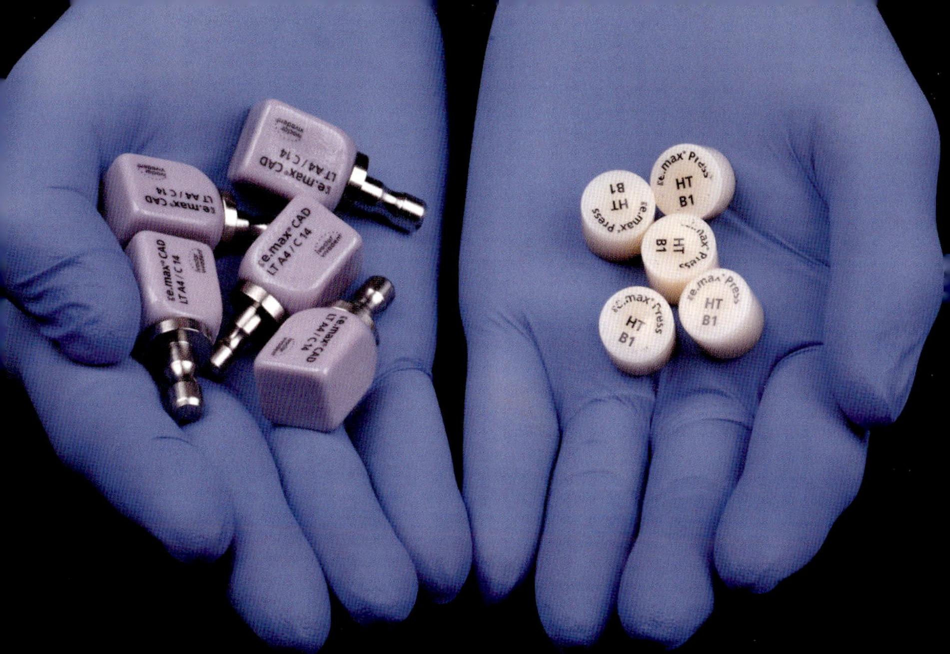

This is key to select **the proper type, shade, and translucency** of the veneer ceramic material

The **greater** the anticipated **color change**, the more **opacity and value** is required of the **ceramic** material

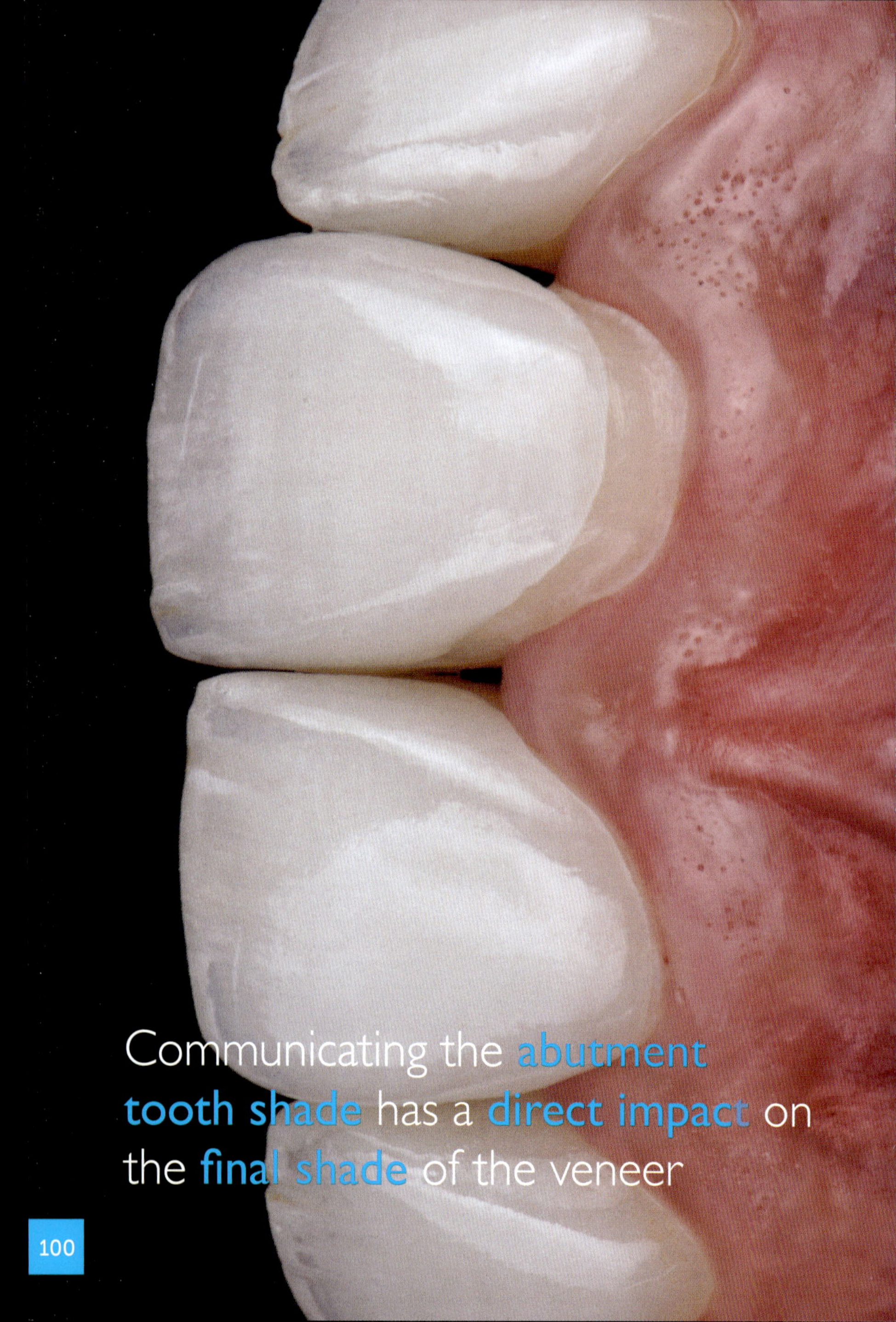

Communicating the abutment tooth shade has a direct impact on the final shade of the veneer

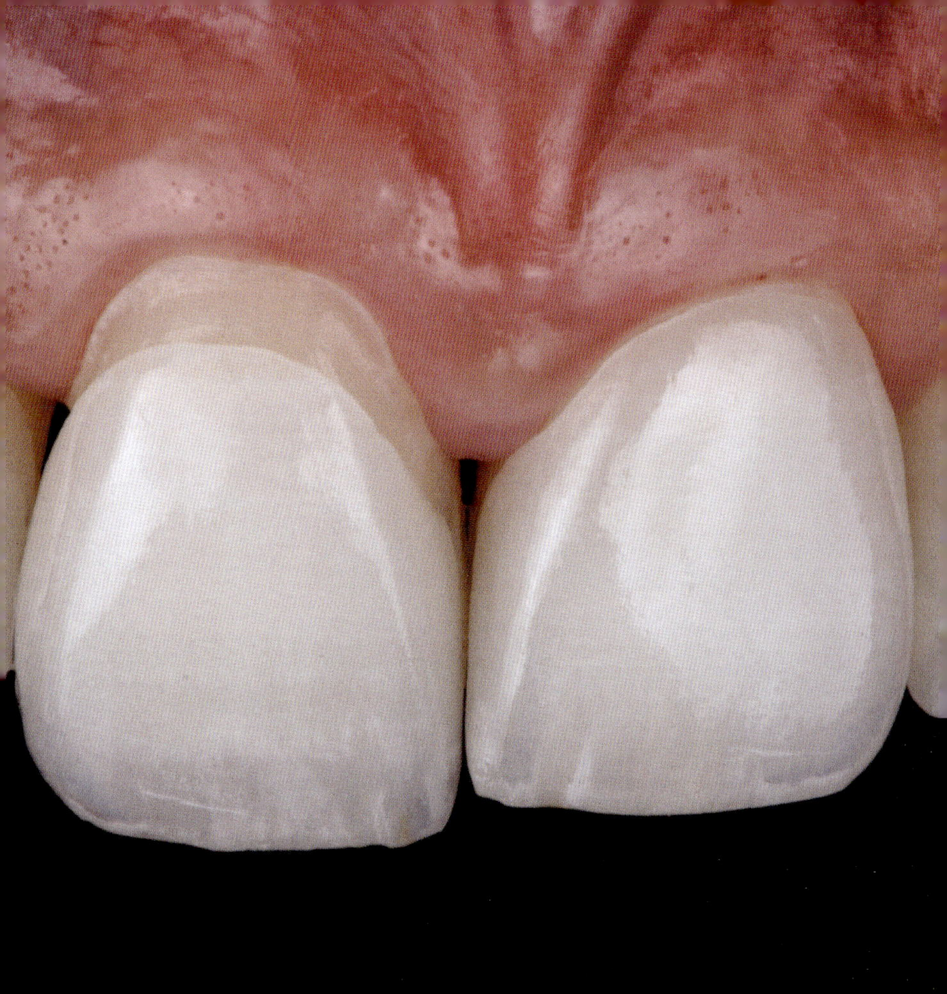

5 FACTORS

DETERMINING THE FINAL SHADE

FACTOR 1

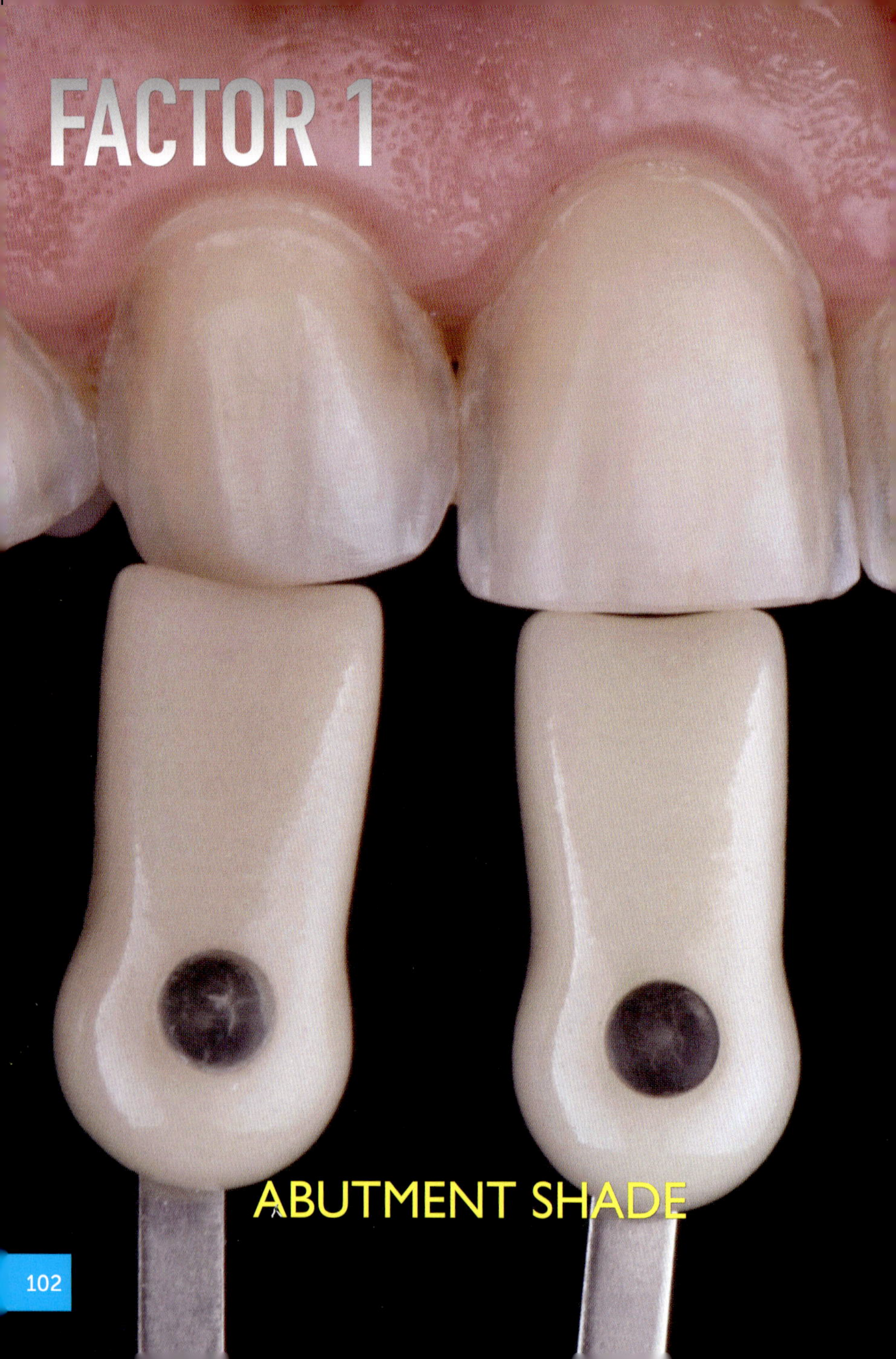

ABUTMENT SHADE

FACTOR 2

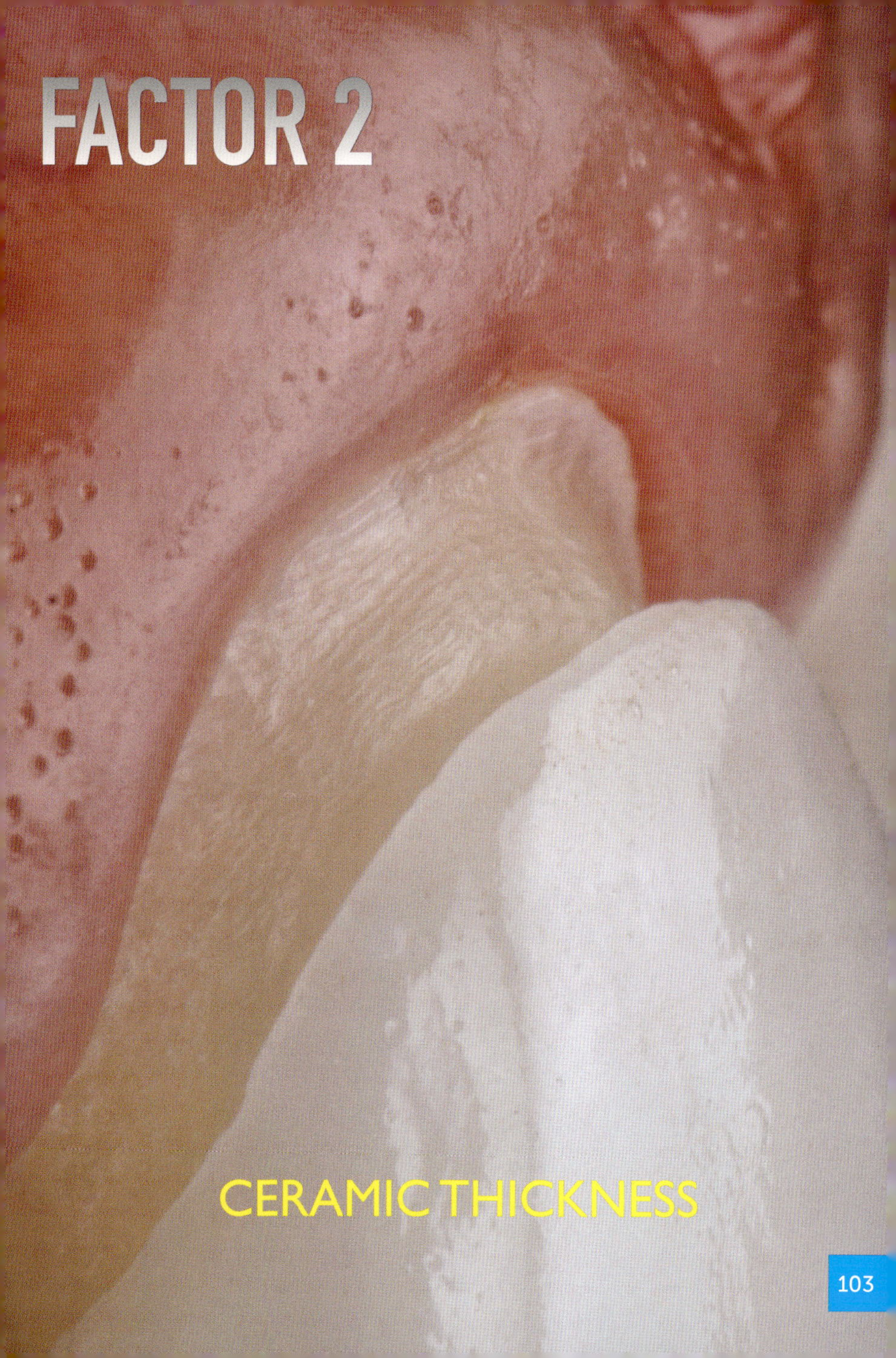

CERAMIC THICKNESS

FACTOR 3

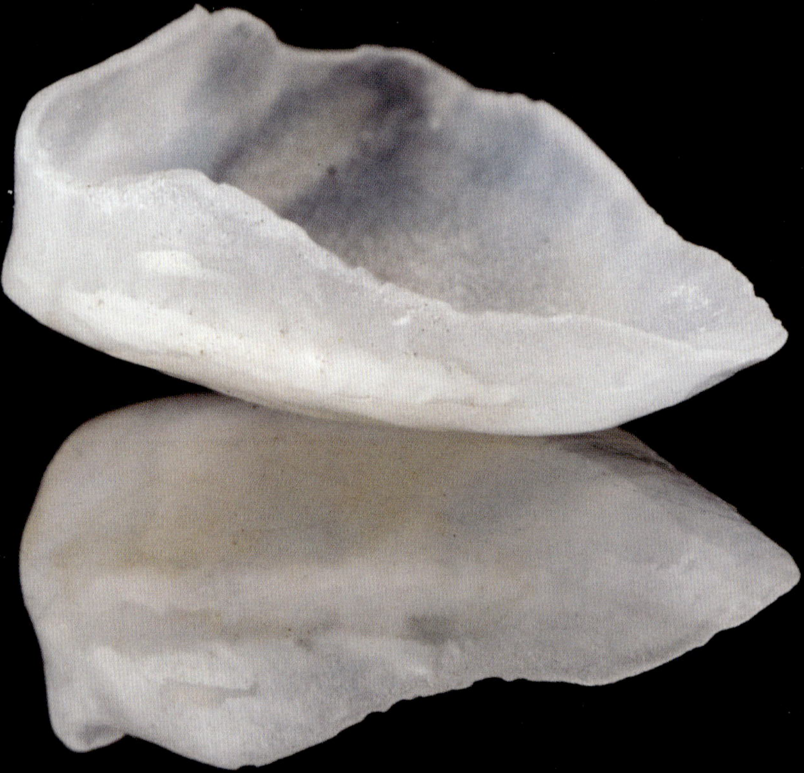

CERAMIC TRANSLUCENCY

FACTOR 4

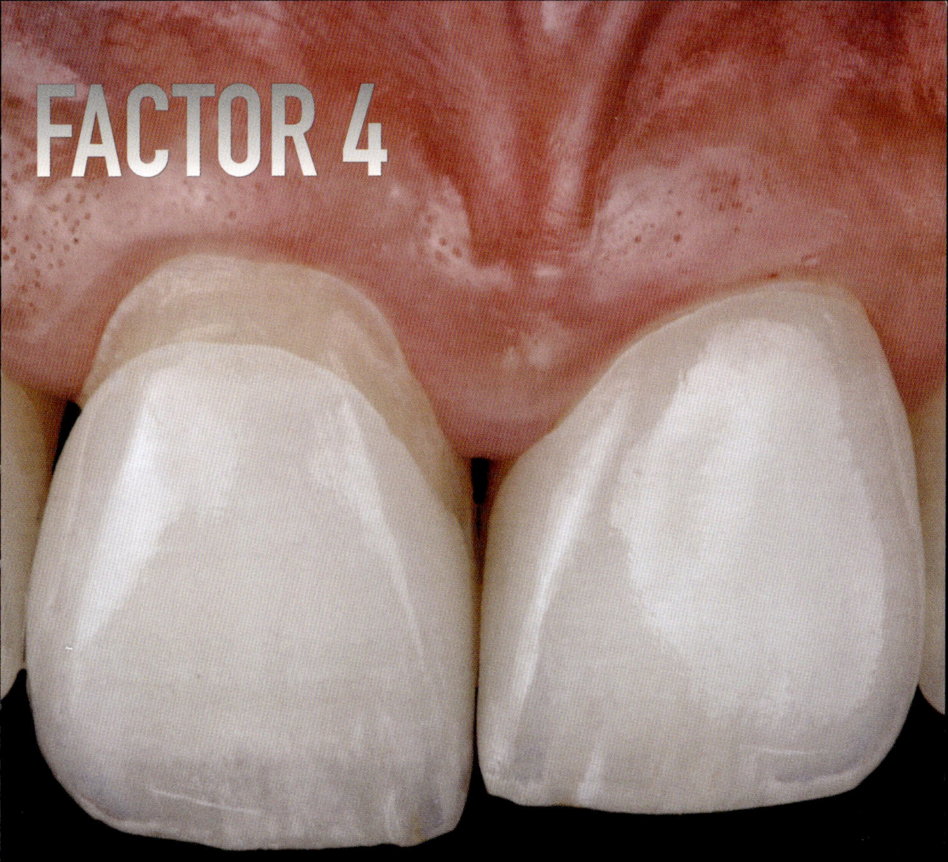

CERAMIC SHADE

FACTOR 5

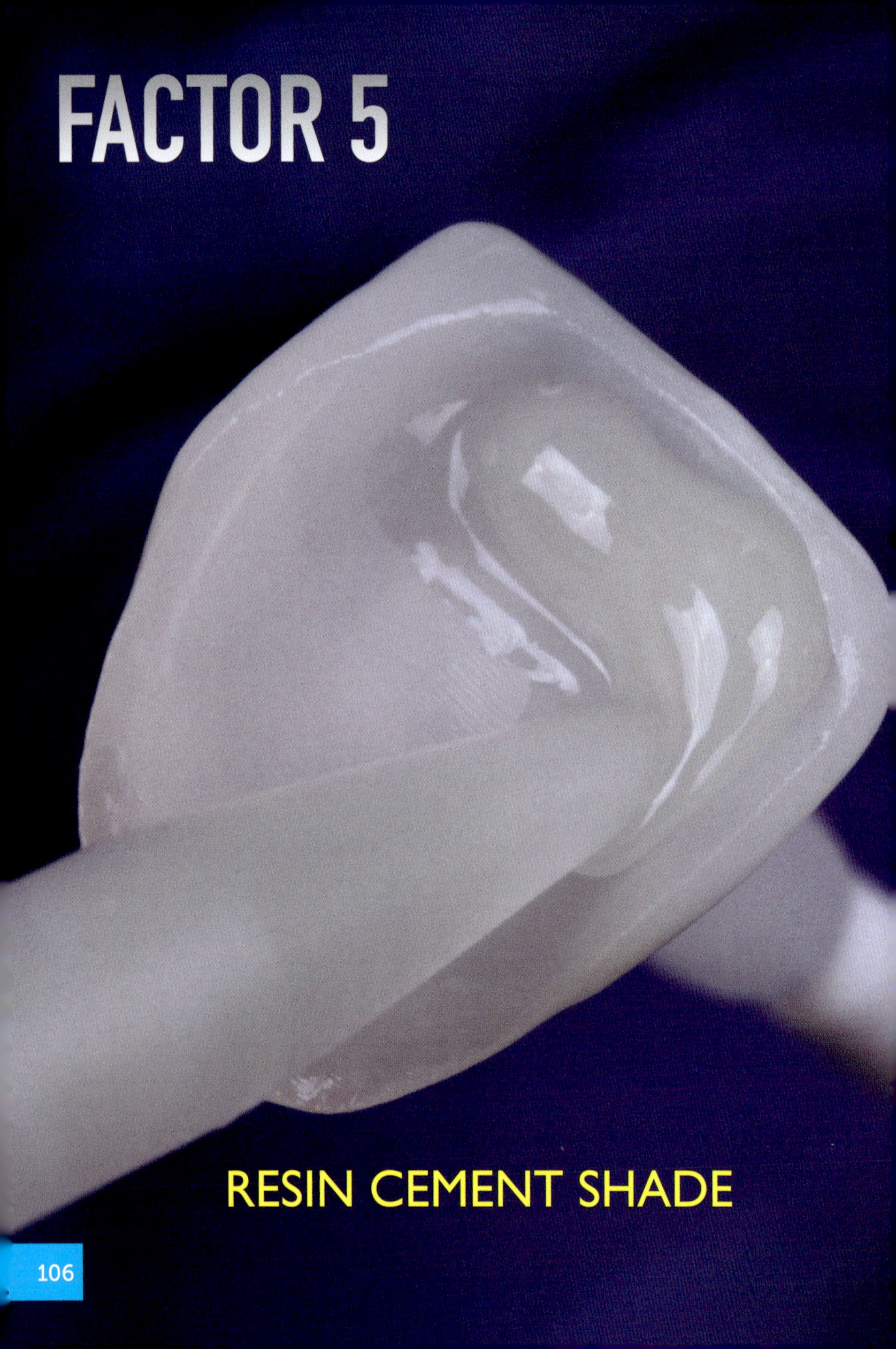

RESIN CEMENT SHADE

IMPRESSION

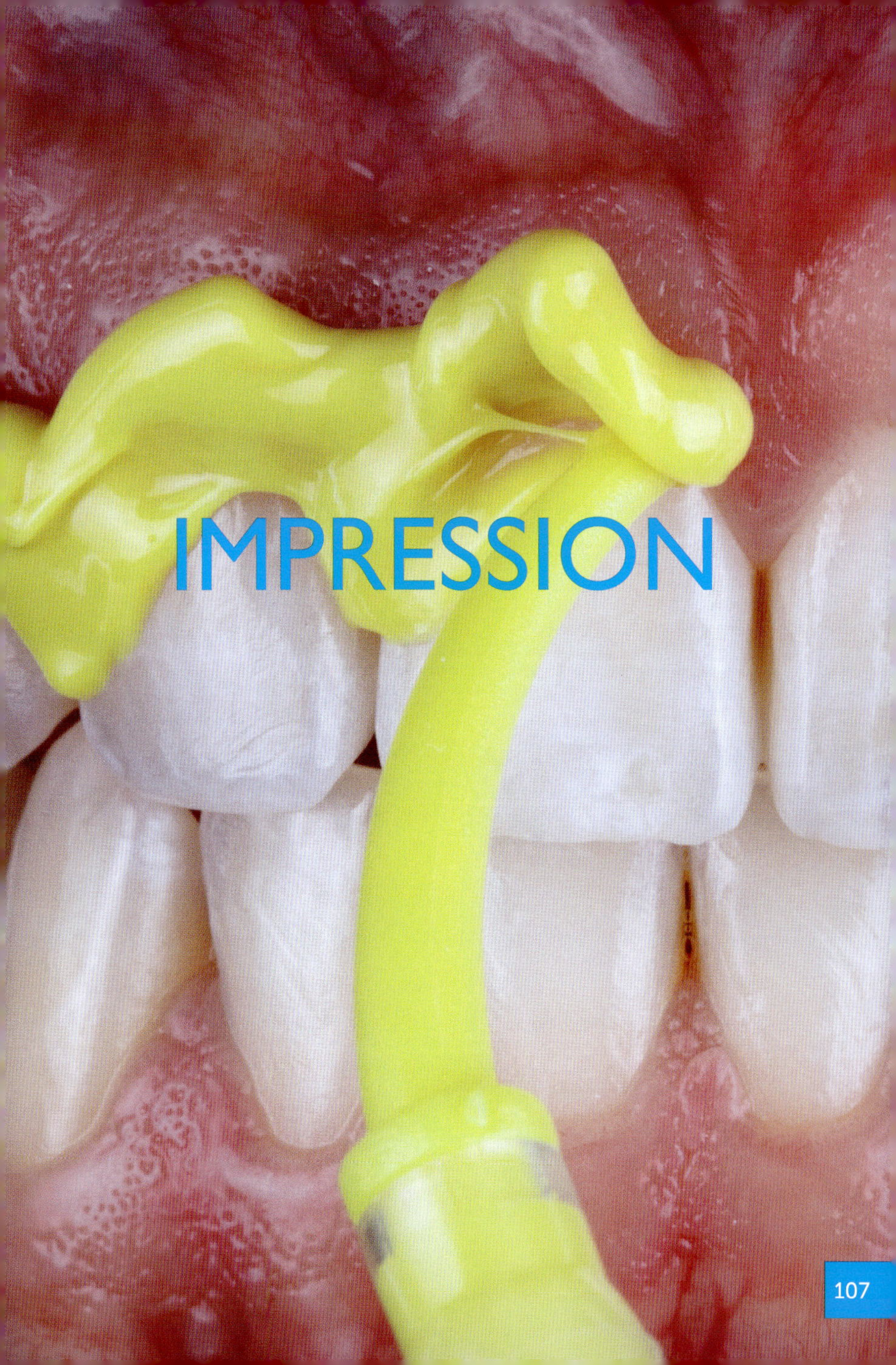

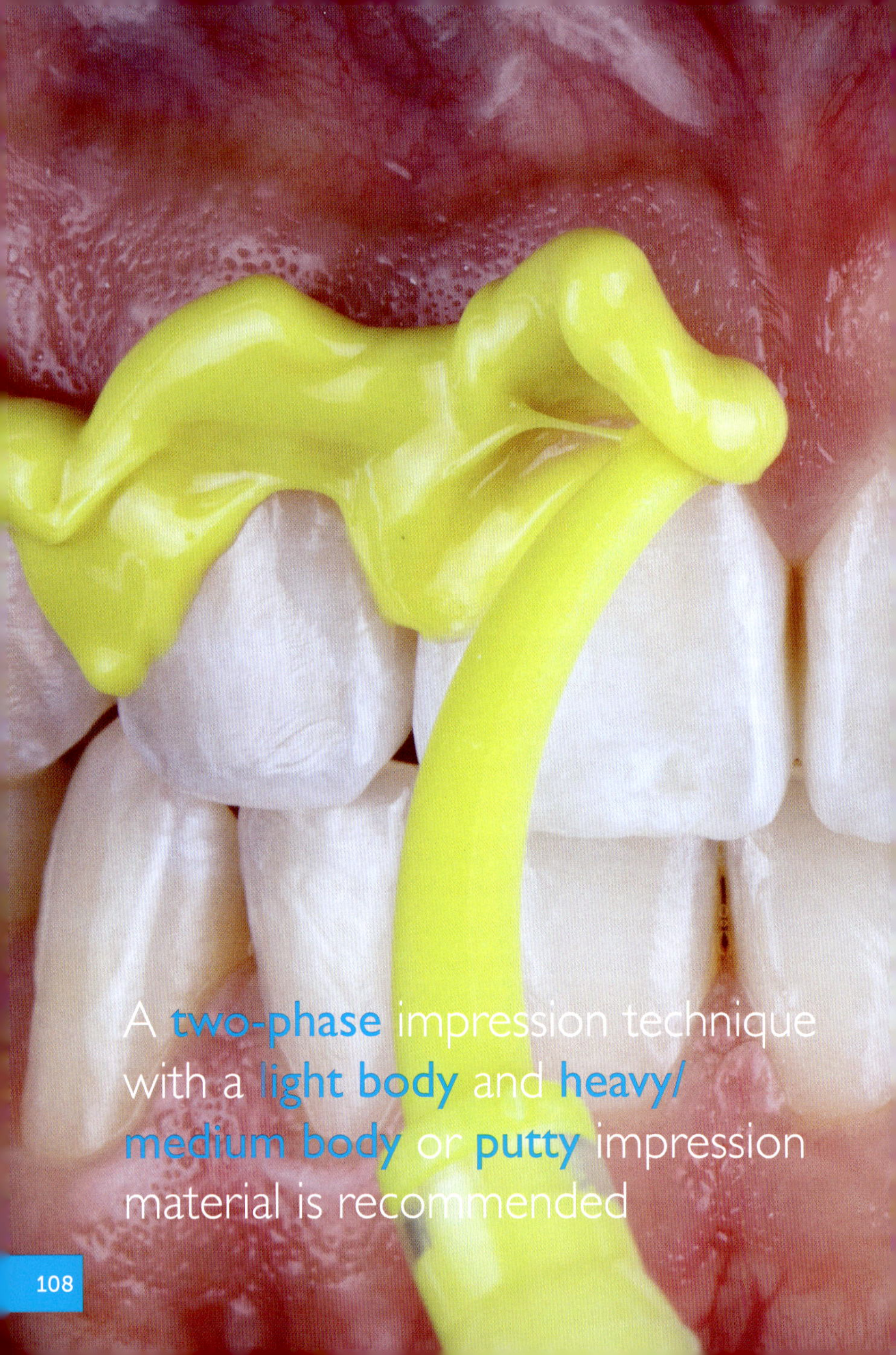

A two-phase impression technique with a light body and heavy/ medium body or putty impression material is recommended

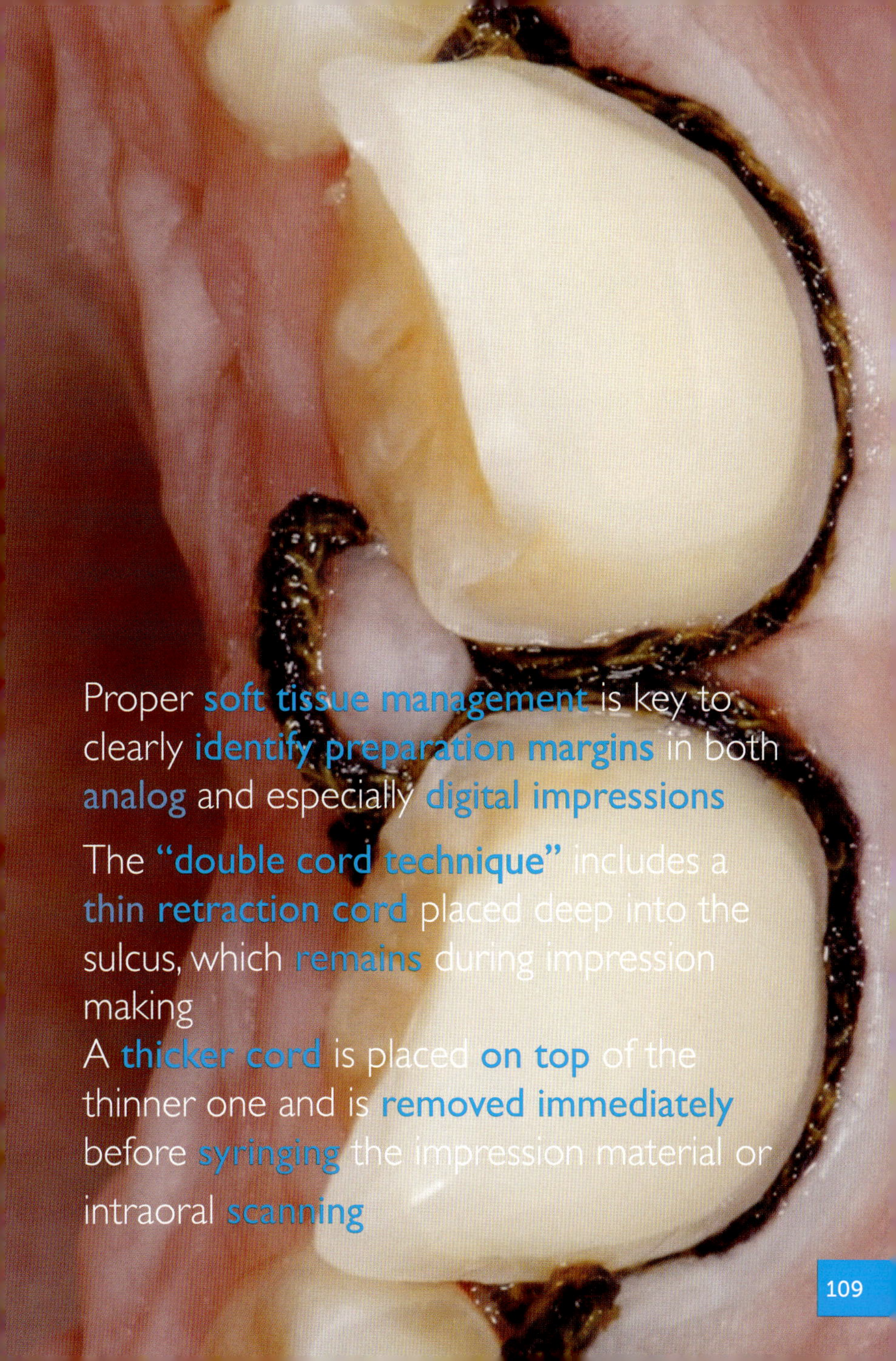

Proper soft tissue management is key to clearly identify preparation margins in both analog and especially digital impressions

The "double cord technique" includes a thin retraction cord placed deep into the sulcus, which remains during impression making

A thicker cord is placed on top of the thinner one and is removed immediately before syringing the impression material or intraoral scanning

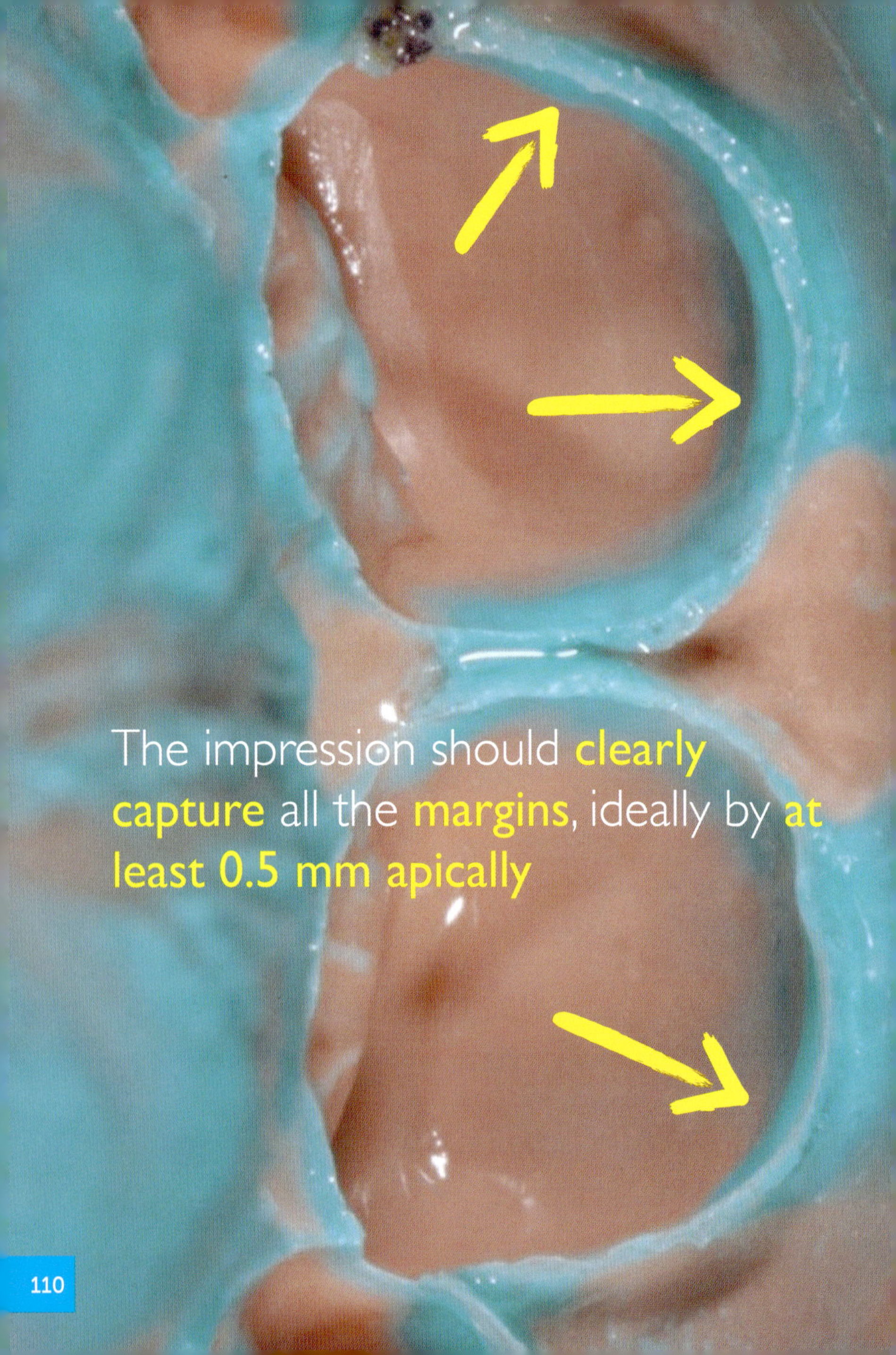

The impression should clearly capture all the margins, ideally by at least 0.5 mm apically

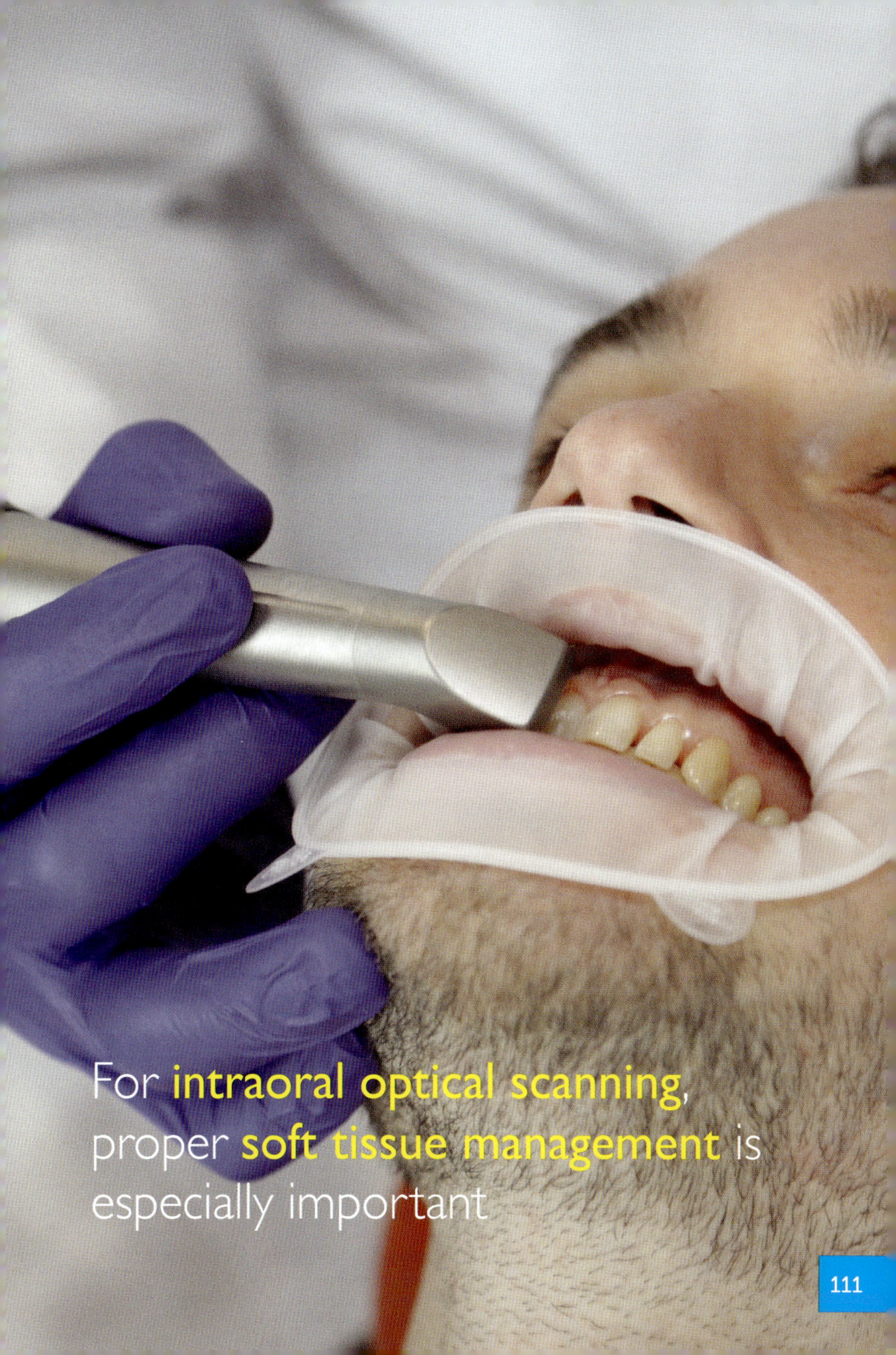

For intraoral optical scanning, proper soft tissue management is especially important

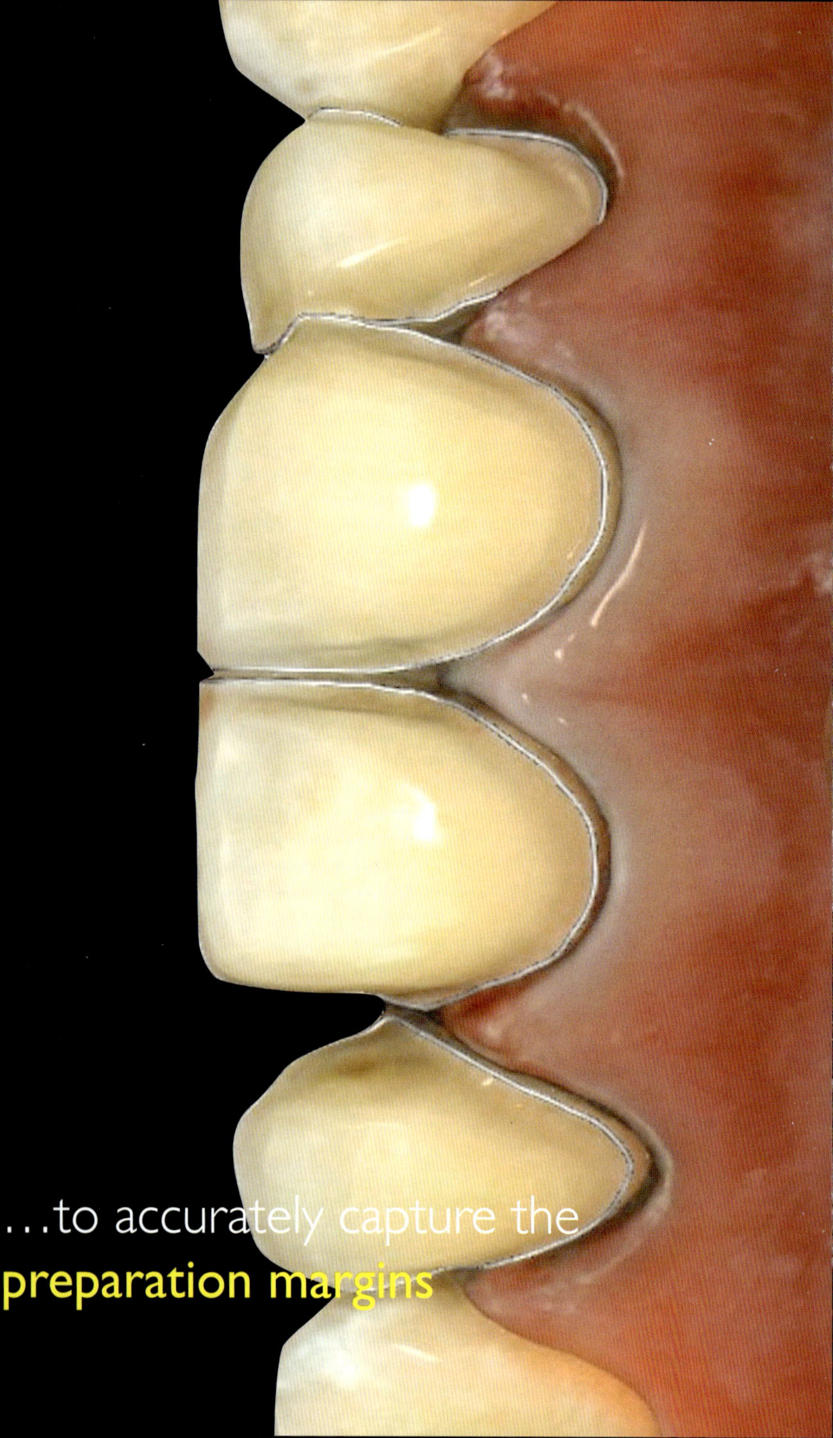

…to accurately capture the
preparation margins

PROVISIONALS

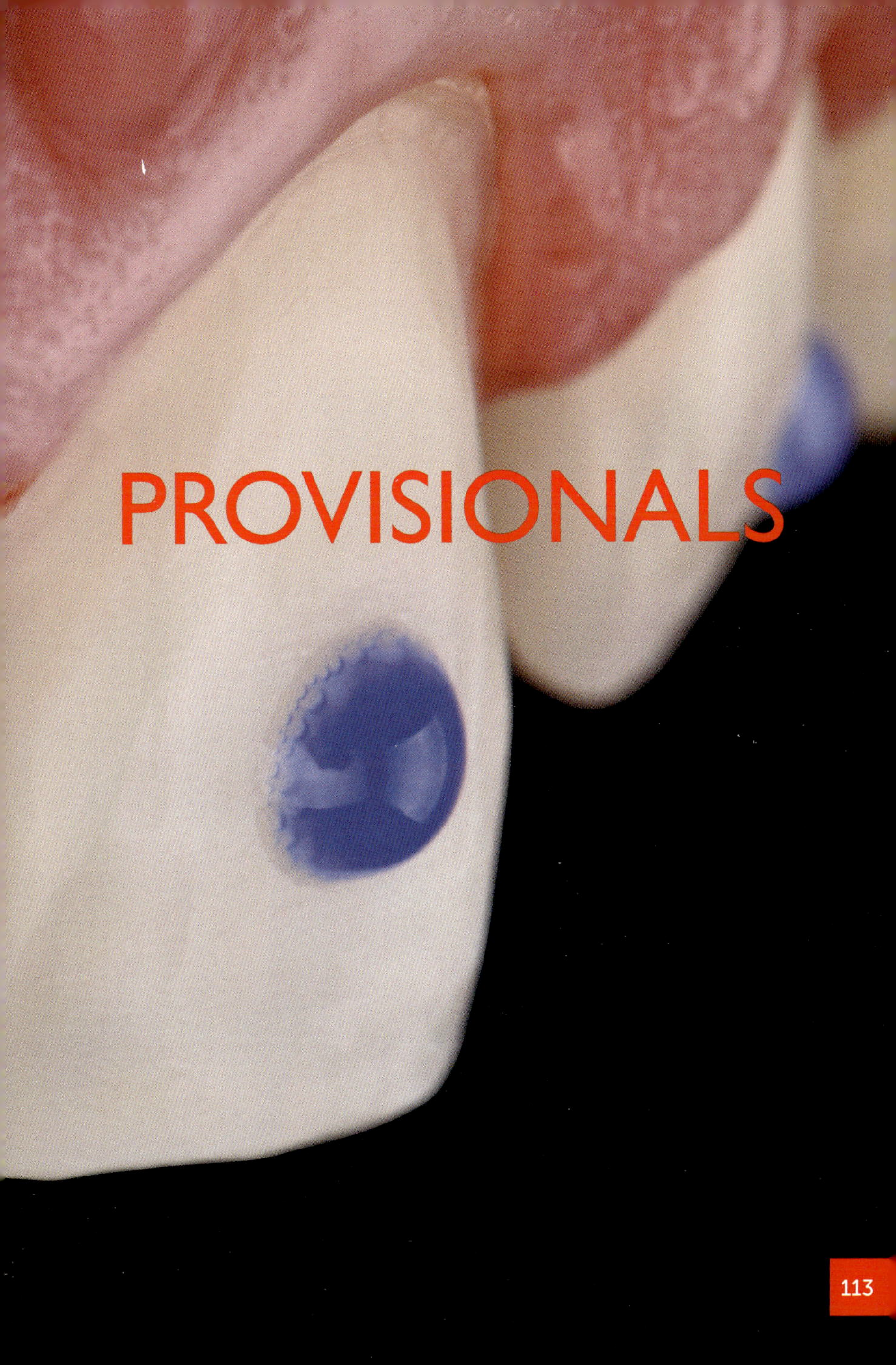

THREE METHODS FOR PROVISIONAL VENEERS

Direct

Spot-etch and **spot bond**

Make a **provisional intraorally** (BisGMA or composite) with a polyvinyl siloxane (**PVS**) **index** or **clear retainer**

Finish and **polish** in situ

Indirect

Make a **scan** or **impression** for the fabrication of an **indirect provisional** in the laboratory

Reline and fit intraorally

Spot-etch and spot **bond**

Insert with **flowable** composite

Semi-direct

Apply **separating agent** on the preparation

Make a **provisional intraorally** (acrylic, BisGMA or composite) with a **PVS index**

Remove from the teeth

Finish and **polish** extraorally

Spot-etch and **spot bond**

Insert with **flowable** composite

DIRECT PROVISIONALS

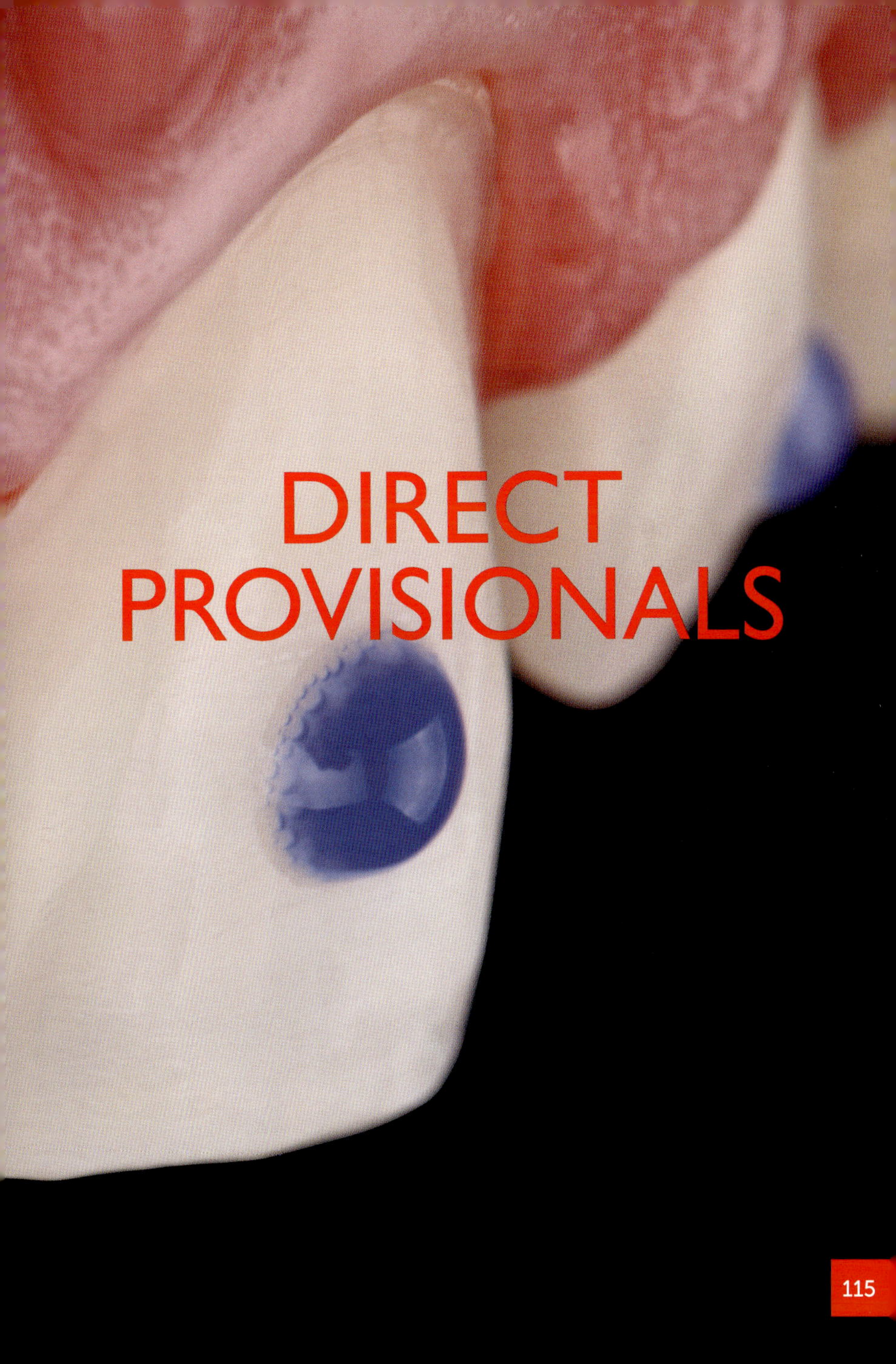

1

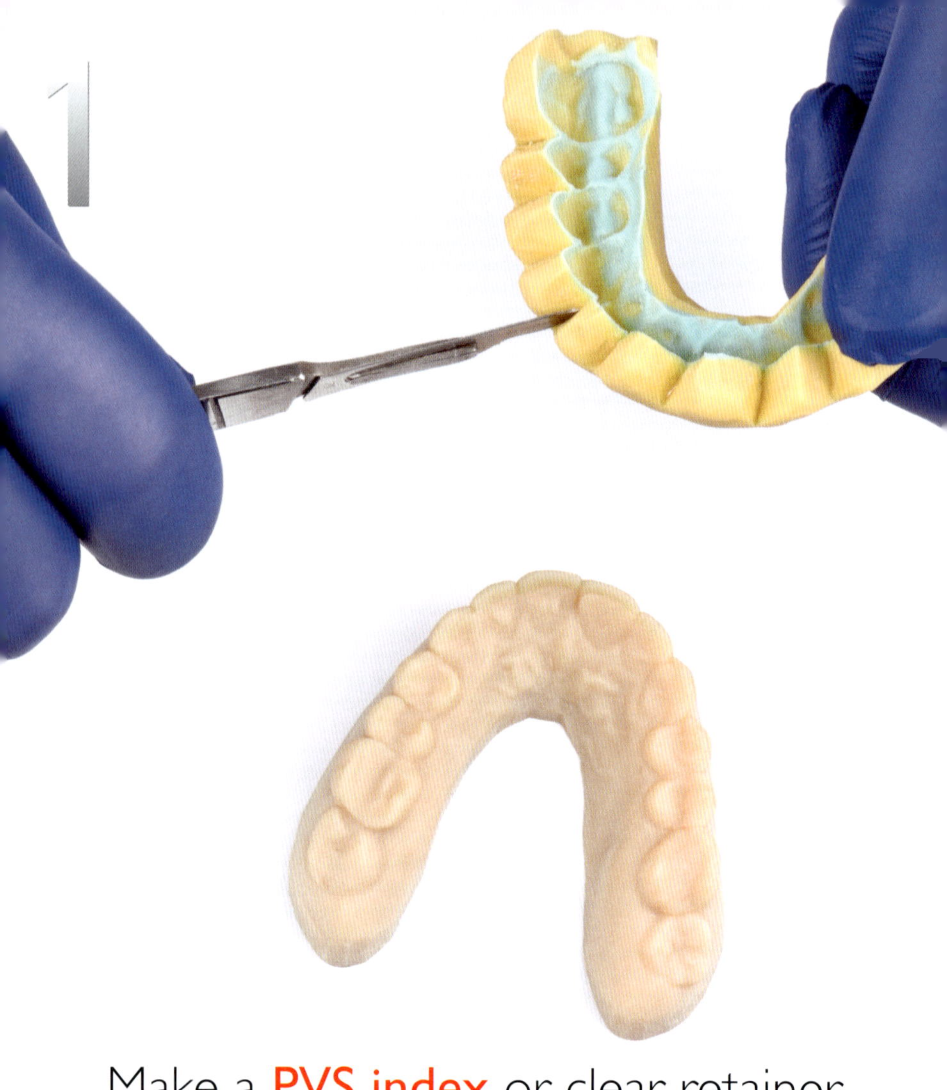

Make a **PVS index** or clear retainer from the wax-up

Trim along the **gingival margins** for easy removal of excess material

2

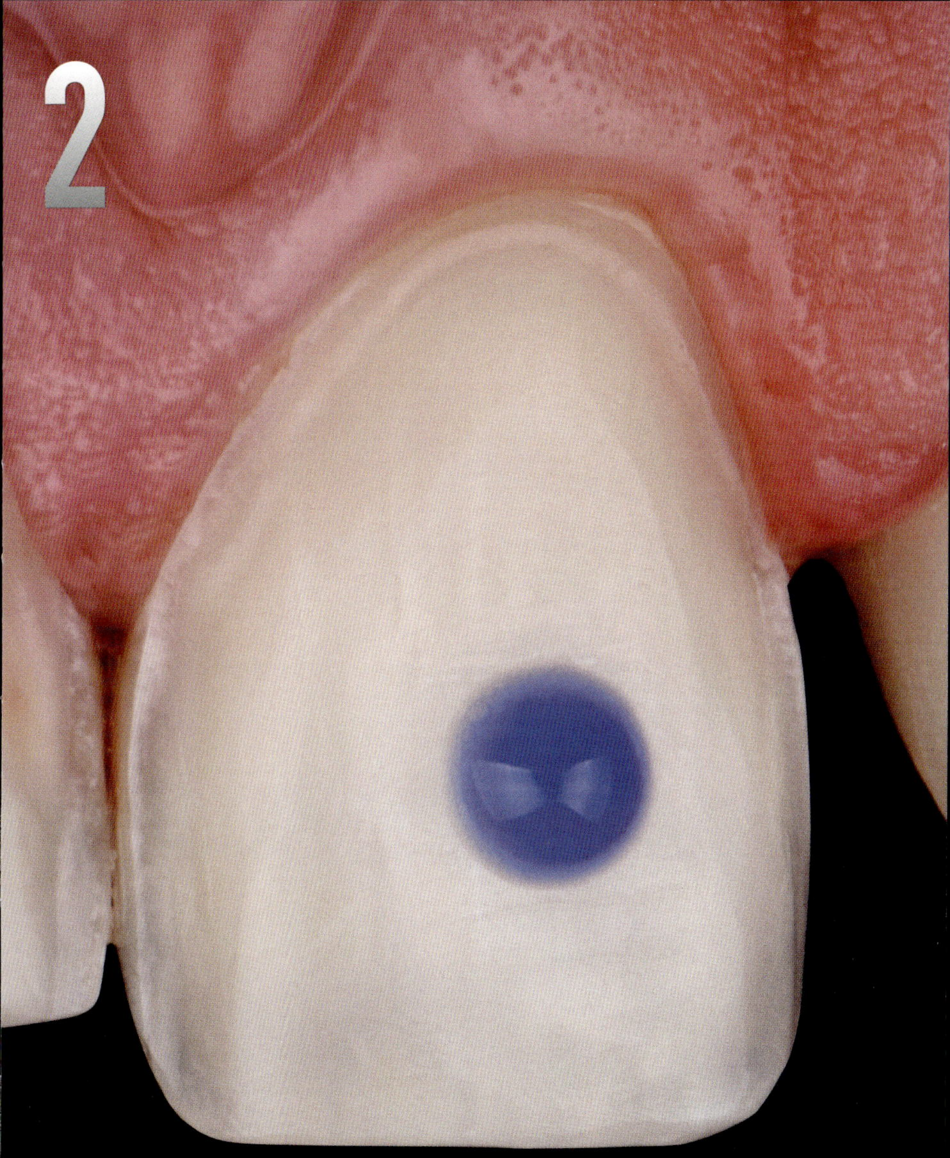

Spot-etch the enamel (H_3PO_4) in a small area and rinse off

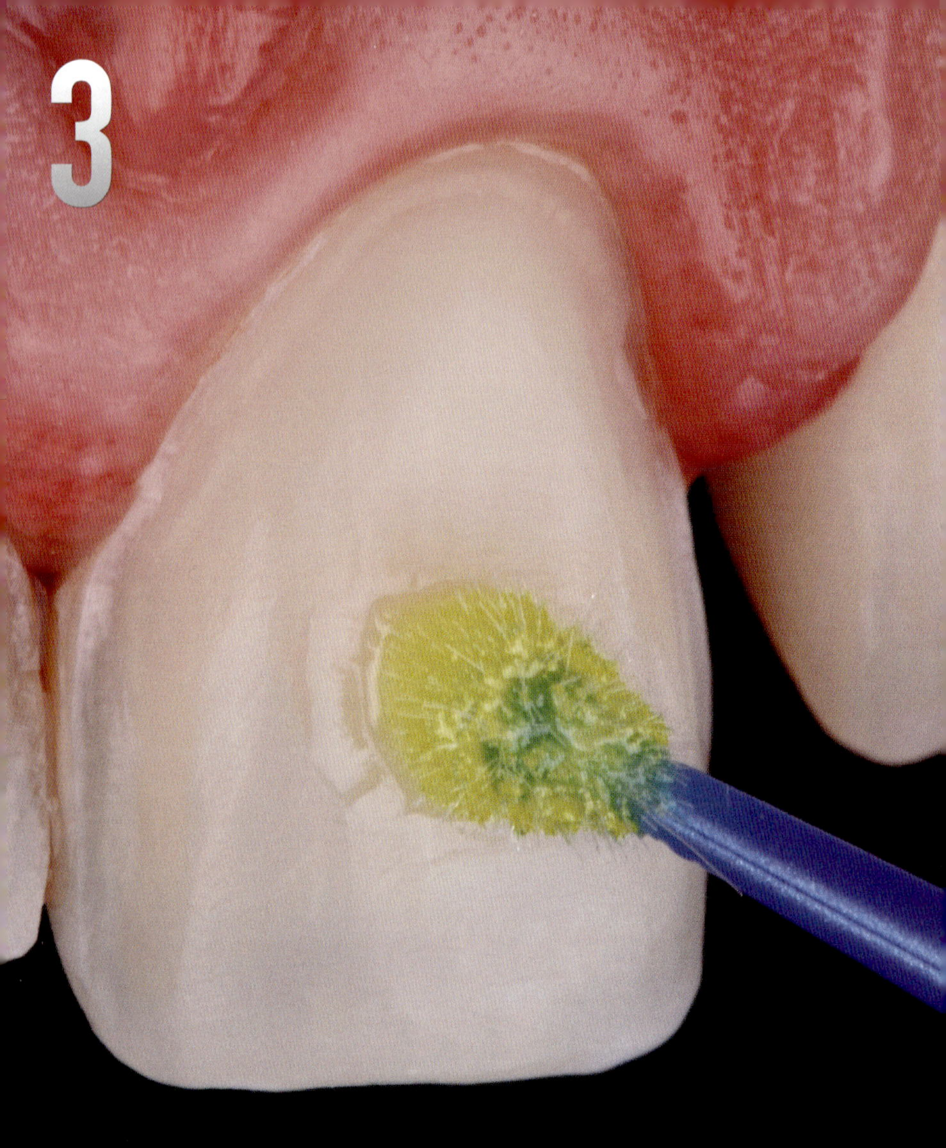

"Spot bond" a small area and light cure

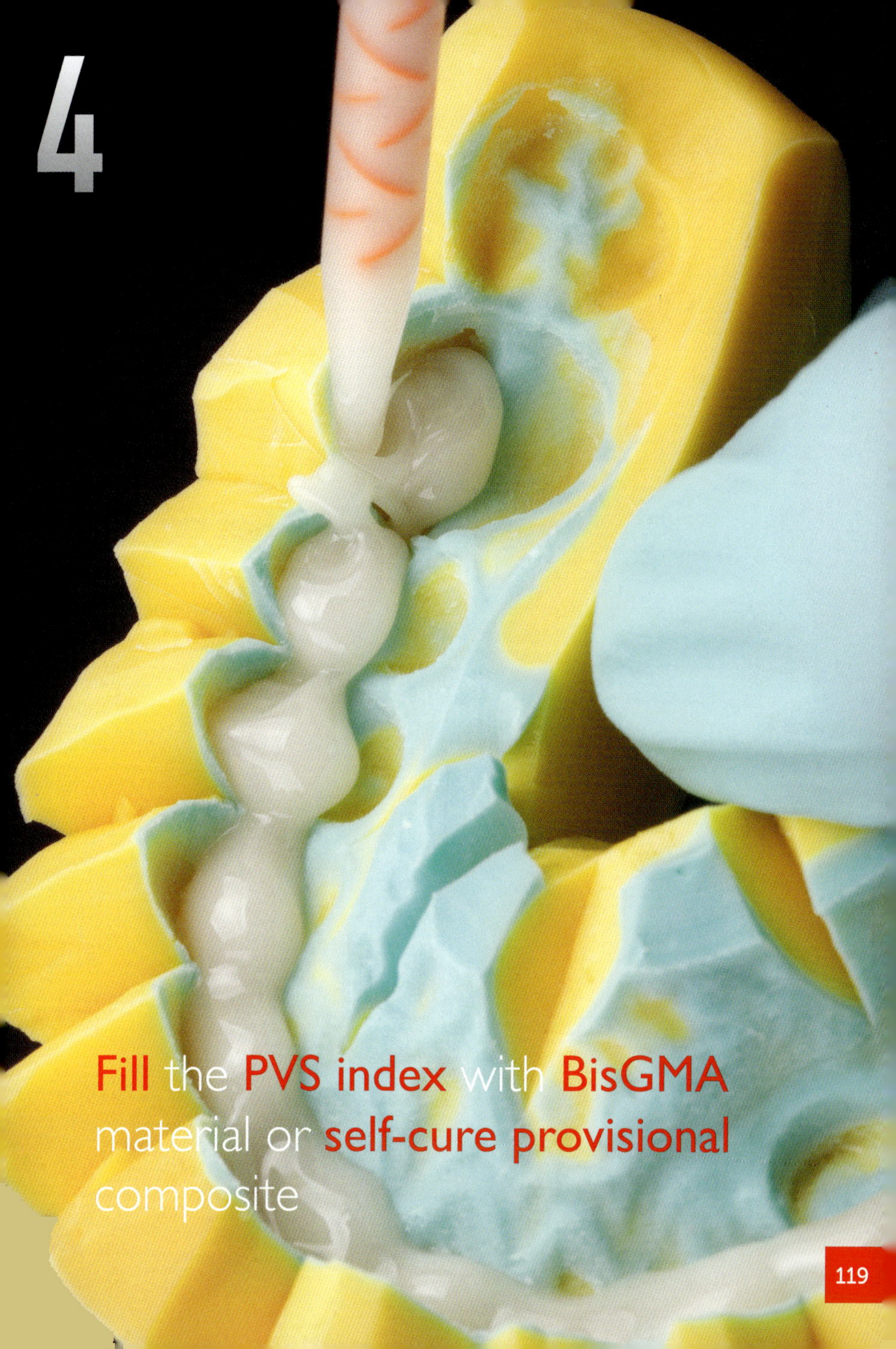

4

Fill the PVS index with BisGMA material or self-cure provisional composite

5

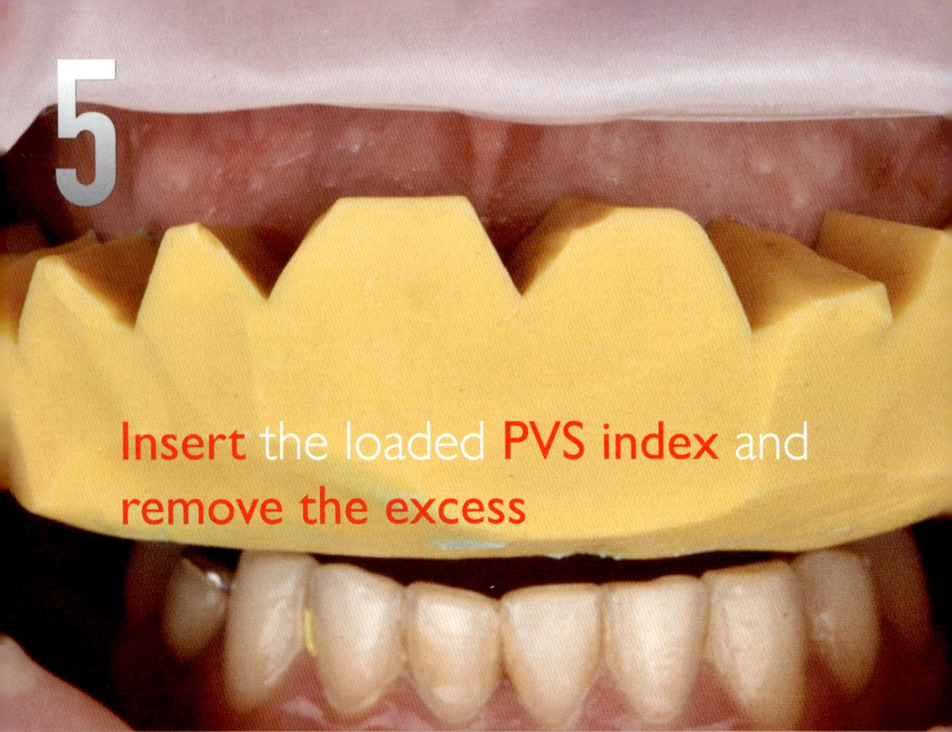

Insert the loaded PVS index and remove the excess

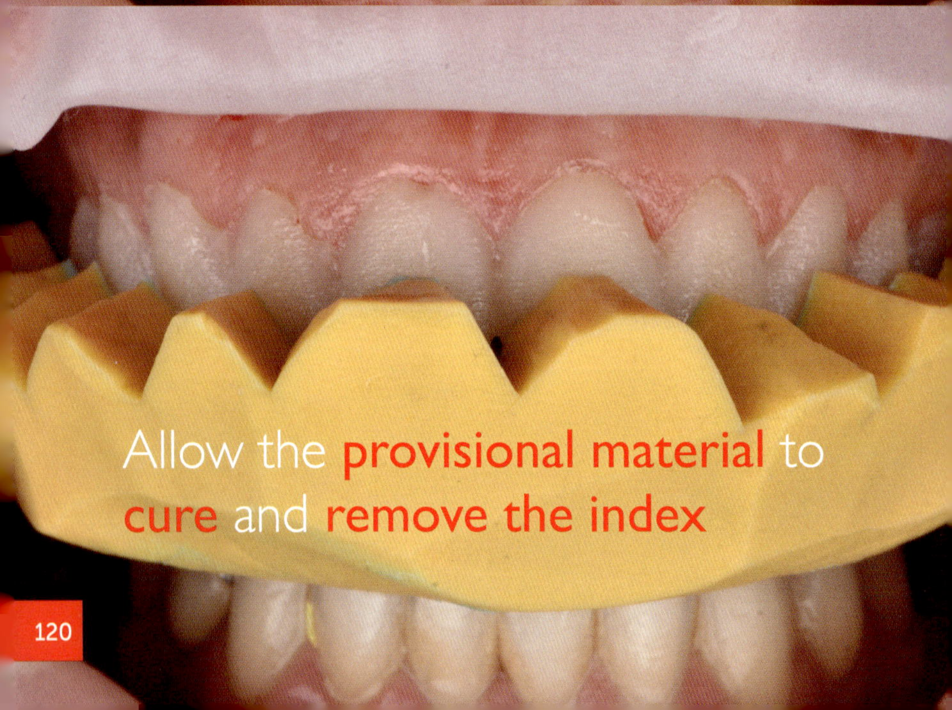

Allow the provisional material to cure and remove the index

6

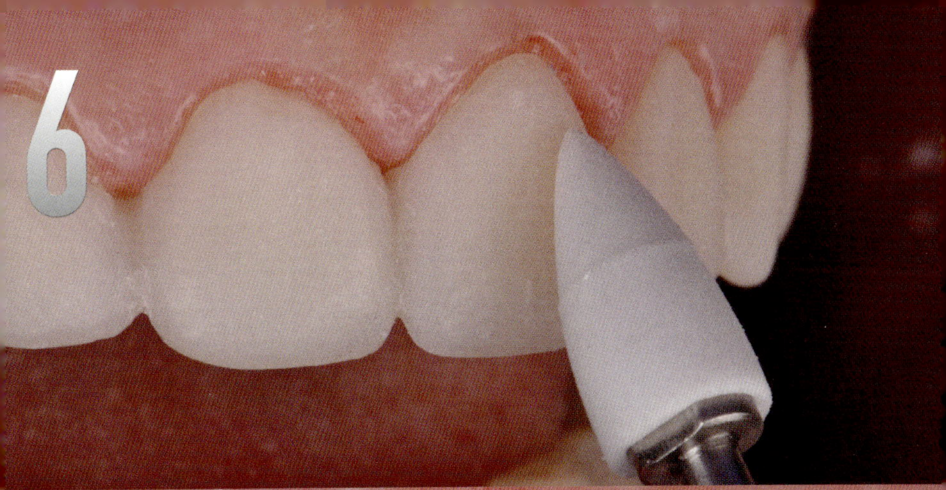

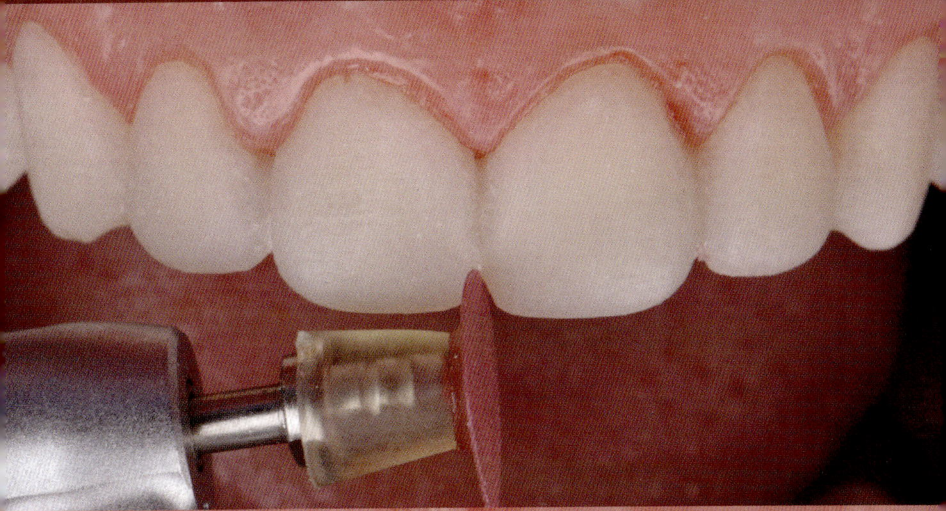

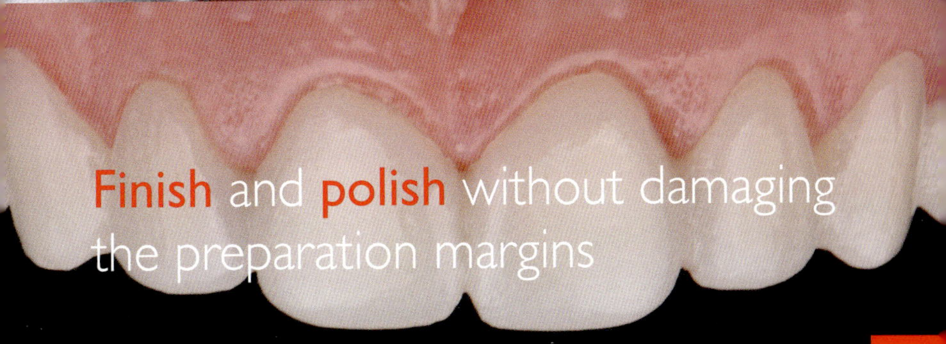

Finish and polish without damaging the preparation margins

DIRECT PROVISIONALS

CHEAT SHEET

1. Make a PVS index from the wax-up
2. Spot-etch the enamel and rinse off
3. Spot bond and light cure
4. Fill the PVS index with self-cure provisional BisGMA or composite
5. Insert the loaded PVS index and remove excess
   Allow the material to cure and remove index
6. Finish and polish

INDIRECT AND SEMI-DIRECT PROVISIONALS

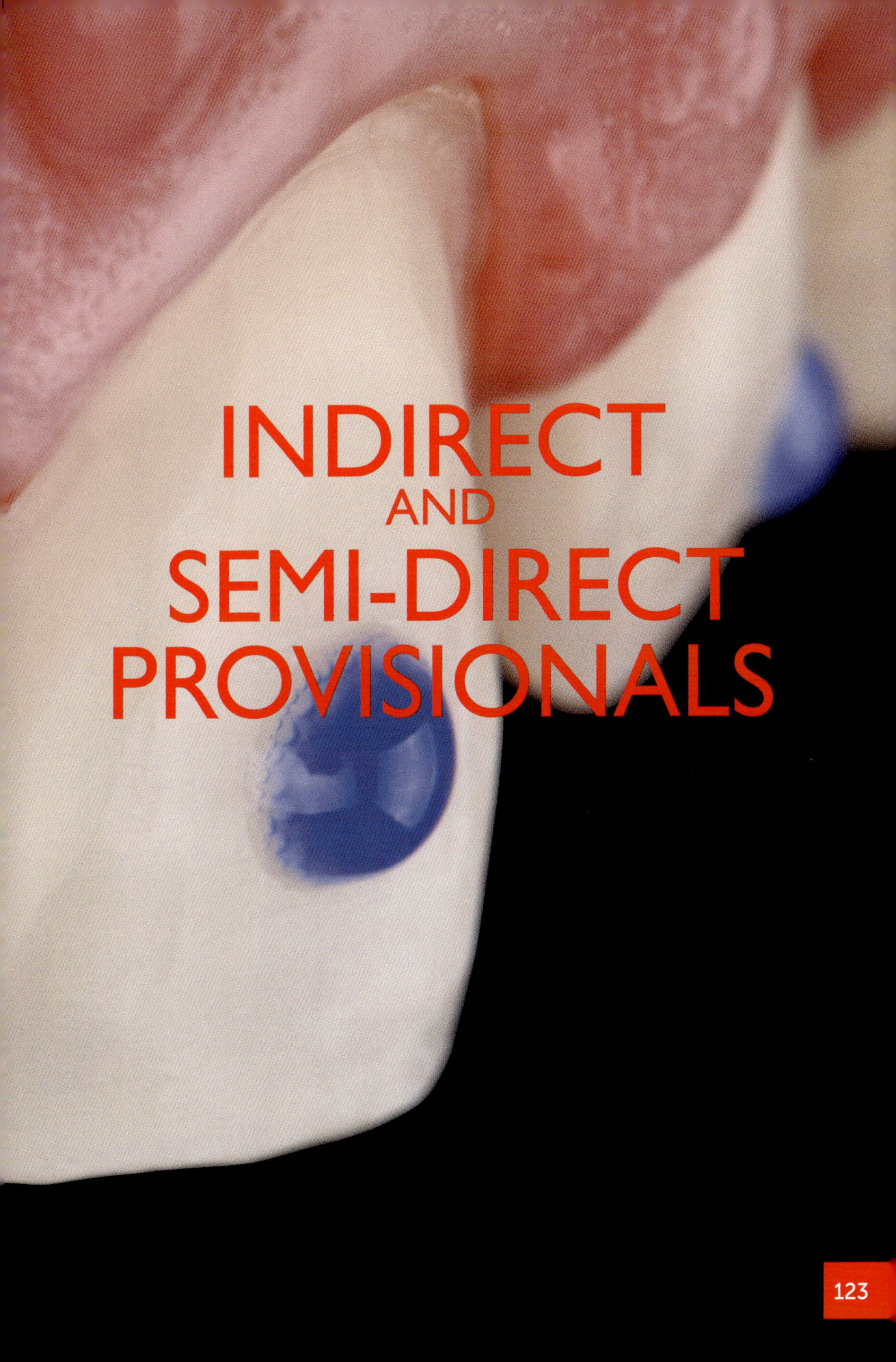

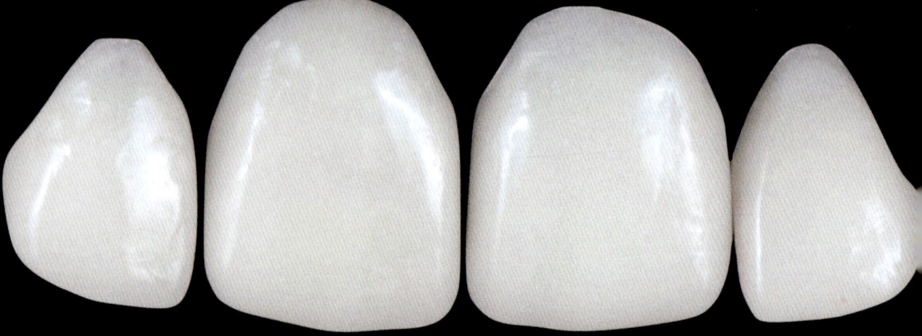

INDIRECT PROVISIONALS are made in the **laboratory** (handmade, milled or 3D printed) and typically **relined** intraorally with acrylic resin, BisGMA or flowable composite, then fitted to the preparation

SEMI-DIRECT PROVISIONALS are made intraorally with a **PVS index** and then removed for adjustment

Both are best **spot bonded**

INDIRECT PROVISIONALS

CHEAT SHEET

1. Make an indirect provisional restoration in the laboratory
2. Reline the indirect provisional and fit it to the preparation
3. Spot-etch the enamel, rinse off, and apply bonding agent in a small spot, then light cure
4. Insert the indirect provisional with flowable composite
5. Light cure
6. Finish and polish

SEMI-DIRECT PROVISIONALS

CHEAT SHEET

1 Apply separating agent on the prepared teeth

2 Make the provisional intraorally with a PVS index
Reline, if needed, and fit to the preparation

3 Spot-etch the enamel, rinse off, apply bonding agent in a small spot, then light cure

4 Insert the provisional with flowable composite

5 Light cure

6 Finish and polish

TIP 1

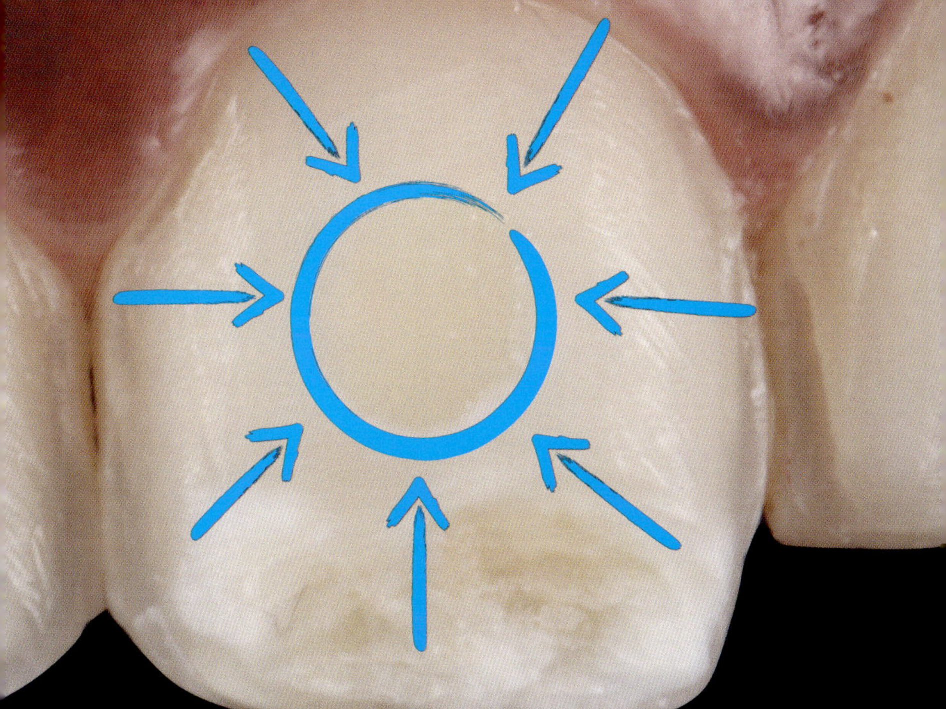

When "spot bonding," keep the **etching/bonding** area very **small** (1 to 2 mm)

DO NOT blow bonding agent over the **entire tooth!**
Light cure immediately!

TIP 2

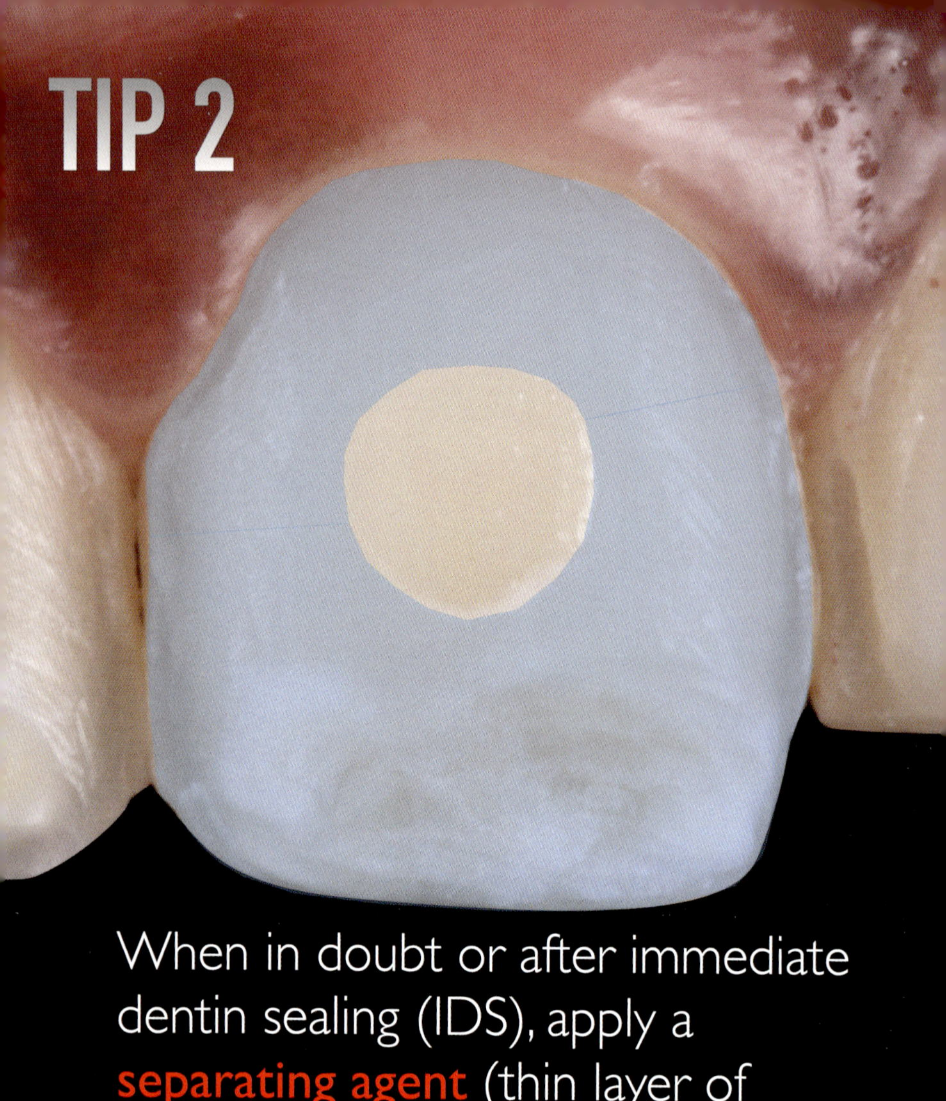

When in doubt or after immediate dentin sealing (IDS), apply a **separating agent** (thin layer of petroleum jelly or cooking oil) to the **remaining tooth structure** for easy removal

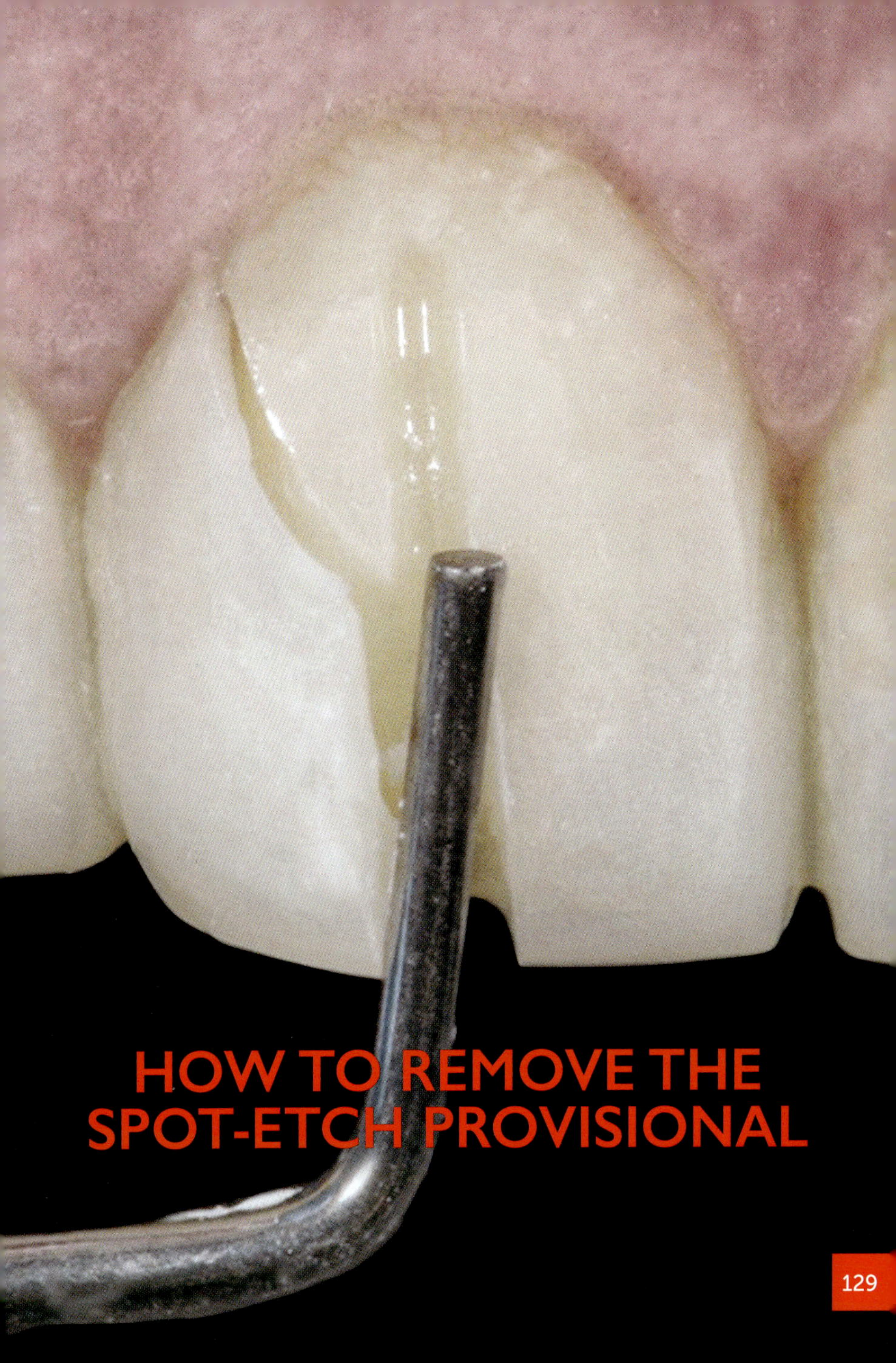

HOW TO REMOVE THE SPOT-ETCH PROVISIONAL

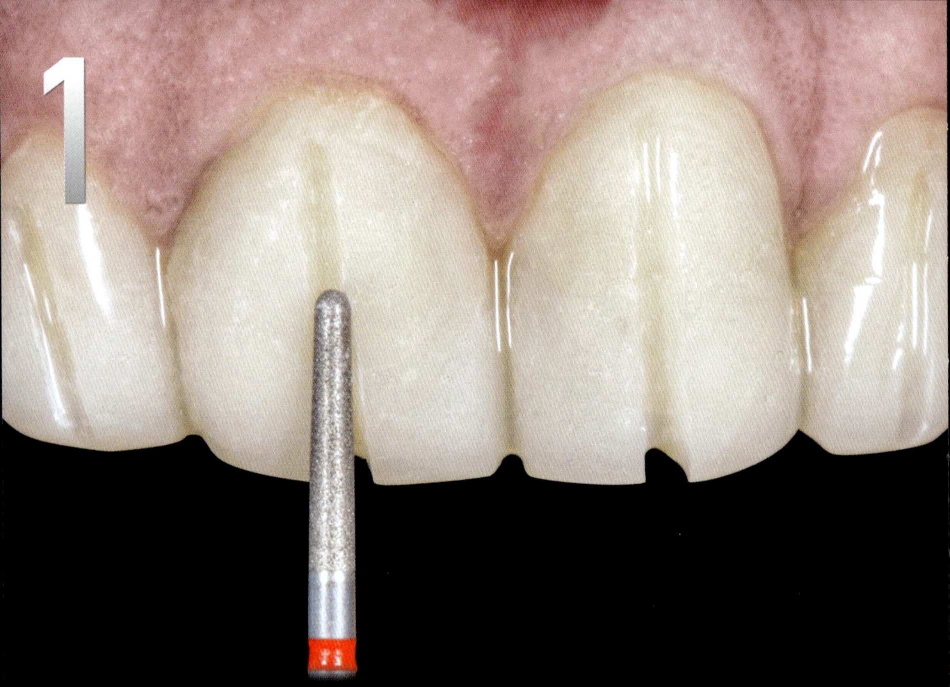

"Slice" provisionals carefully with a diamond bur

Do not damage the tooth
Stop short of the preparation finish line

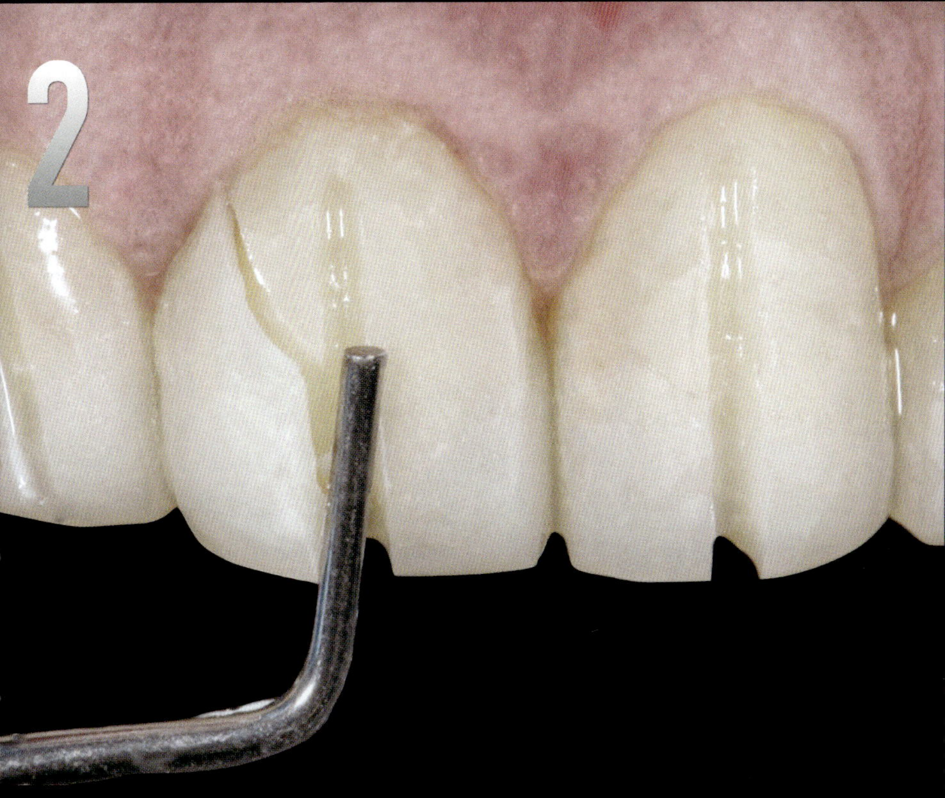

"Pry" and break off the pieces with a sturdy instrument

If the bond was applied only in a small spot and contacts are not too tight, the pieces will come out easily

3

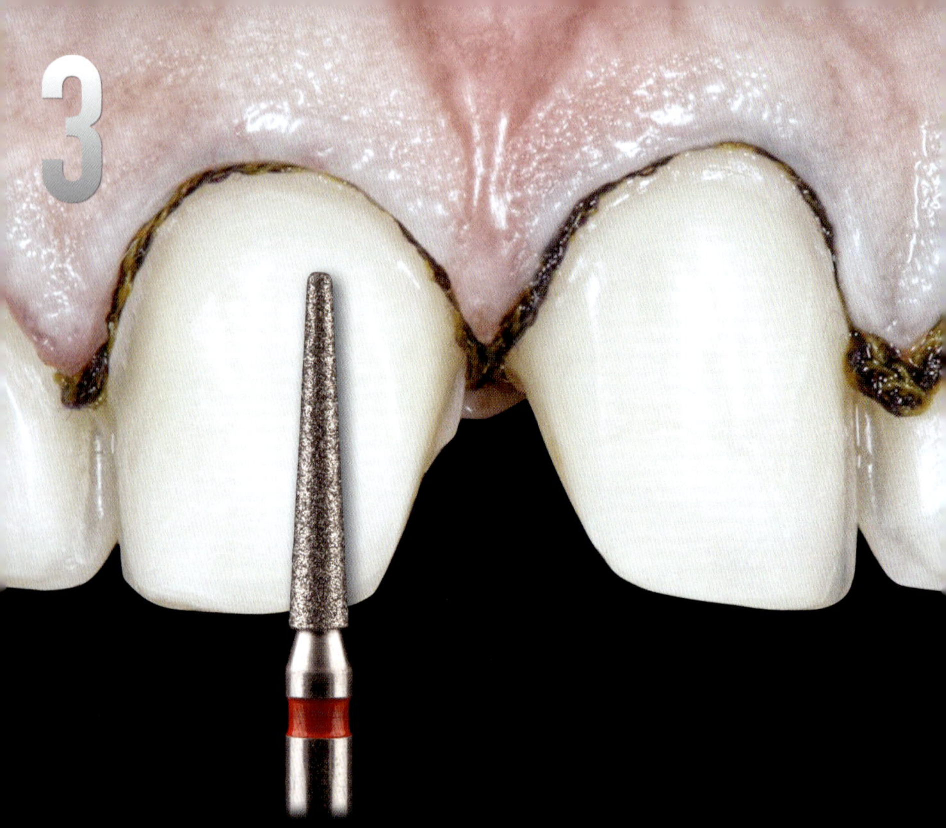

Carefully **"level"** the small spot-bonded area and carefully **remove** any remaining bonded **composite before** the veneer try-in

TIP: Use a **UV light** to make the composite more visible

REMOVE SPOT-ETCH PROVISIONALS

CHEAT SHEET

1. Slice carefully with a diamond bur
2. Pry and break off with a sturdy instrument
3. Level the composite remnants in the bonded area to ensure proper fit of the definitive veneer

VENEER BONDING

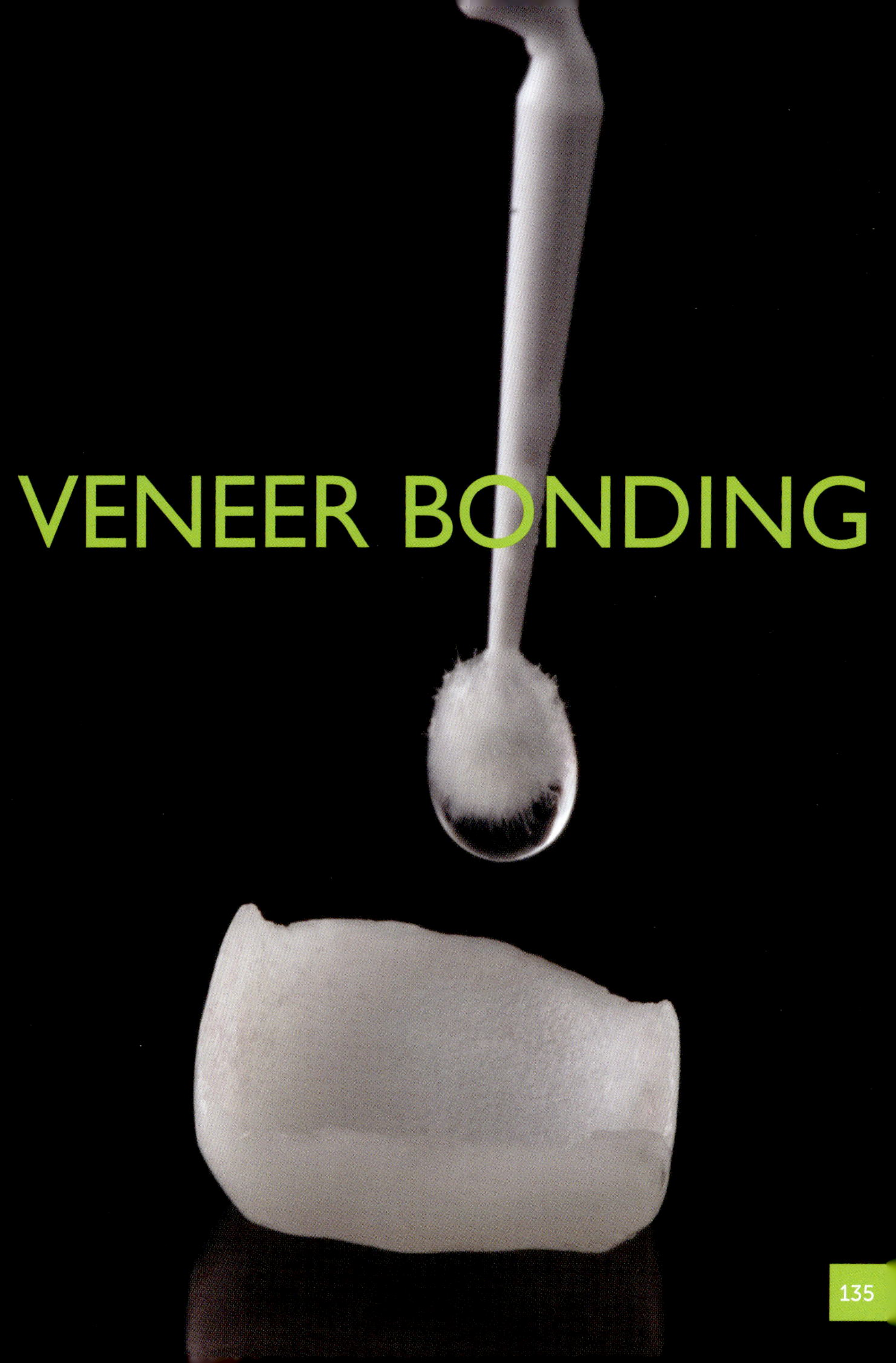

RUBBER DAM

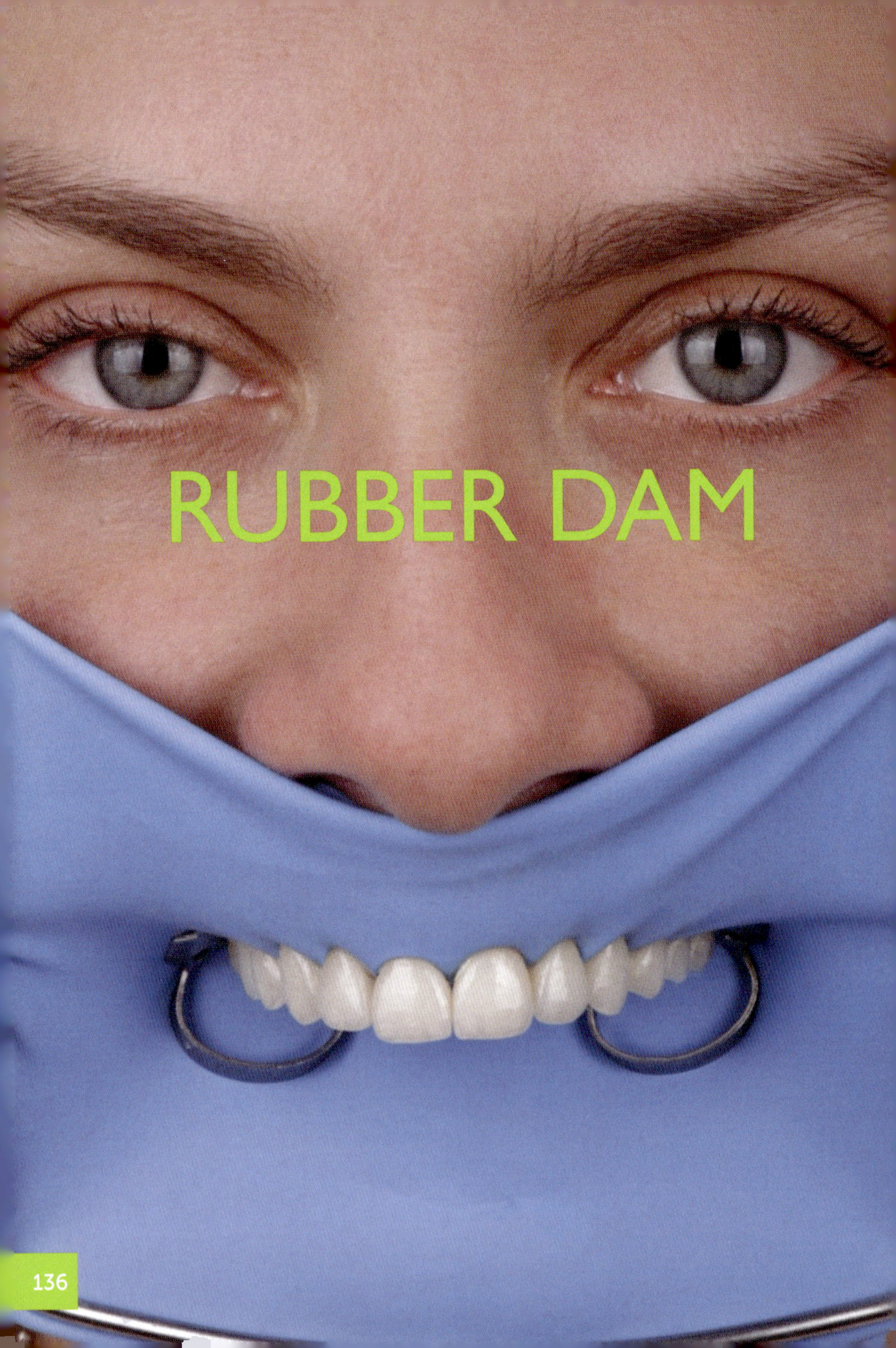

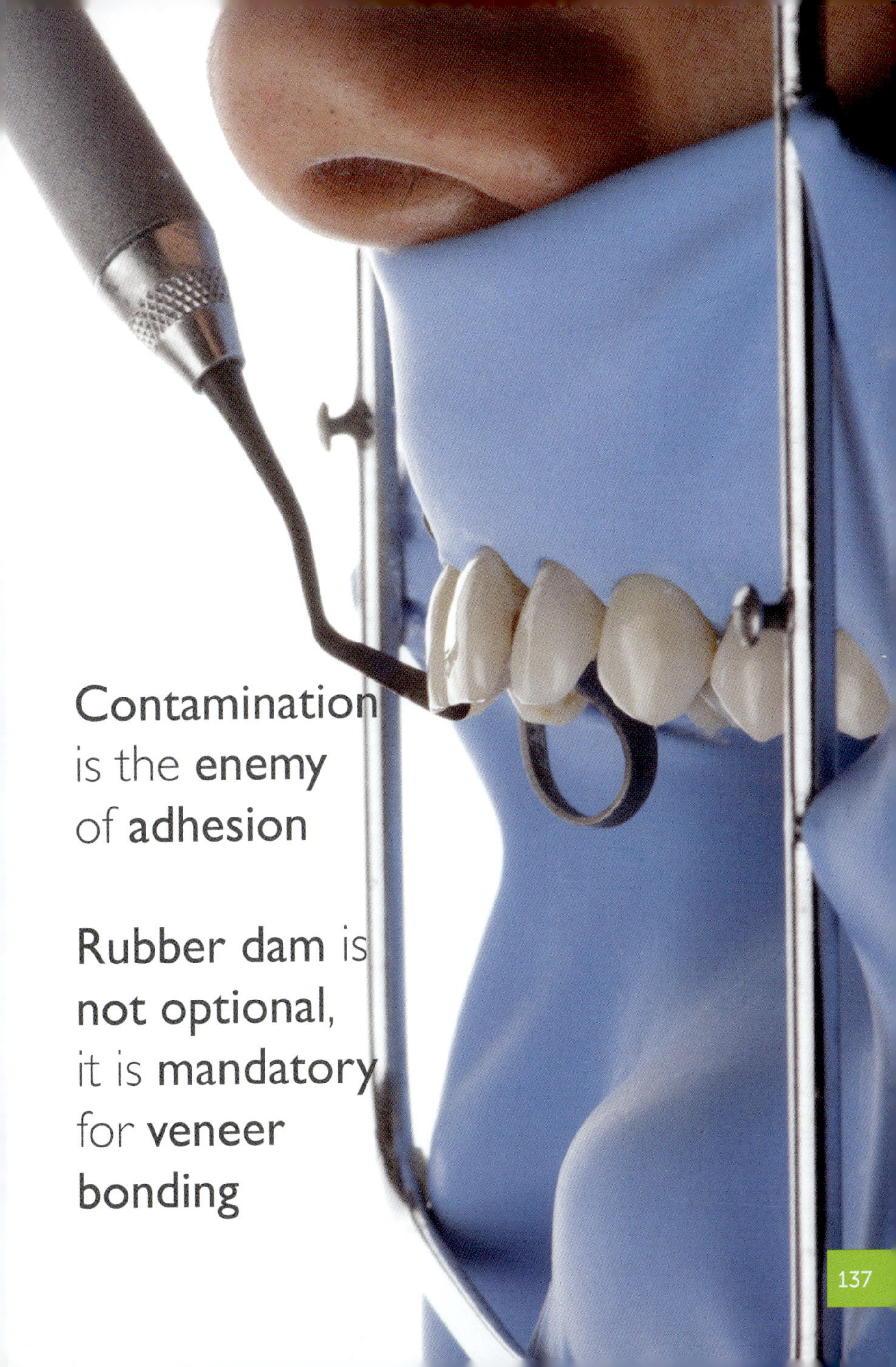

Contamination is the **enemy** of **adhesion**

Rubber dam is **not optional**, it is **mandatory** for **veneer bonding**

J Esthet Restor Dent 2023;35:48–55

Clinical in-situ evaluation of the effect of rubber dam isolation on bond strength to enamel

Falacho RI, Melo EA, Marques JA, Ramos JC, Guerra F, Blatz MB

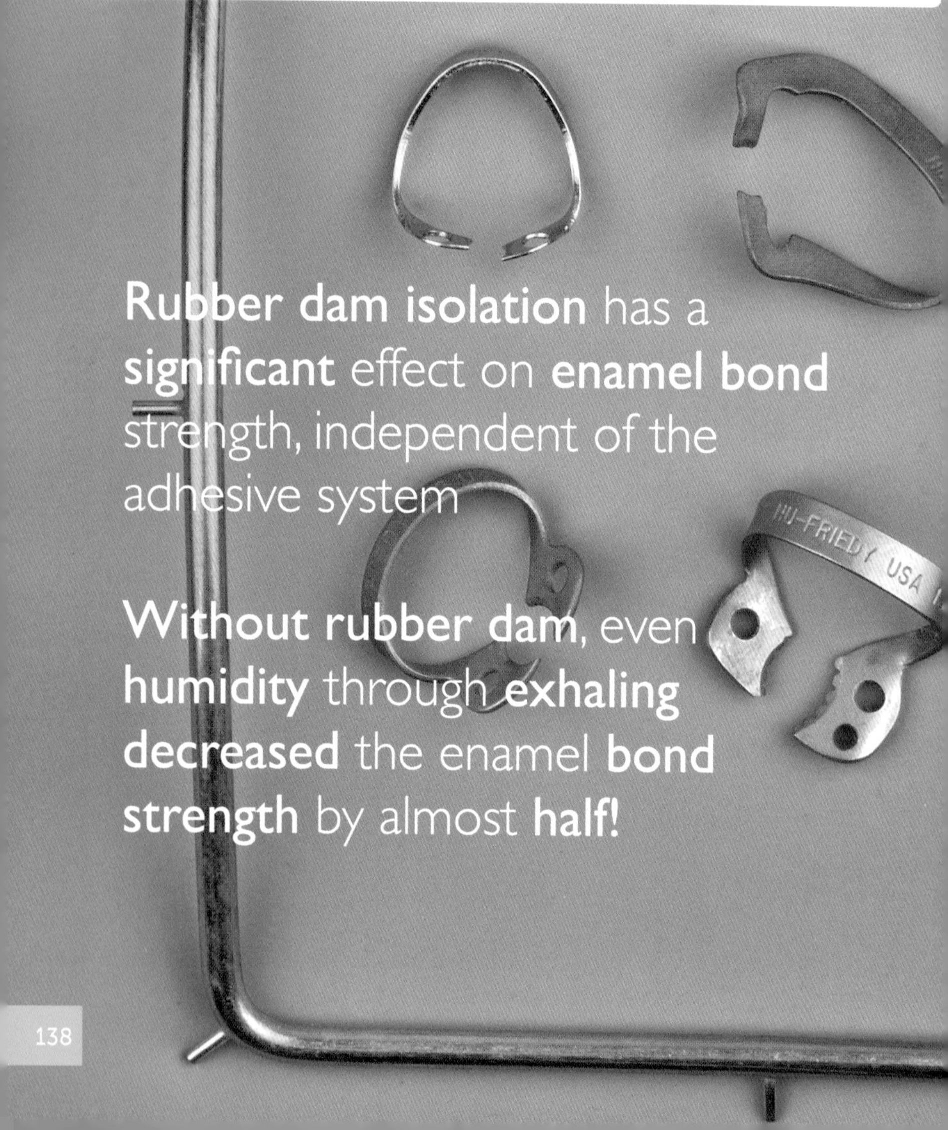

Rubber dam isolation has a **significant** effect on **enamel bond** strength, independent of the adhesive system

Without rubber dam, even **humidity** through **exhaling decreased** the enamel **bond strength** by almost **half!**

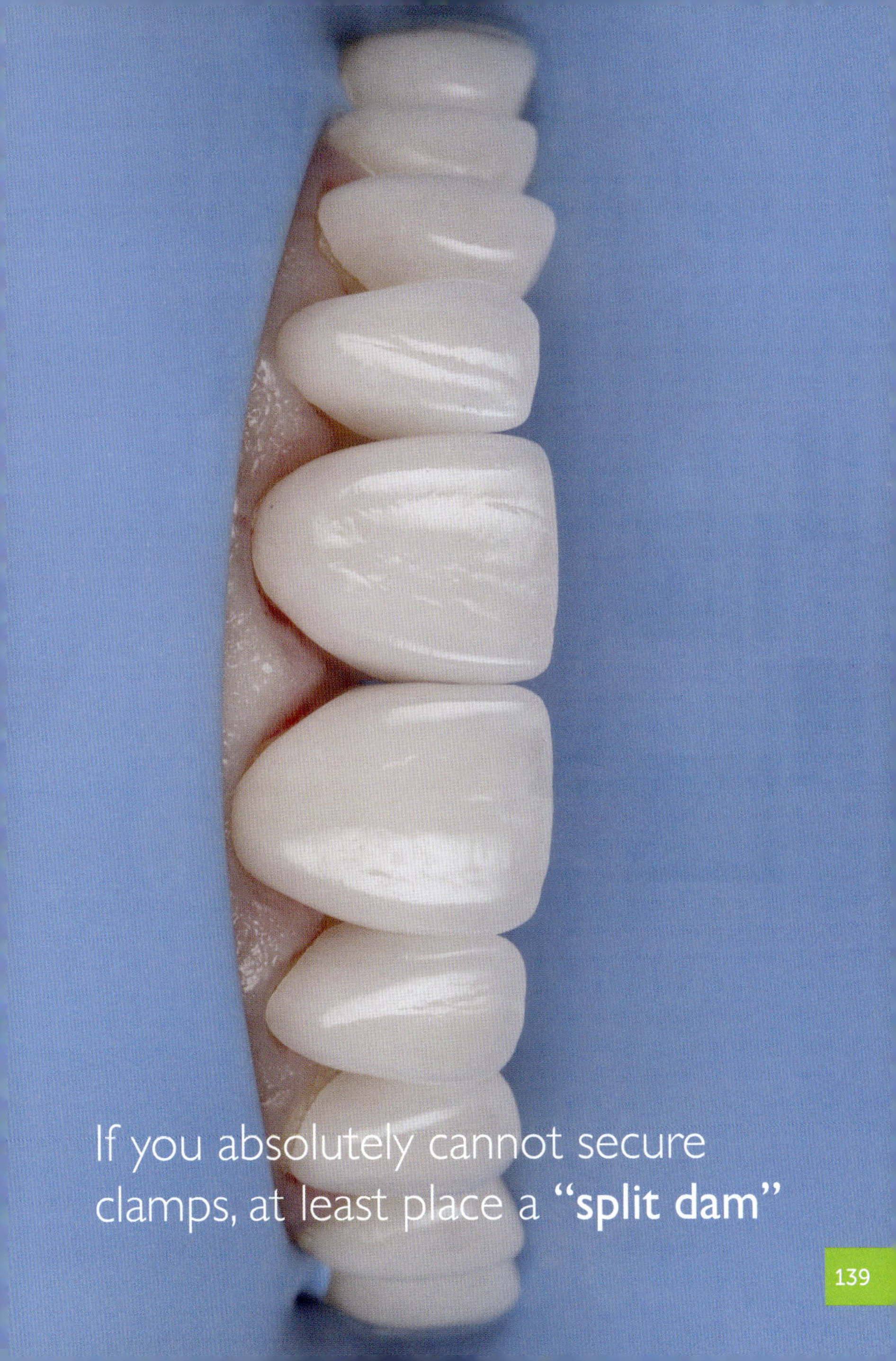

If you absolutely cannot secure clamps, at least place a “**split dam**”

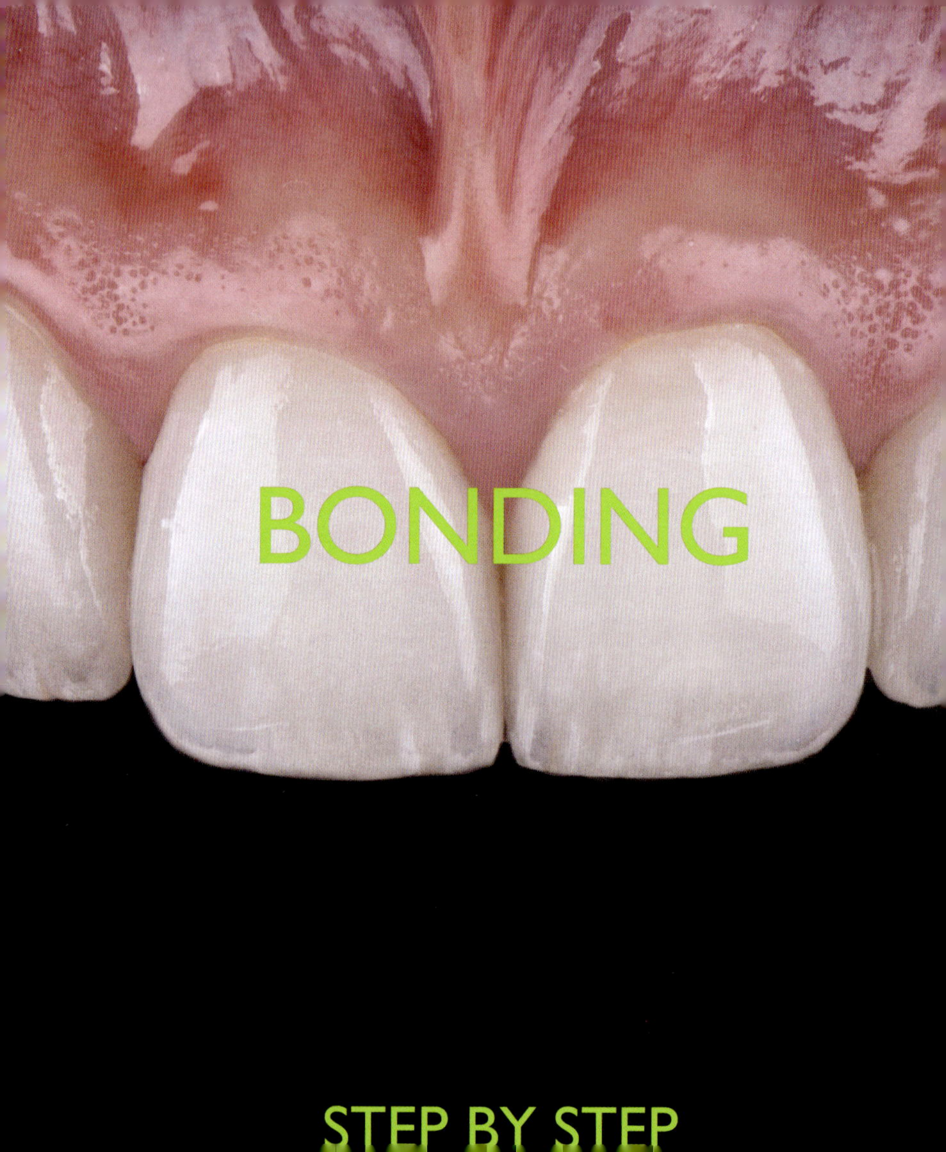
BONDING
STEP BY STEP

Hydrofluoric acid (HF) etch veneer 1

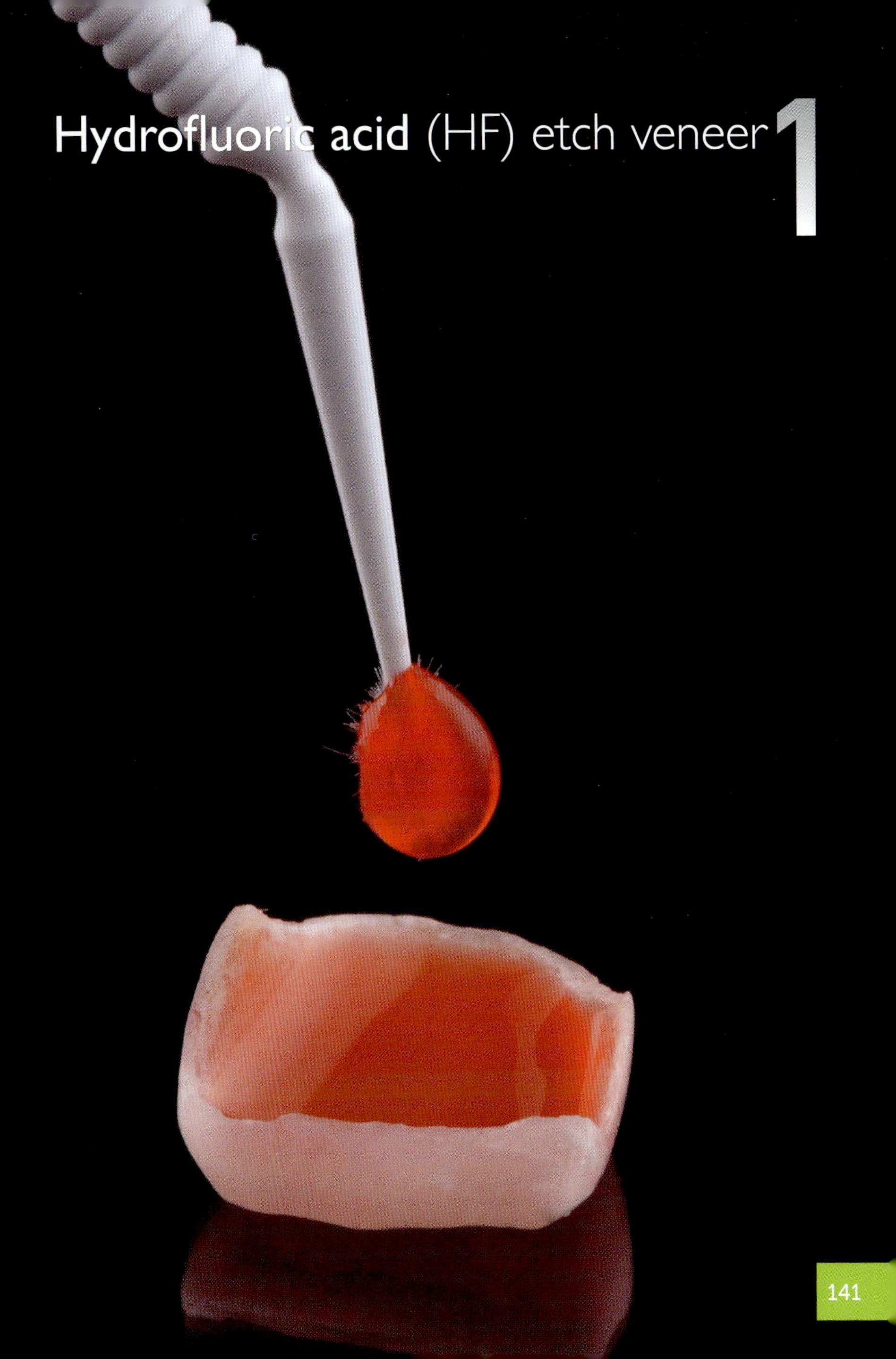

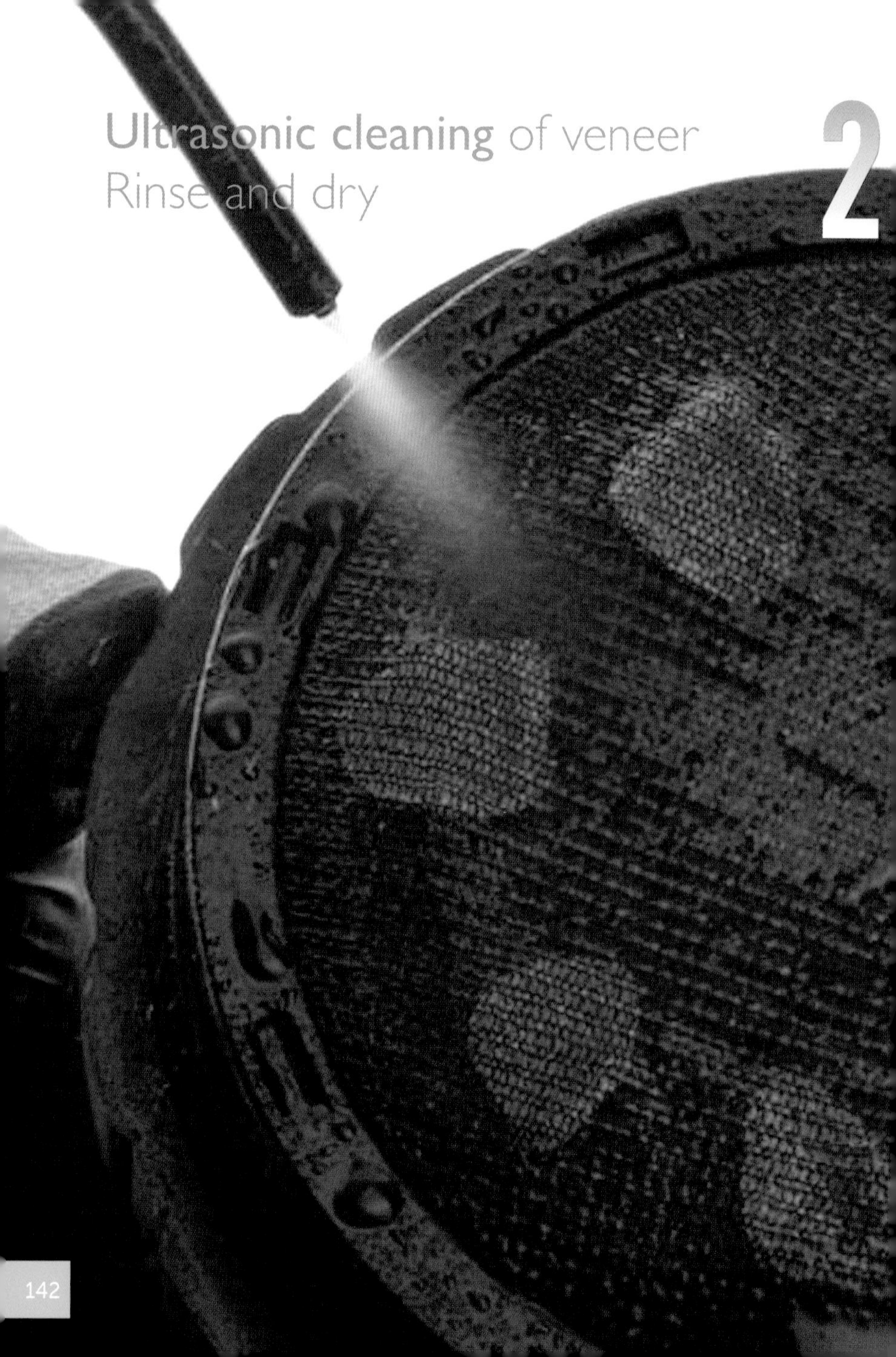

Ultrasonic cleaning of veneer
Rinse and dry

2

Apply a **silane** coupling agent

3

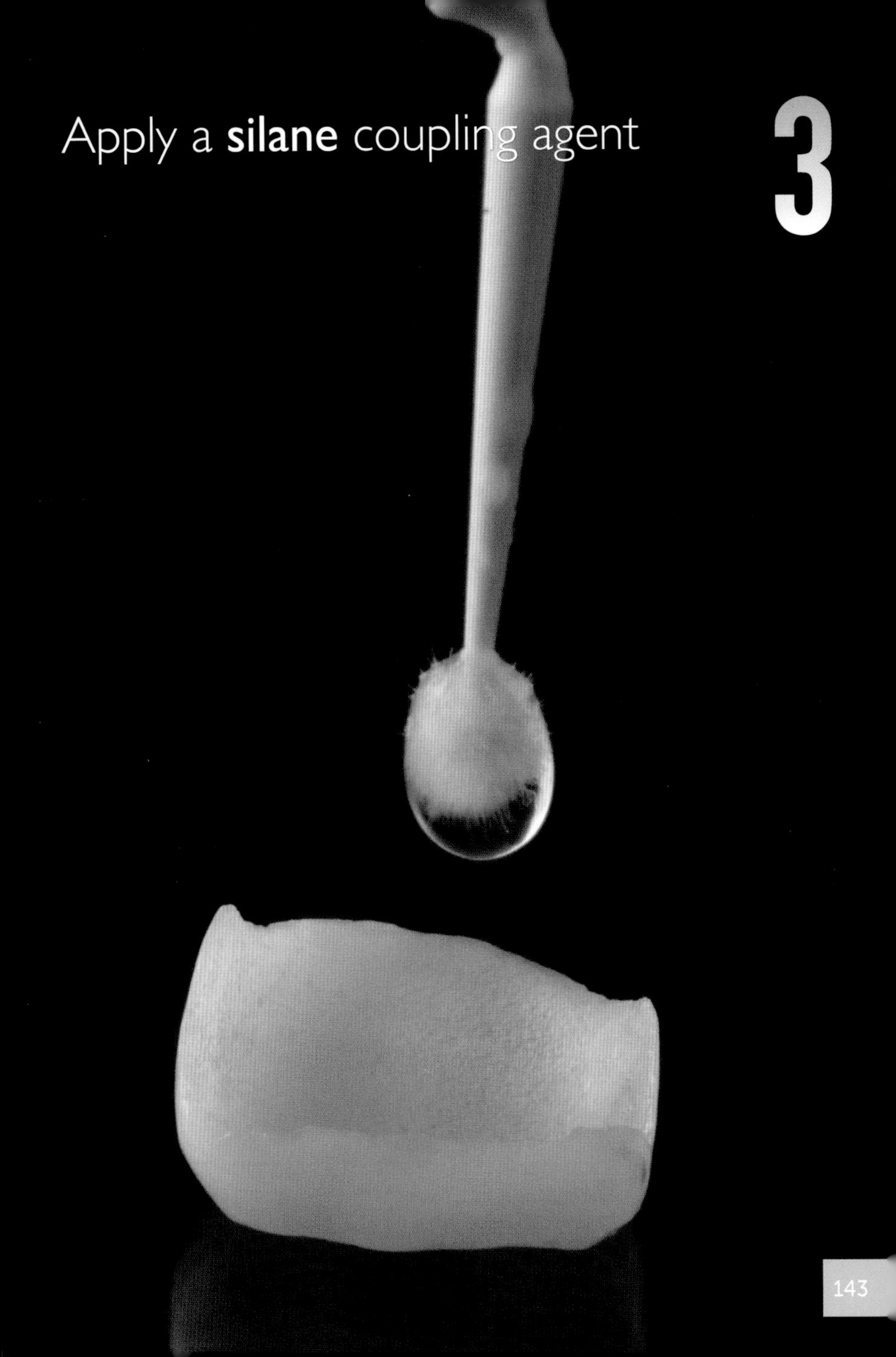

Phosphoric acid etching of **enamel**
Rinse and dry

4

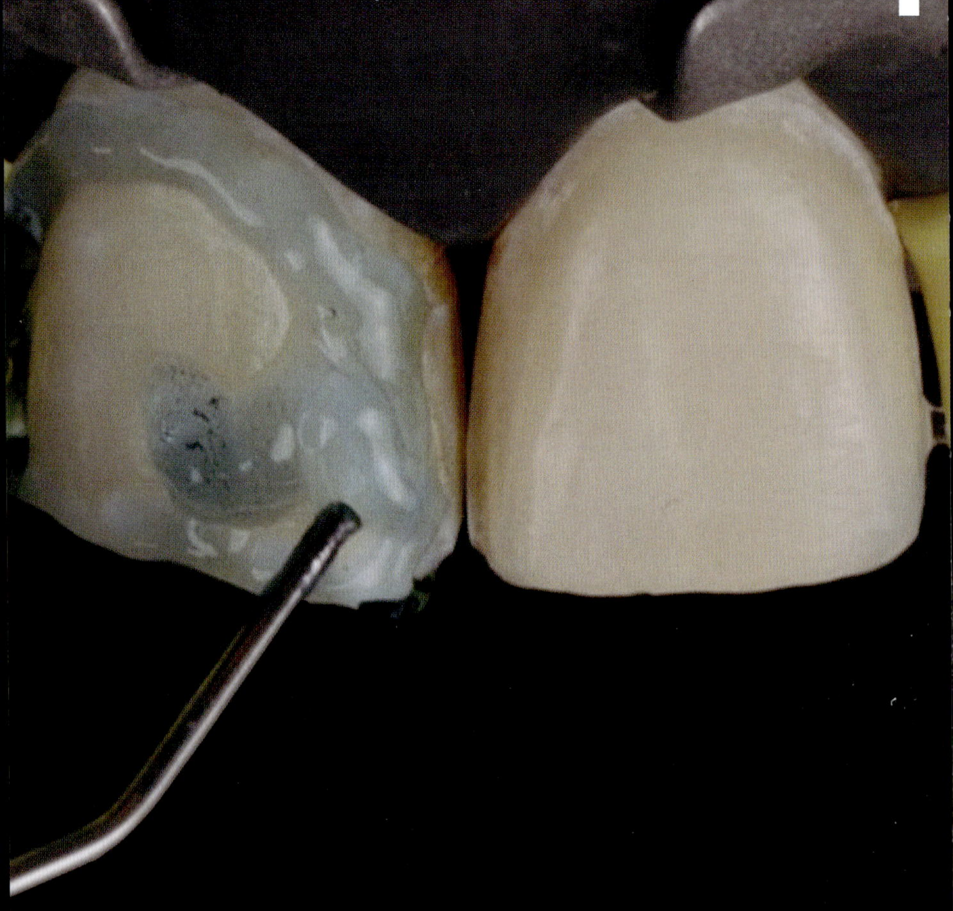

Always follow the **manufacturer** instructions

5

Apply **bonding agent** to the etched enamel
Light cure separately or **co-cure** with resin cement after veneer insertion

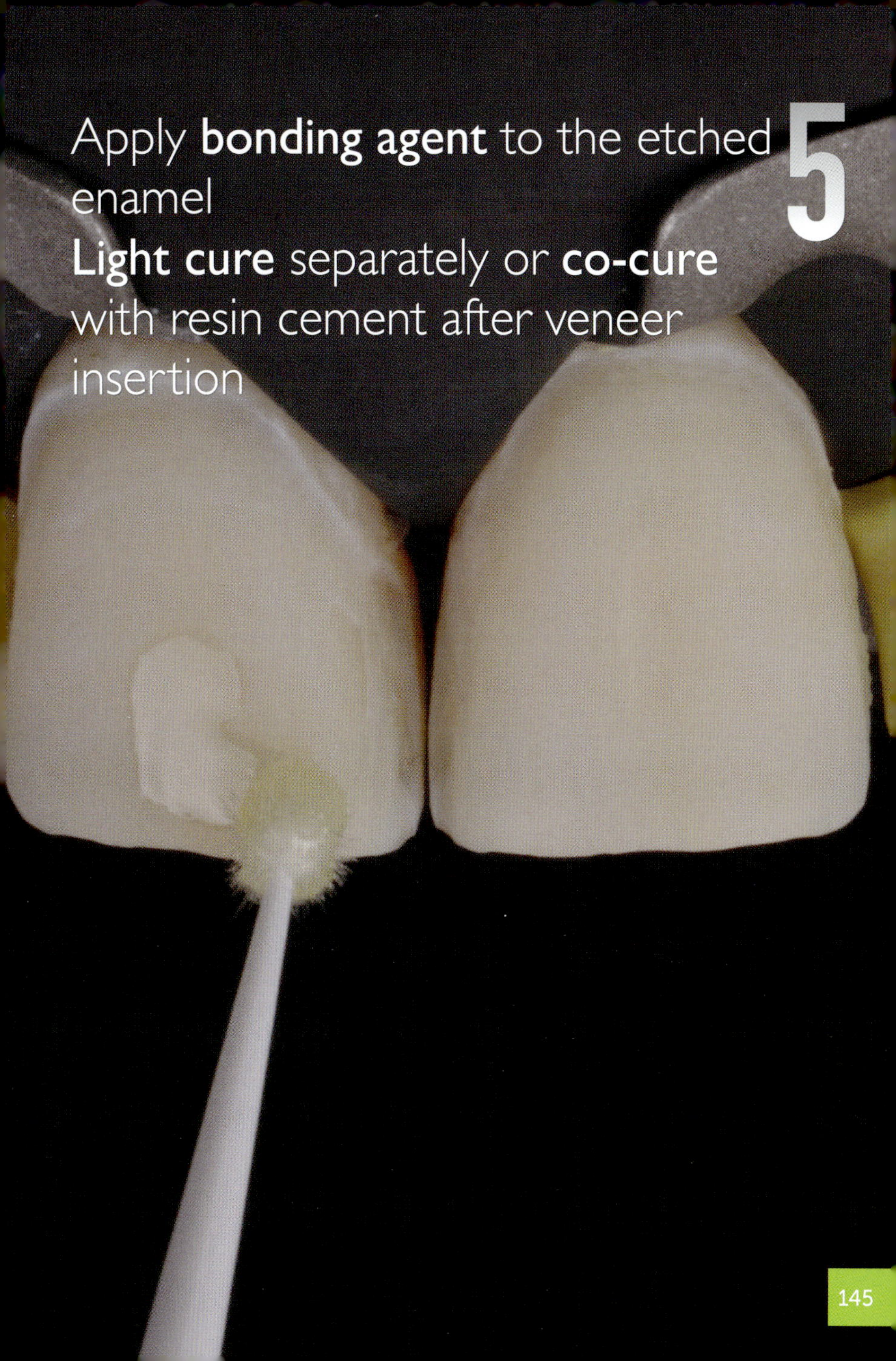

Apply **resin cement** to the bonding surface of the veneer

6

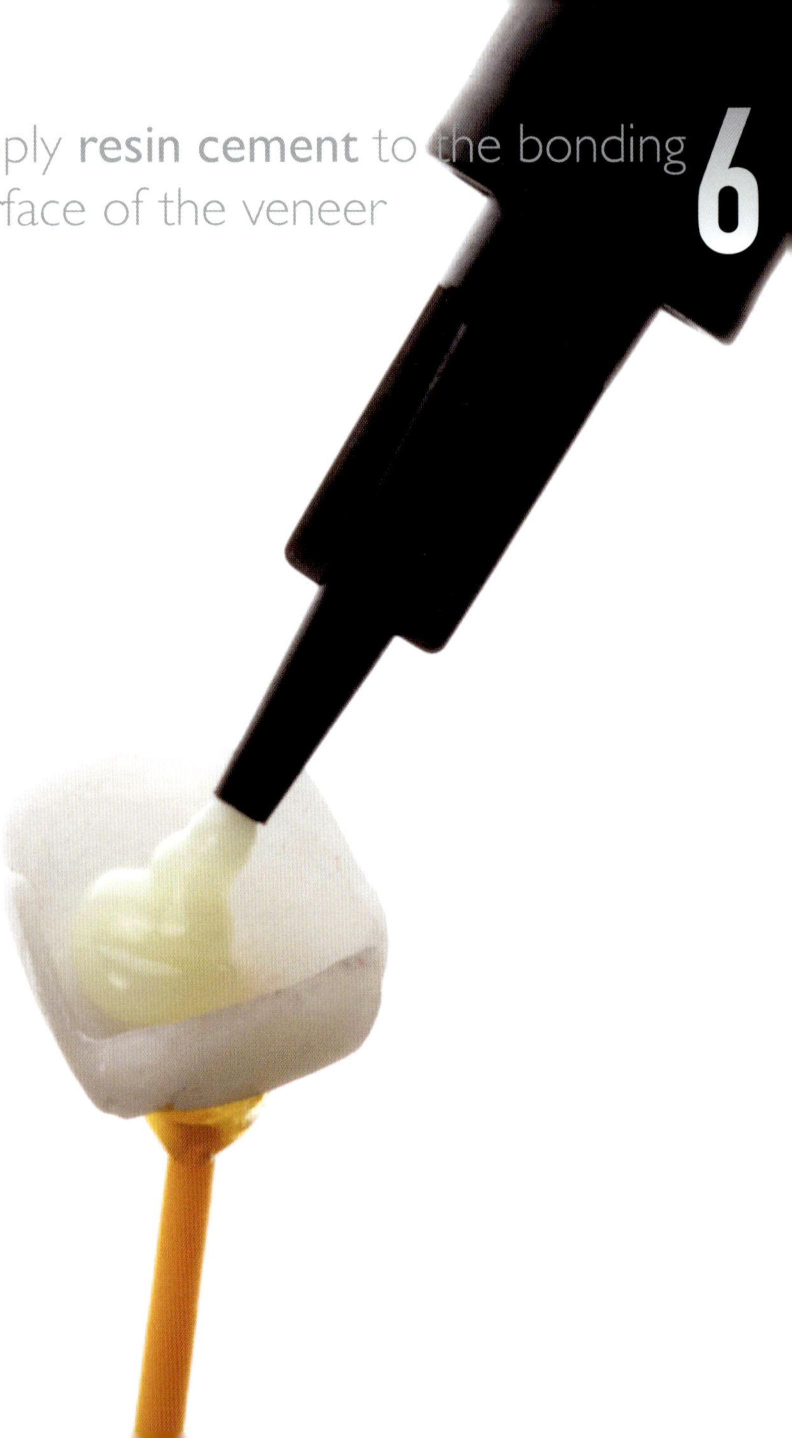

Insert the veneer

7

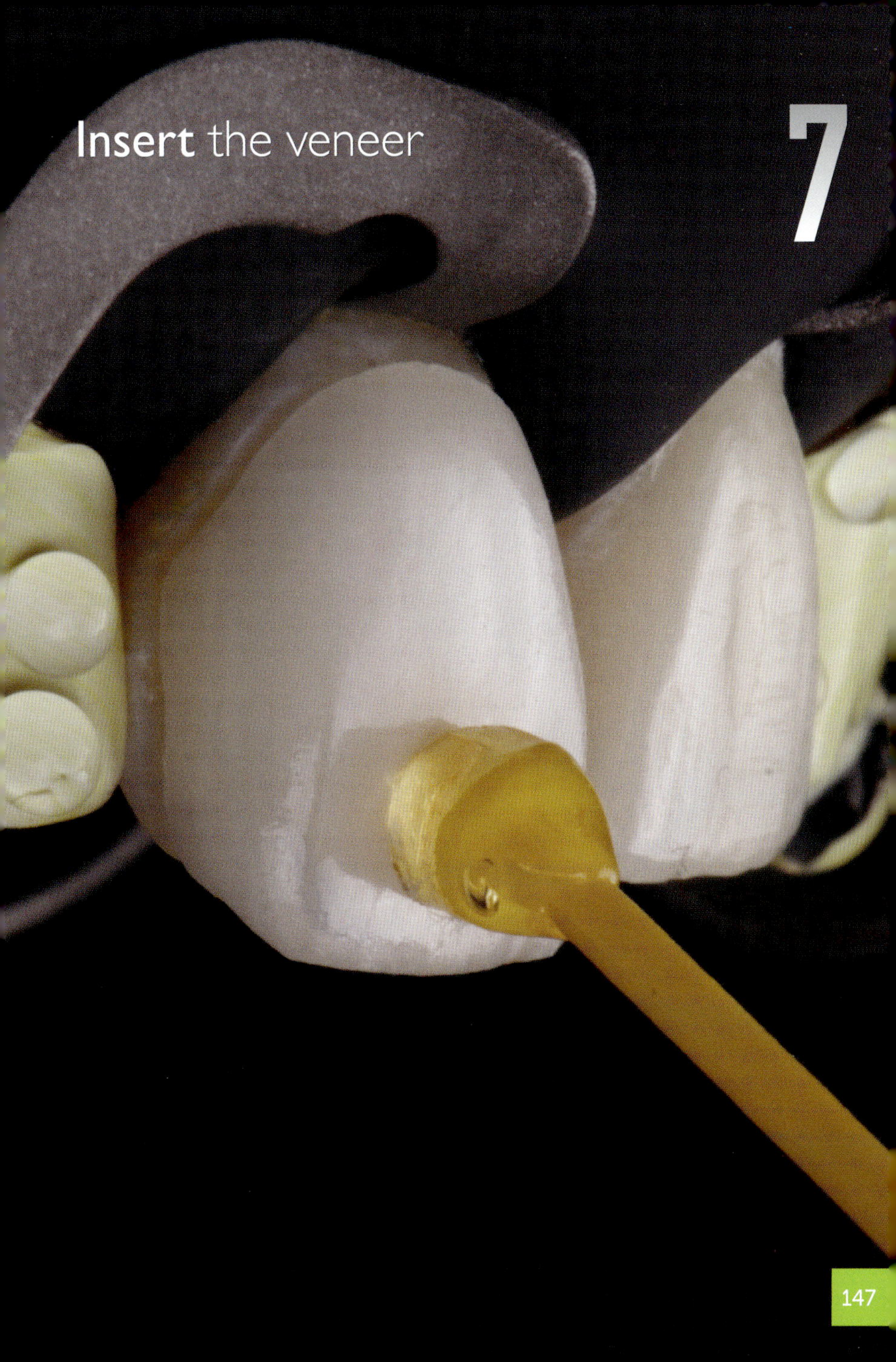

Remove excess resin cement
Light cure from all sides for 60 s

8

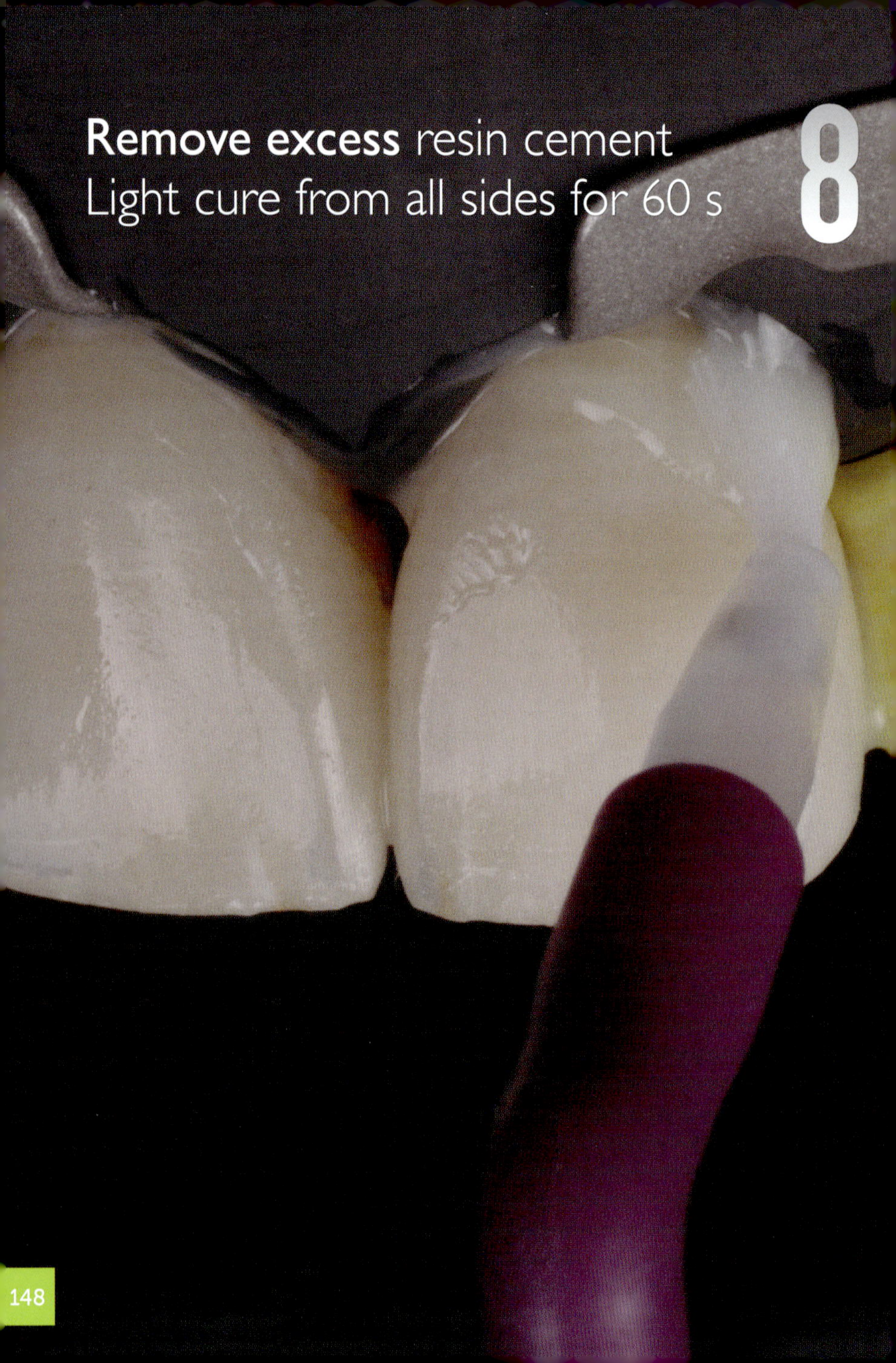

9 Finish and polish

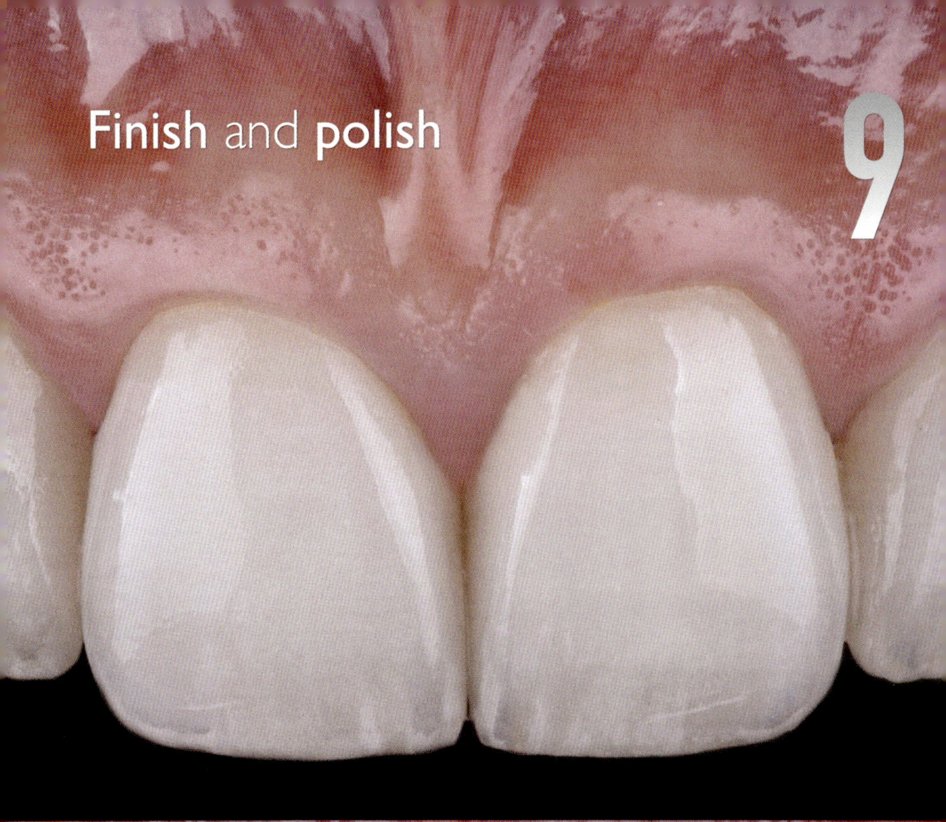

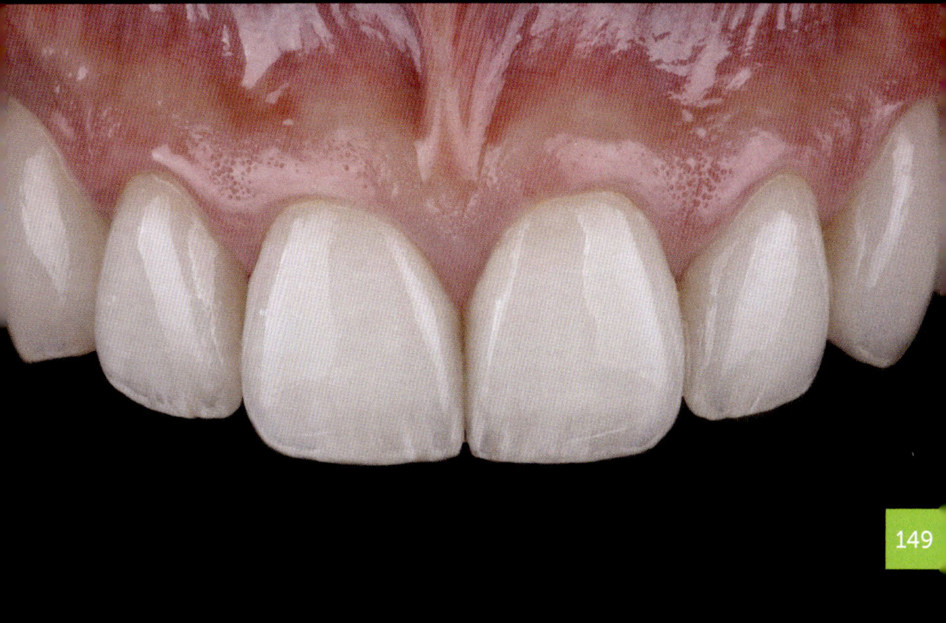

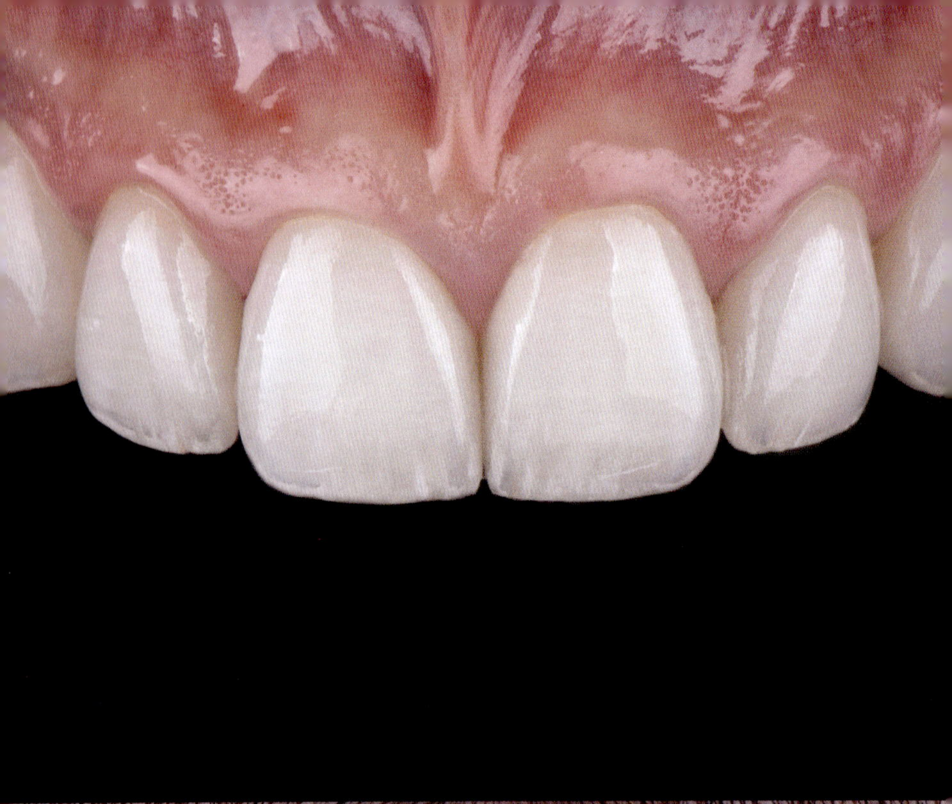

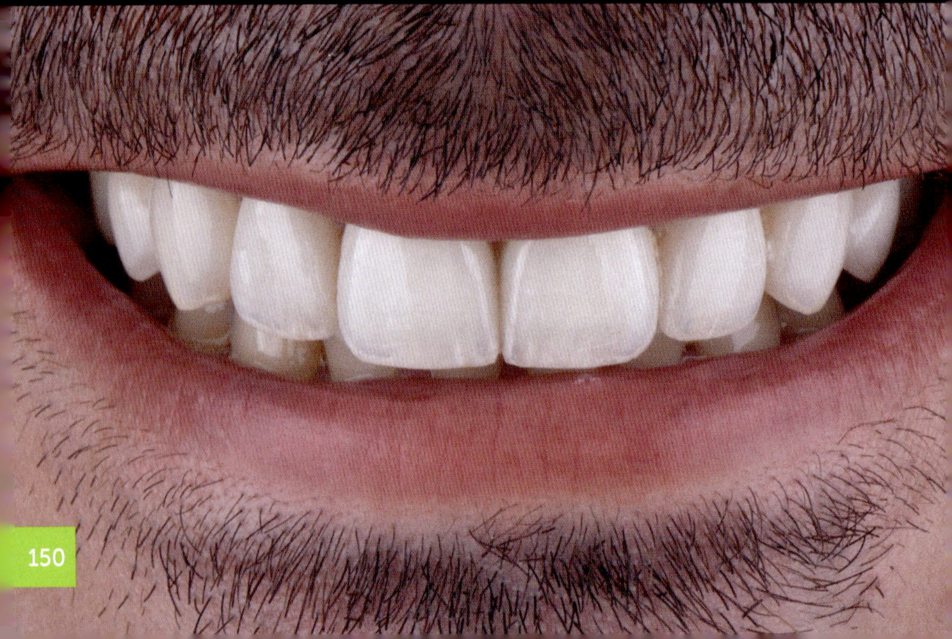

BONDING

CHEAT SHEET

1 HF etch veneer

2 Clean veneer ultrasonically in alcohol
Dry

3 Apply a silane coupling agent to the veneer

4 Etch the enamel with phosphoric acid
Rinse and dry

5 Apply a bonding agent to the etched enamel
Light cure or co-cure with composite cement

6 Apply a composite cement to the bonding surface of the veneer

7 Insert the veneer

8 Remove excess composite
Light cure

9 Finish and polish

Braz Oral Res 2019;33:e095

Bond strengths of various resin cements to different ceramics

Farias DCS, Gonçalves LM, Walter R, Chung Y, Blatz MB

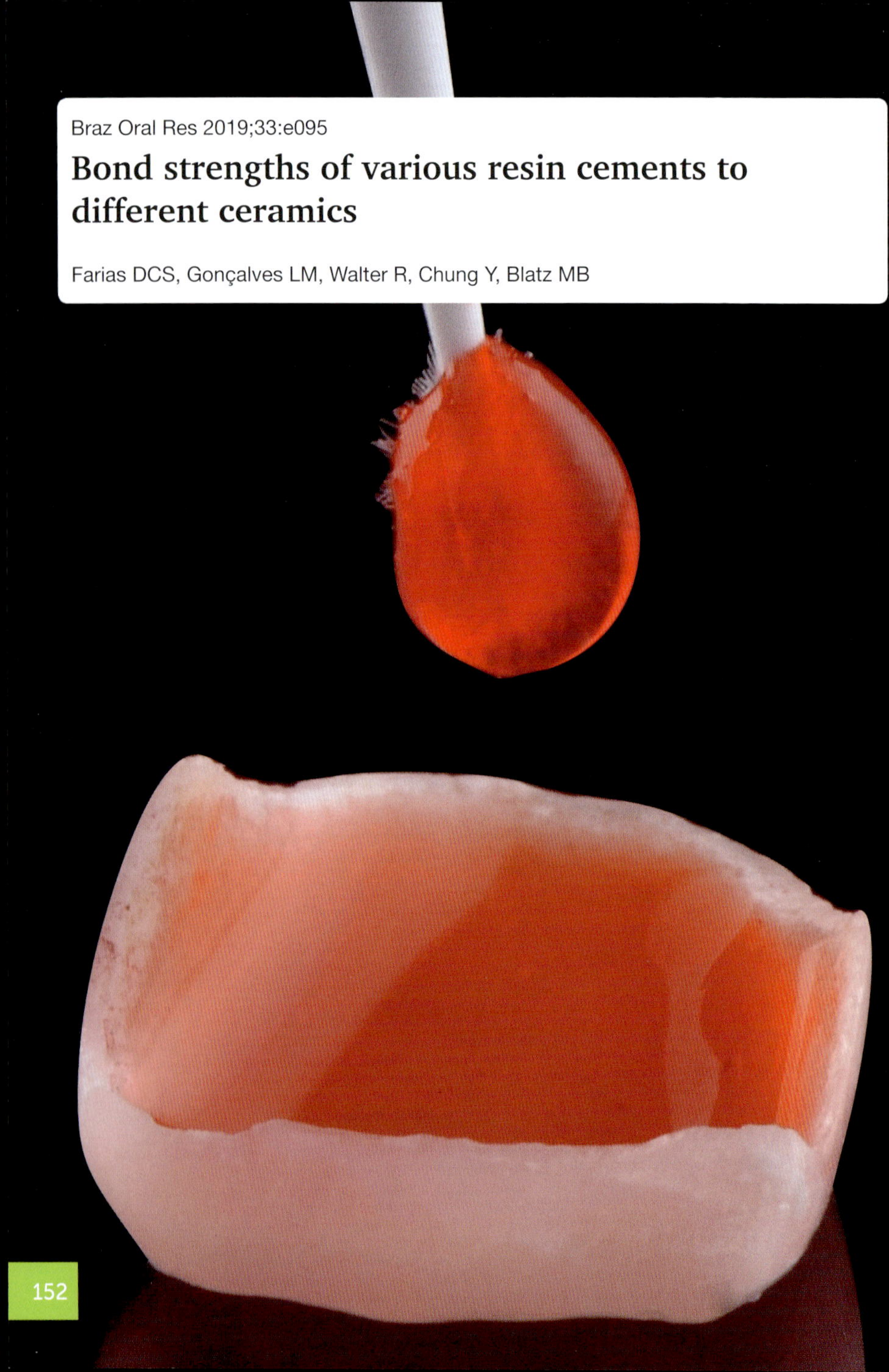

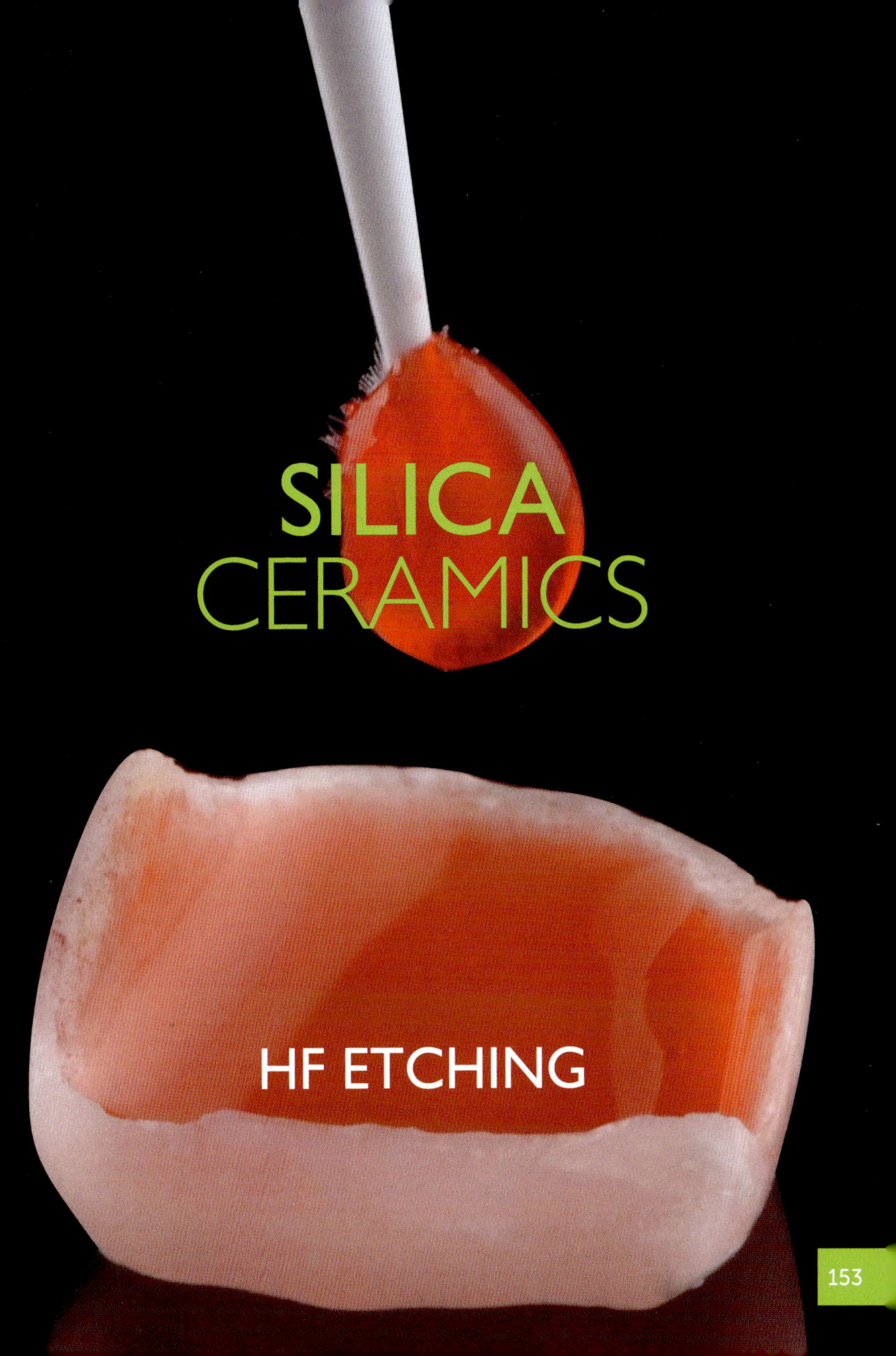

SILICA CERAMICS

HF ETCHING

HF ETCHING

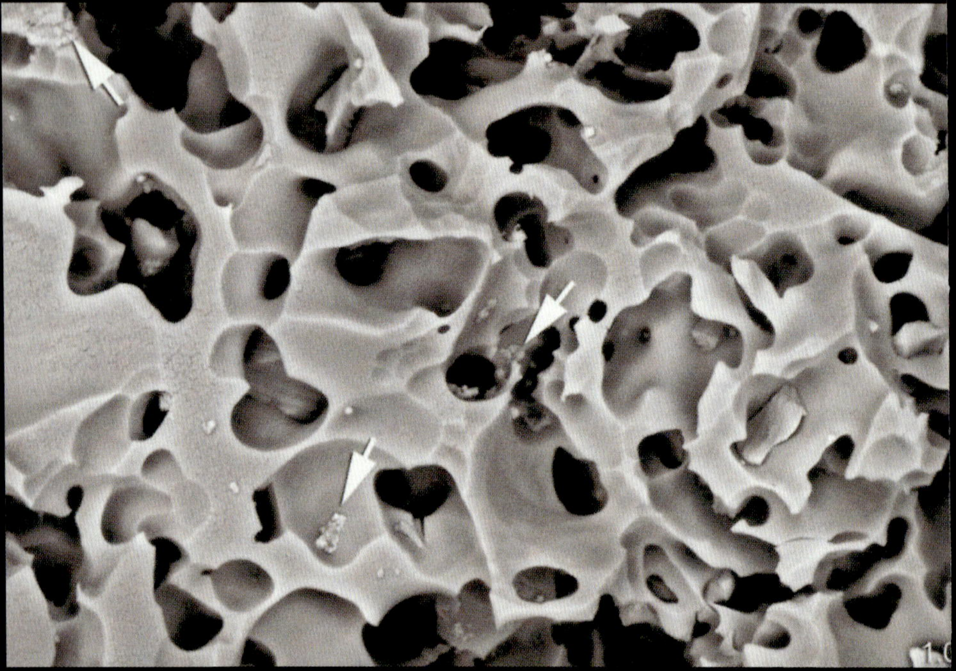

HF "dissolves" the glassy matrix between the crystals in **silica-based ceramics**

Duarte, Phark, Blatz, Sadan. Quint Dent Technol 2010;33:41–60

HF ETCHING

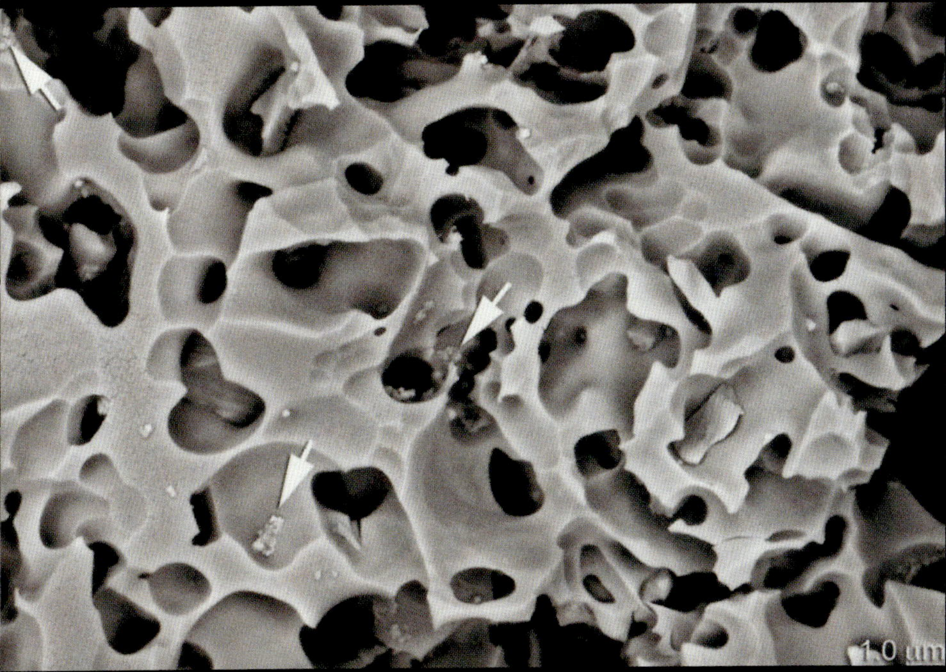

Therefore, **silica-based ceramics** with different **crystal content** require different **HF concentration** and **etching times!**

Duarte, Phark, Blatz, Sadan. Quint Dent Technol 2010;33:41–60

HF ETCHING

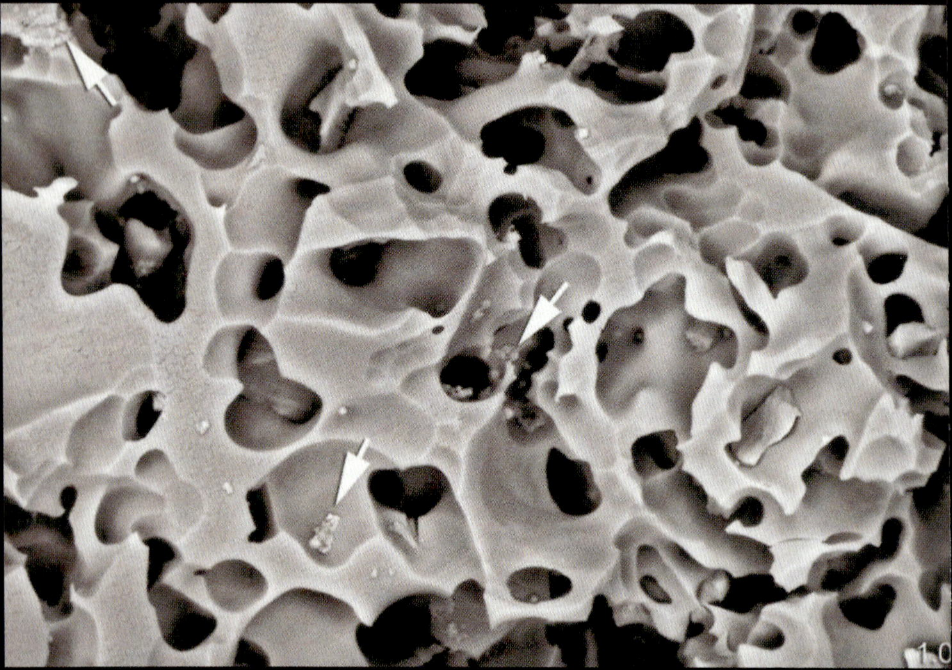

Feldspathic porcelain (FP)	9% HF for 2 min
CAD/CAM FP	9% HF for 1 min
Leucite-reinforced FP	9% HF for 1 min
Lithium disilicate	5% HF for 20 s

Duarte, Phark, Blatz, Sadan. Quint Dent Technol 2010;33:41–60

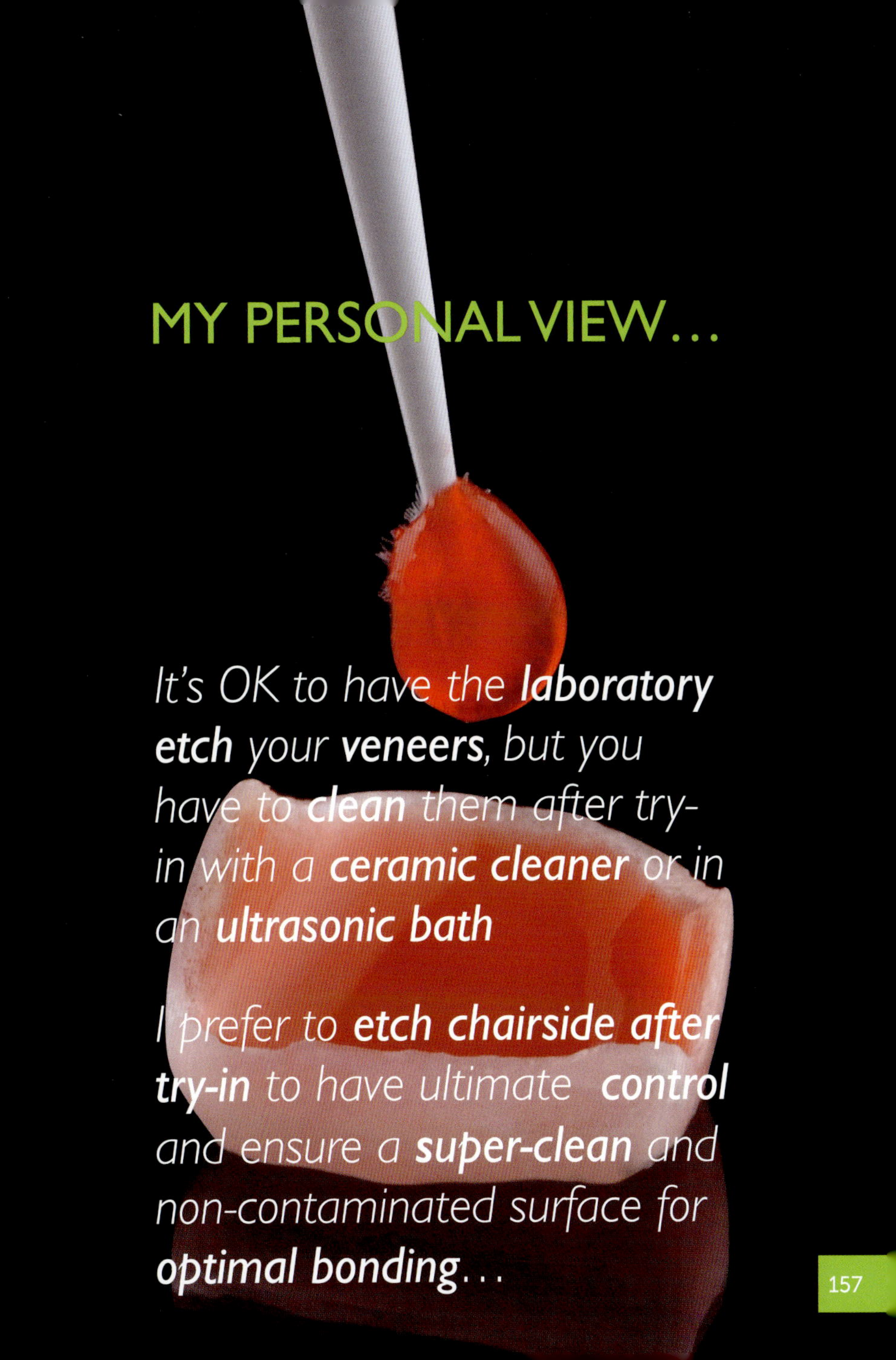

MY PERSONAL VIEW…

It's OK to have the ***laboratory etch*** *your* ***veneers****, but you have to* ***clean*** *them after try-in with a* ***ceramic cleaner*** *or in an* ***ultrasonic bath***

I prefer to ***etch chairside after try-in*** *to have ultimate* ***control*** *and ensure a* ***super-clean*** *and non-contaminated surface for* ***optimal bonding****…*

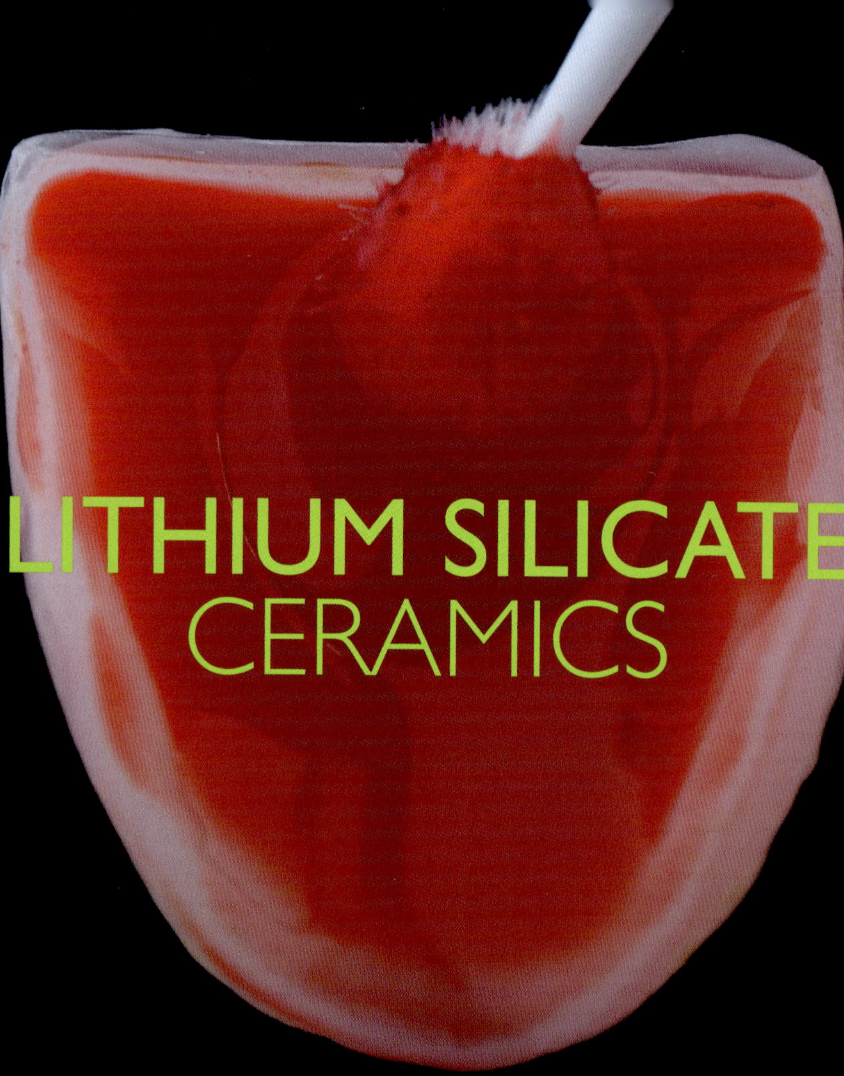

LITHIUM SILICATE CERAMICS

HF ETCHING TIMES and CONCENTRATION

J Adhes Dent 2020;22:175–182

Influence of acid concentration and etching time on composite cement adhesion to lithium-silicate glass ceramics

Fabian Fonzar R, Goracci C, Carrabba M, Louca C, Ferrari M, Vichi A

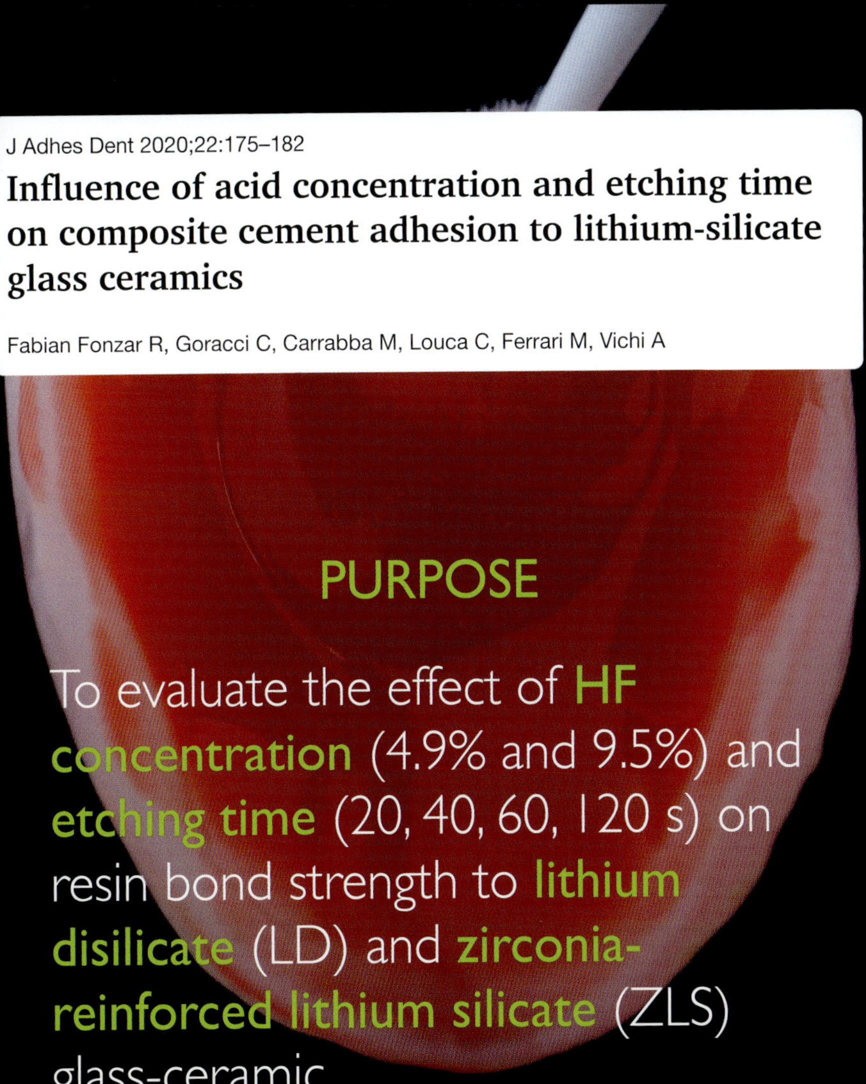

PURPOSE

To evaluate the effect of **HF concentration** (4.9% and 9.5%) and **etching time** (20, 40, 60, 120 s) on resin bond strength to **lithium disilicate** (LD) and **zirconia-reinforced lithium silicate** (ZLS) glass-ceramic

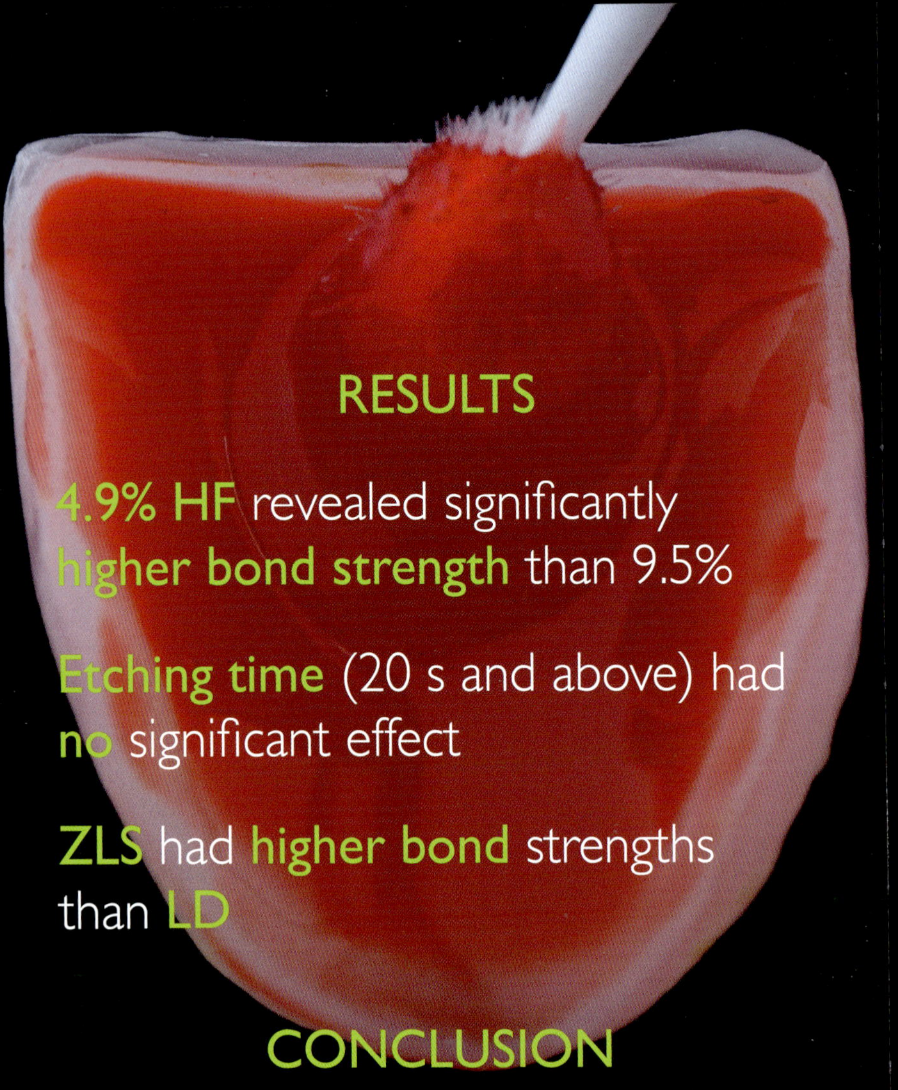

RESULTS

4.9% HF revealed significantly higher bond strength than 9.5%

Etching time (20 s and above) had no significant effect

ZLS had higher bond strengths than LD

CONCLUSION

4.9% HF for 20 s is most effective for lithium silicate ceramics

Fabian Fonzar et al. | Adhes Dent 2020;22:175–182

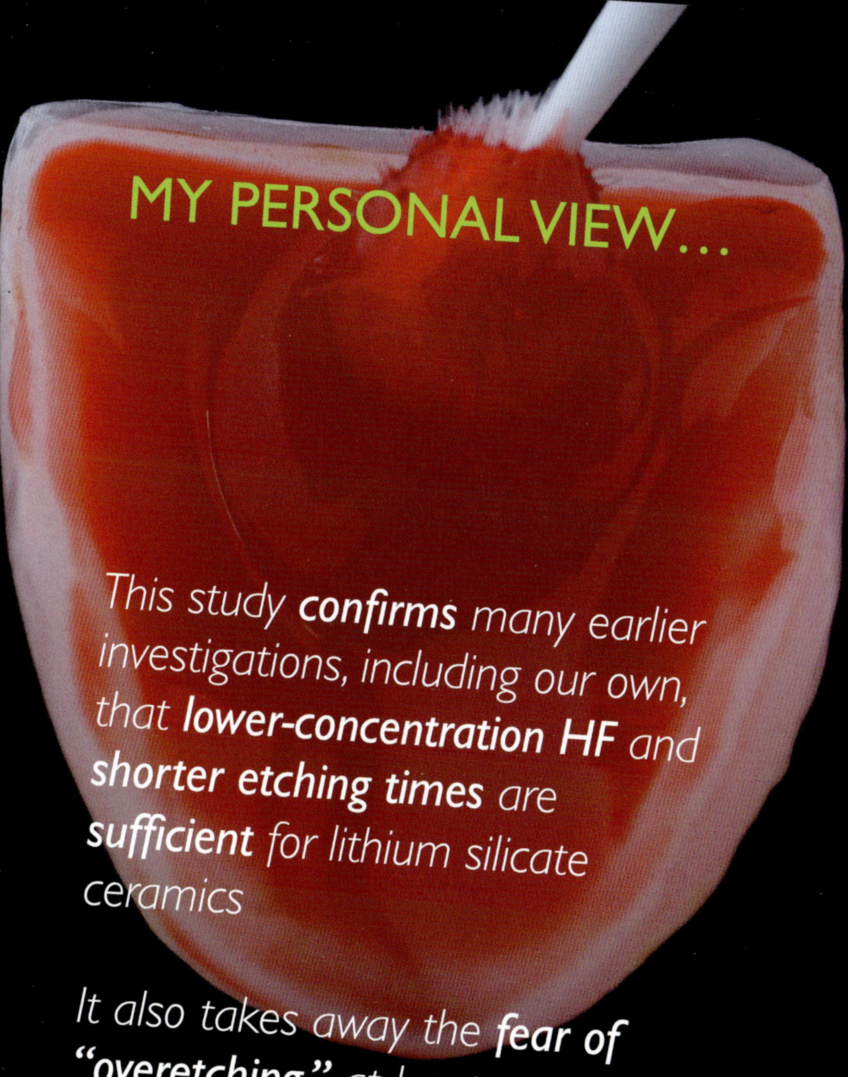

MY PERSONAL VIEW…

This study ***confirms*** *many earlier investigations, including our own, that* ***lower-concentration HF*** *and* ***shorter etching times*** *are* ***sufficient*** *for lithium silicate ceramics*

It also takes away the ***fear of "overetching,"*** *at least up to 2 min, since* ***longer etching times*** *had* ***no effect*** *on bond strength*

SILICA CERAMICS

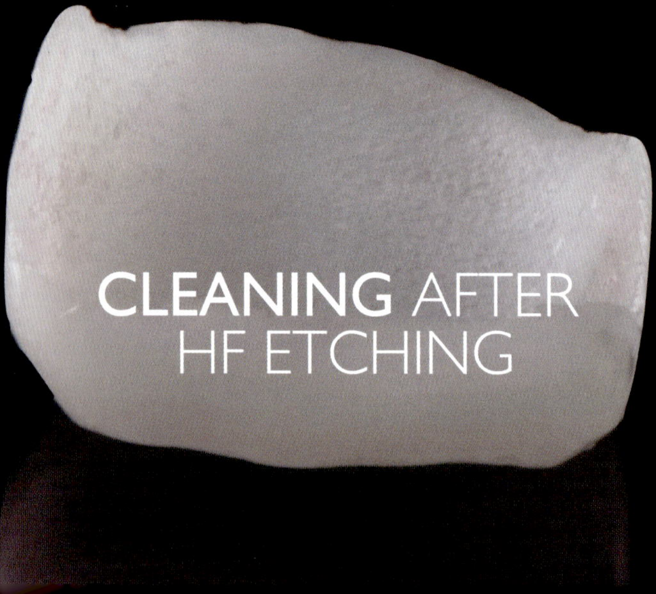

CLEANING AFTER HF ETCHING

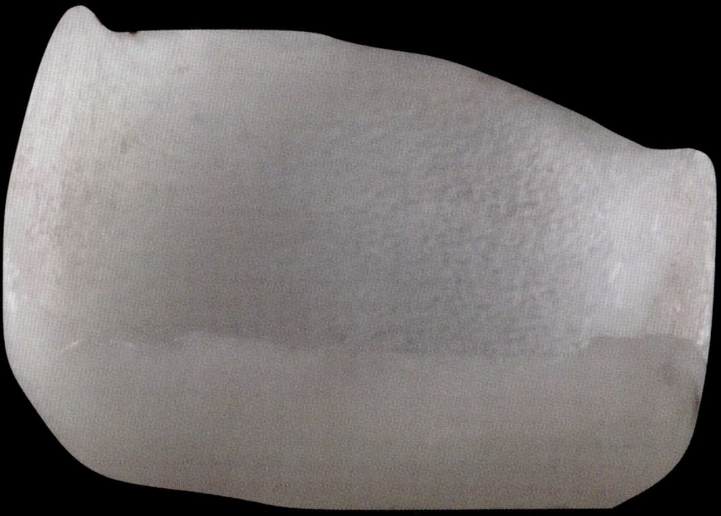

AFTER HF etching, rinse thoroughly with water and allow drying until the entire intaglio ceramic surface looks "dull" again

Duarte, Phark, Blatz, Sadan. Quint Dent Technol 2010;33:41–60

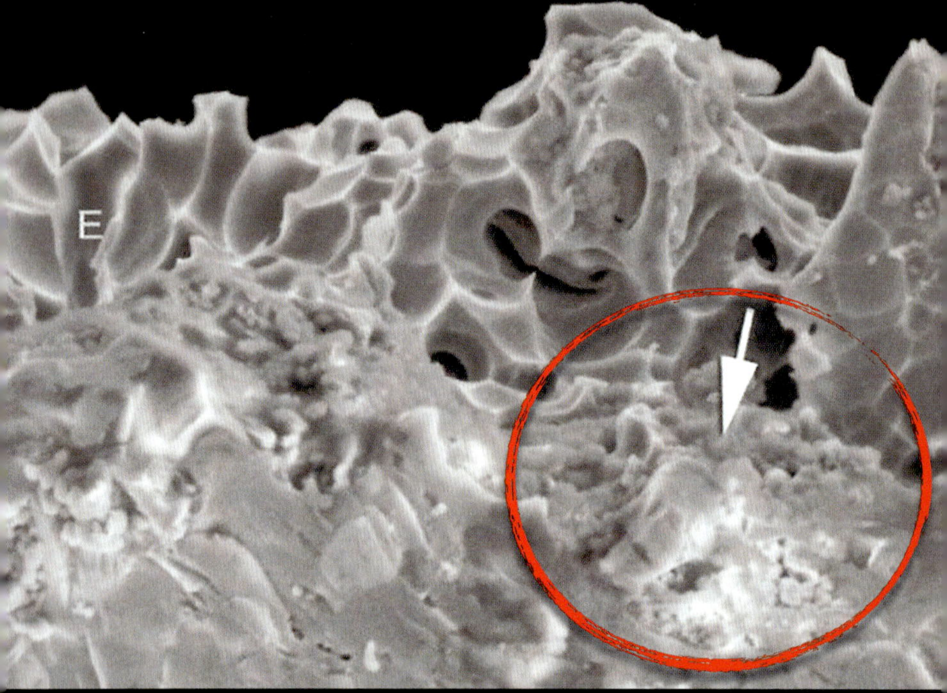

A white layer of residual acids, crystalline precipitates, and remineralized salts is often found and may block some of the created grooves and undercuts

Duarte, Phark, Blatz, Sadan. Quint Dent Technol 2010;33:41–60

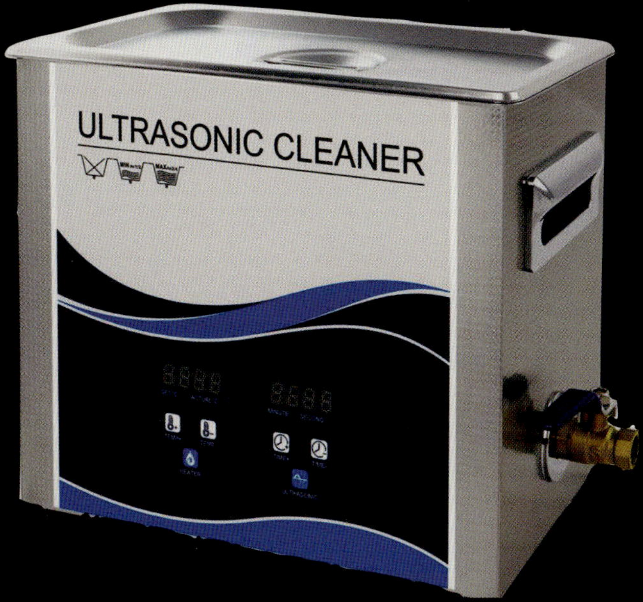

TO IMPROVE THE BOND, remove this layer in an **ultrasonic cleaning** bath for **2 to 5 min** (alcohol) before silane application

Duarte, Phark, Blatz, Sadan, Quint Dent Technol 2010;33:41–60

SILICA CERAMICS

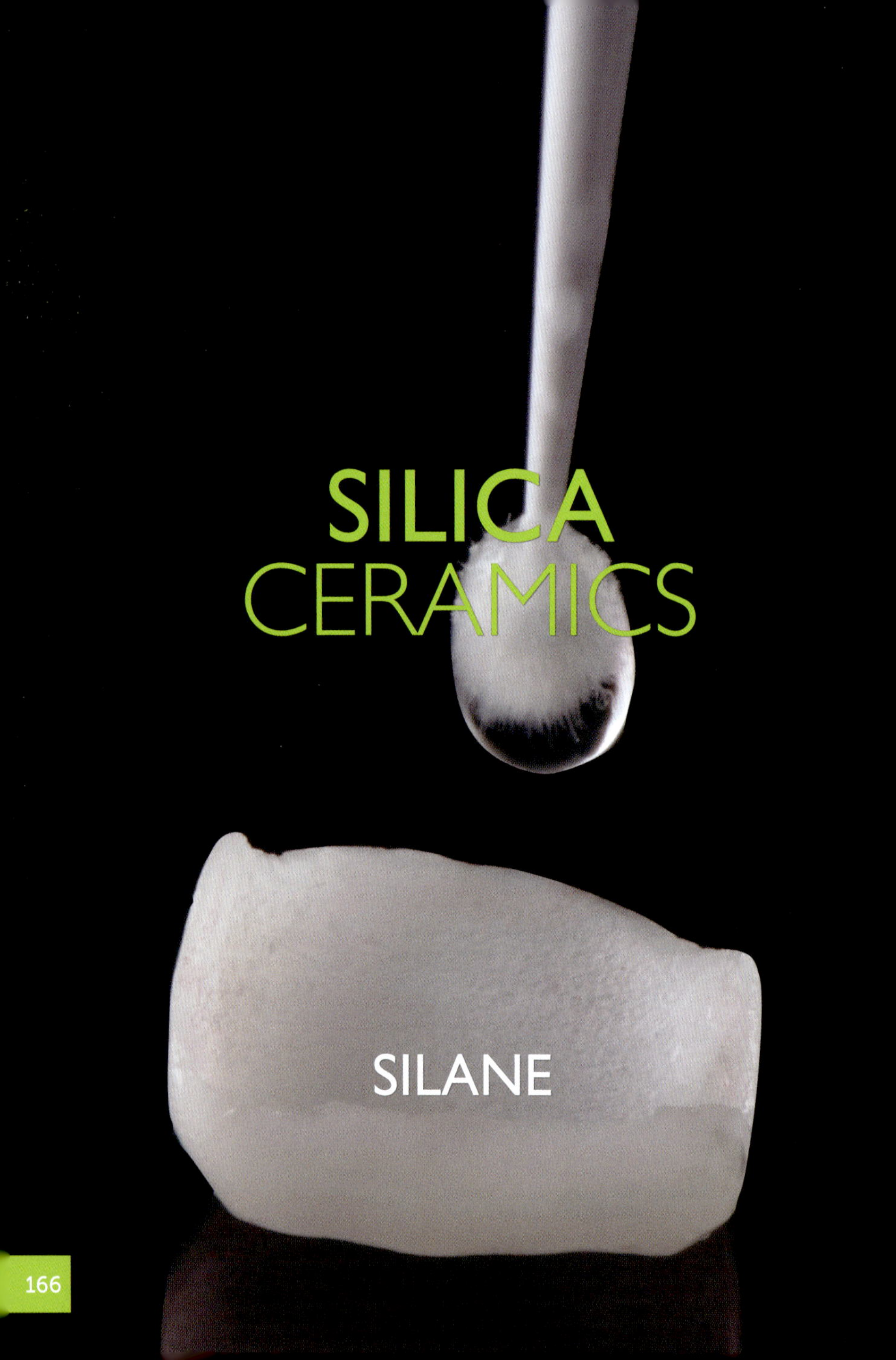

SILANE

SILANE

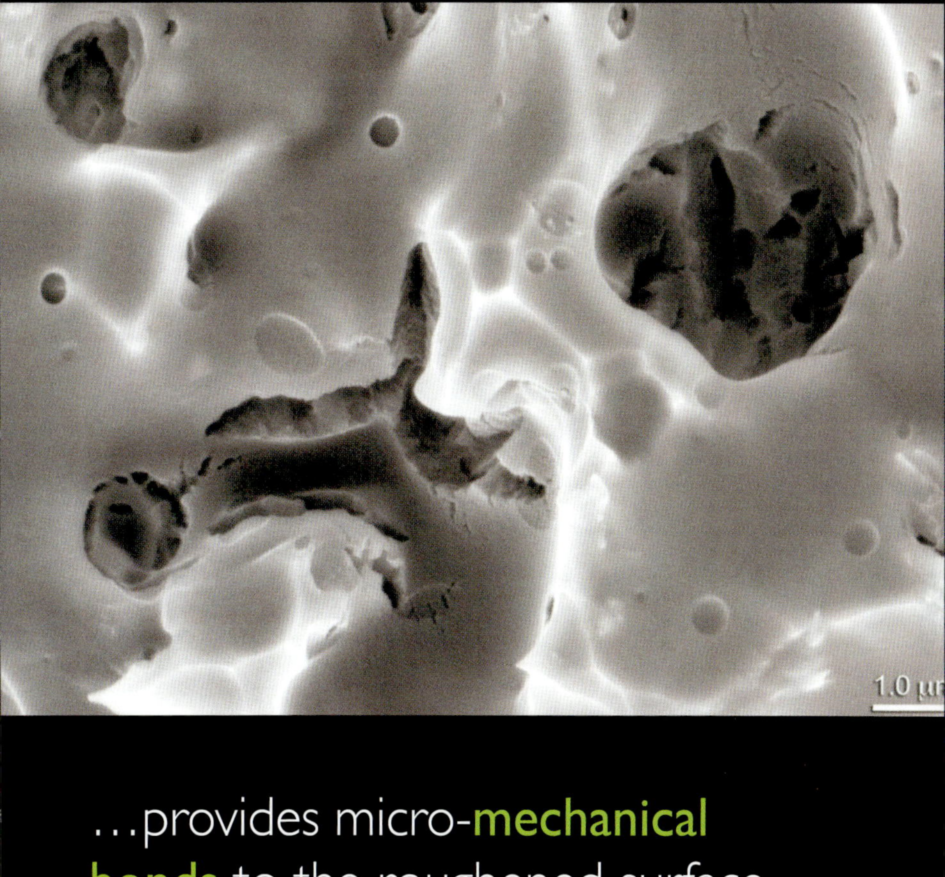

...provides micro-**mechanical bonds** to the roughened surface, but also true **chemical bonds** to the **silica** in the ceramic

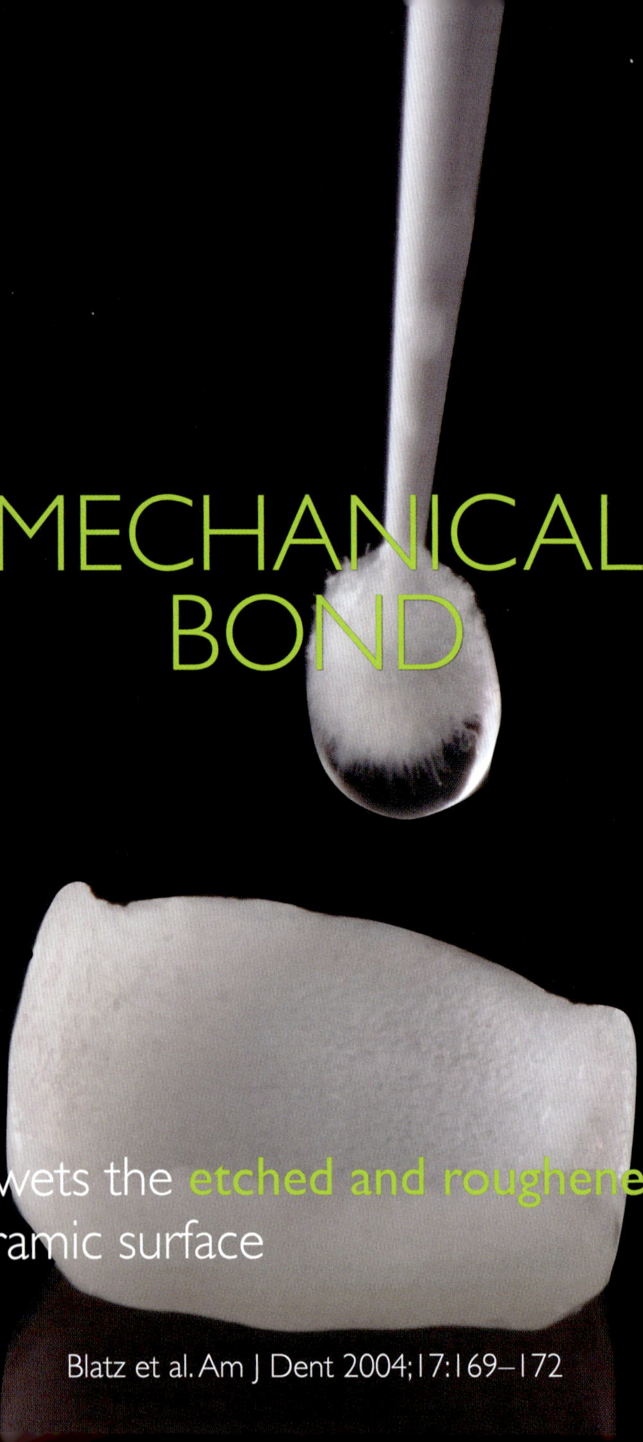

MECHANICAL BOND

...wets the **etched and roughened** ceramic surface

Blatz et al. Am J Dent 2004;17:169–172

CHEMICAL BOND

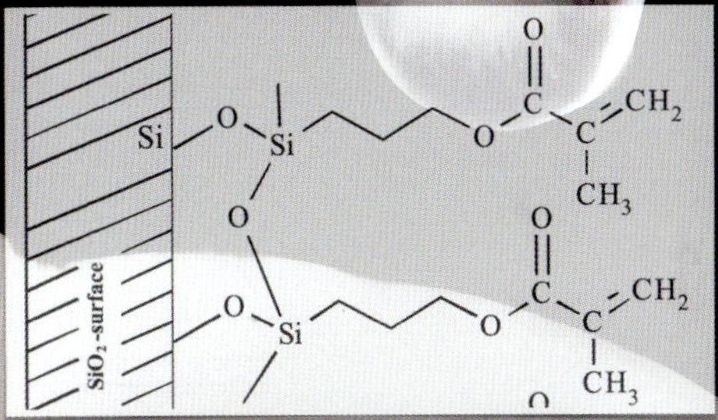

…forms **siloxane bonds** to the **silica** in the ceramic and **copolymerizes** with the **organic matrix** (composite)

Blatz et al. Am J Dent 2004;17:169–172

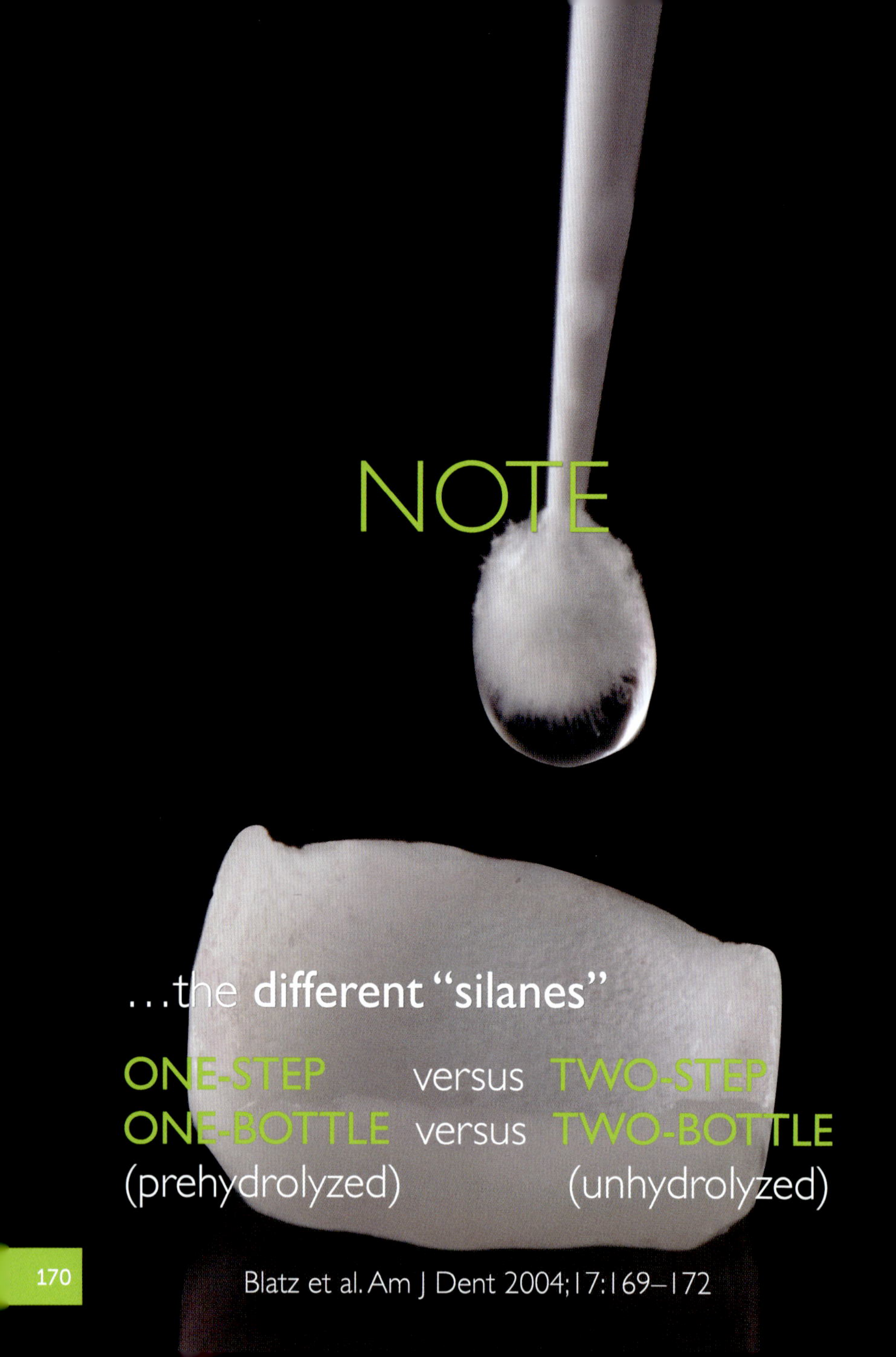

NOTE

…the **different "silanes"**

ONE-STEP versus **TWO-STEP**
ONE-BOTTLE versus **TWO-BOTTLE**
(prehydrolyzed) (unhydrolyzed)

Blatz et al. Am J Dent 2004;17:169–172

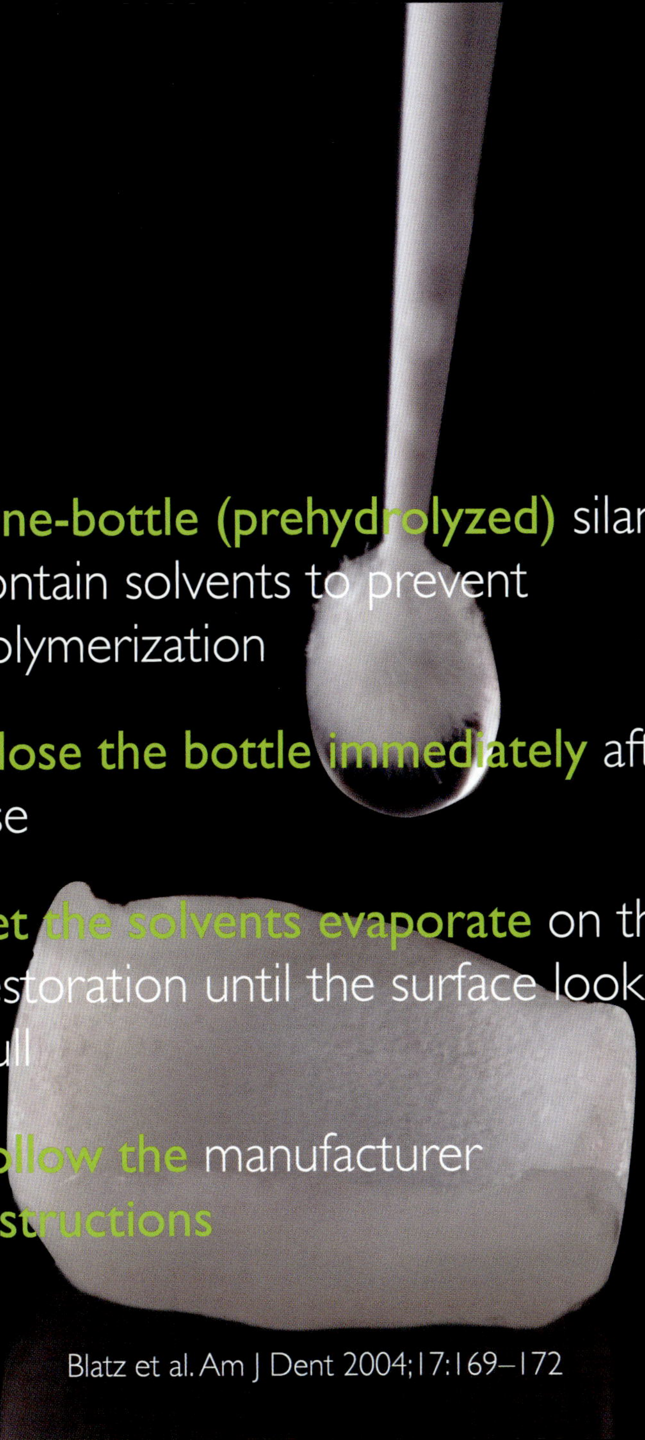

One-bottle (prehydrolyzed) silanes contain solvents to prevent polymerization

Close the bottle immediately after use

Let the solvents evaporate on the restoration until the surface looks dull

Follow the manufacturer **instructions**

Blatz et al. Am J Dent 2004;17:169–172

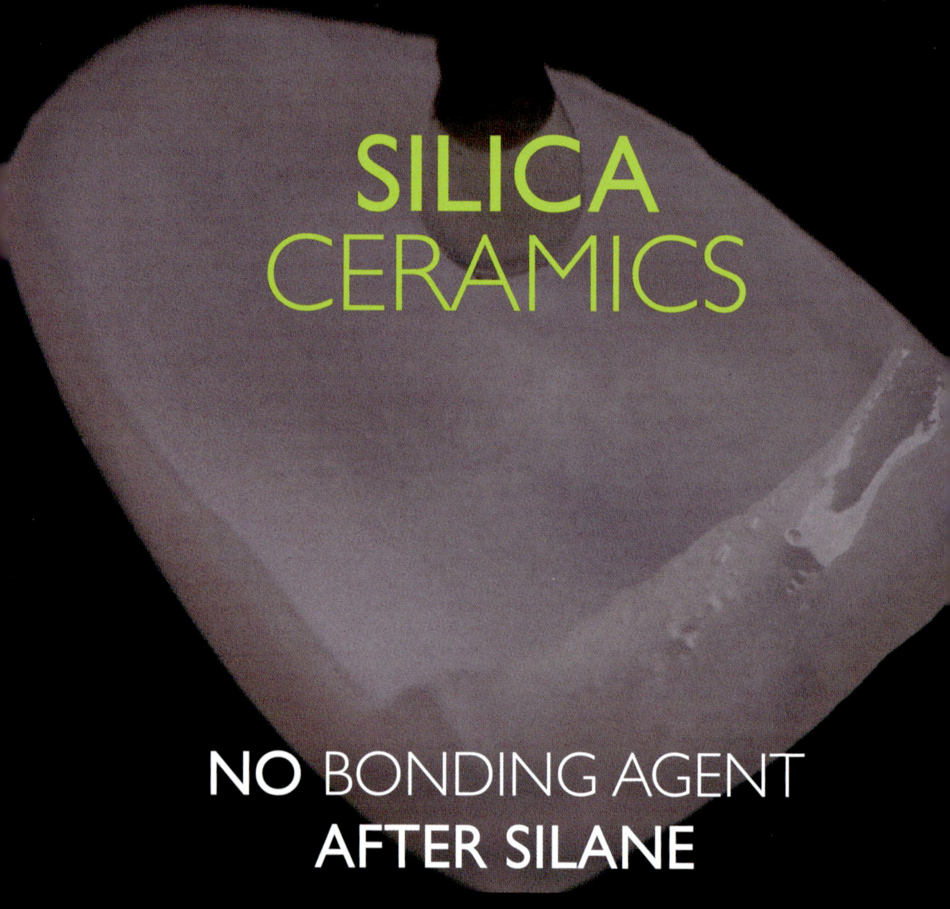

SILICA CERAMICS

NO BONDING AGENT **AFTER SILANE**

J Prosthet Dent 2021;125:56–64

Does the application of an adhesive layer improve the bond strength of etched and silanized glass-ceramics to resin-based materials? A systematic review and meta-analysis

Nogueira IO, Oliveira PFG, Magno MB, Ferreira DMTP, Maia LC, Rabello TB

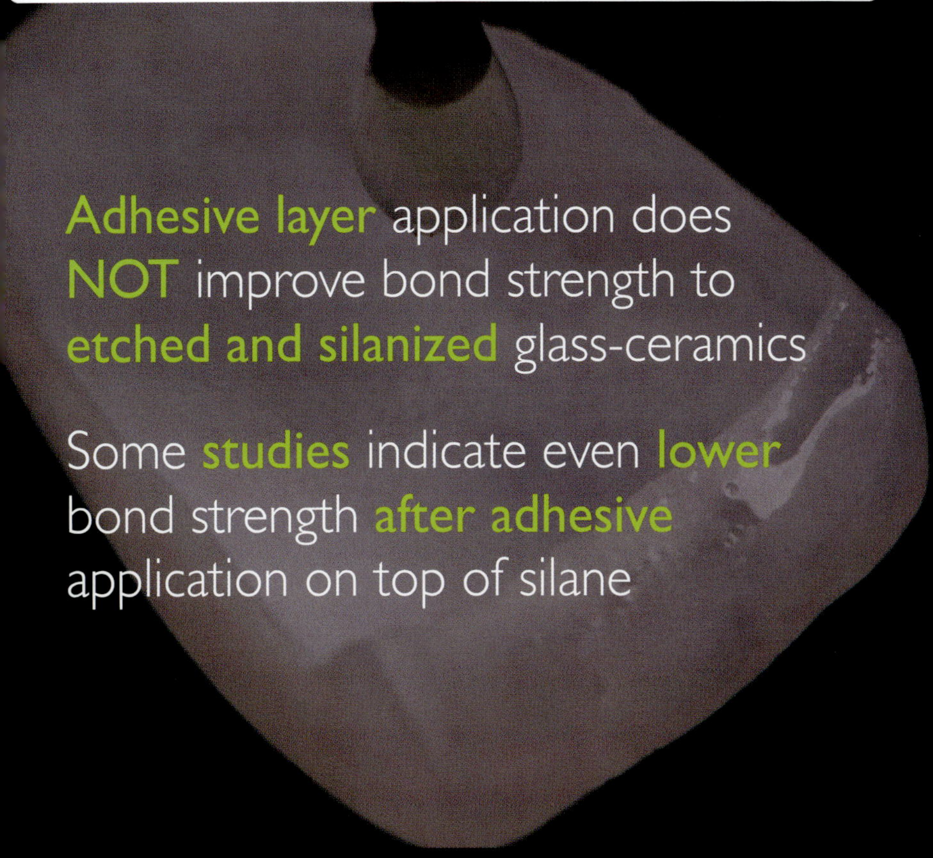

Adhesive layer application does **NOT** improve bond strength to **etched and silanized** glass-ceramics

Some **studies** indicate even **lower** bond strength **after adhesive** application on top of silane

ENAMEL BOND

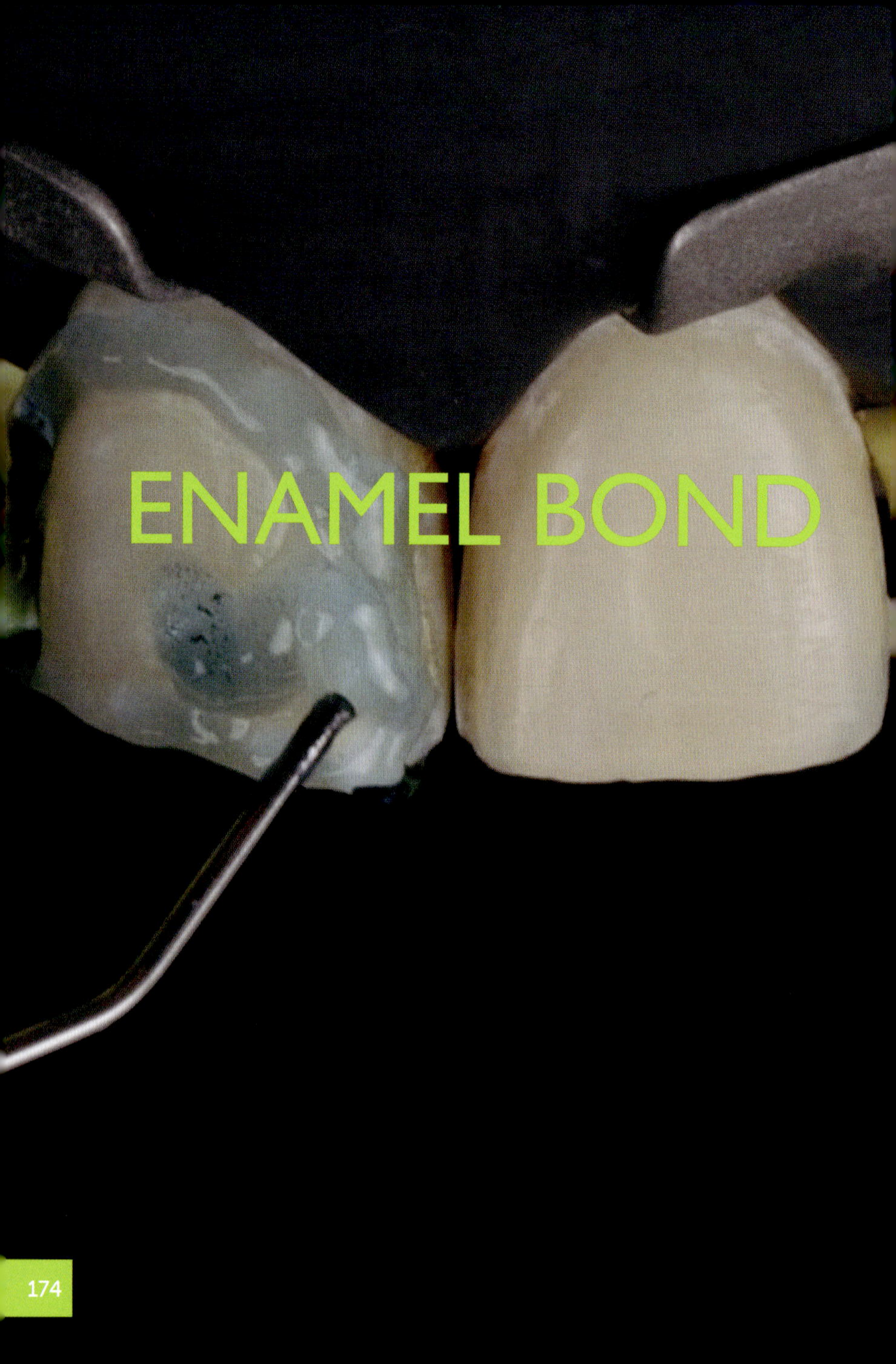

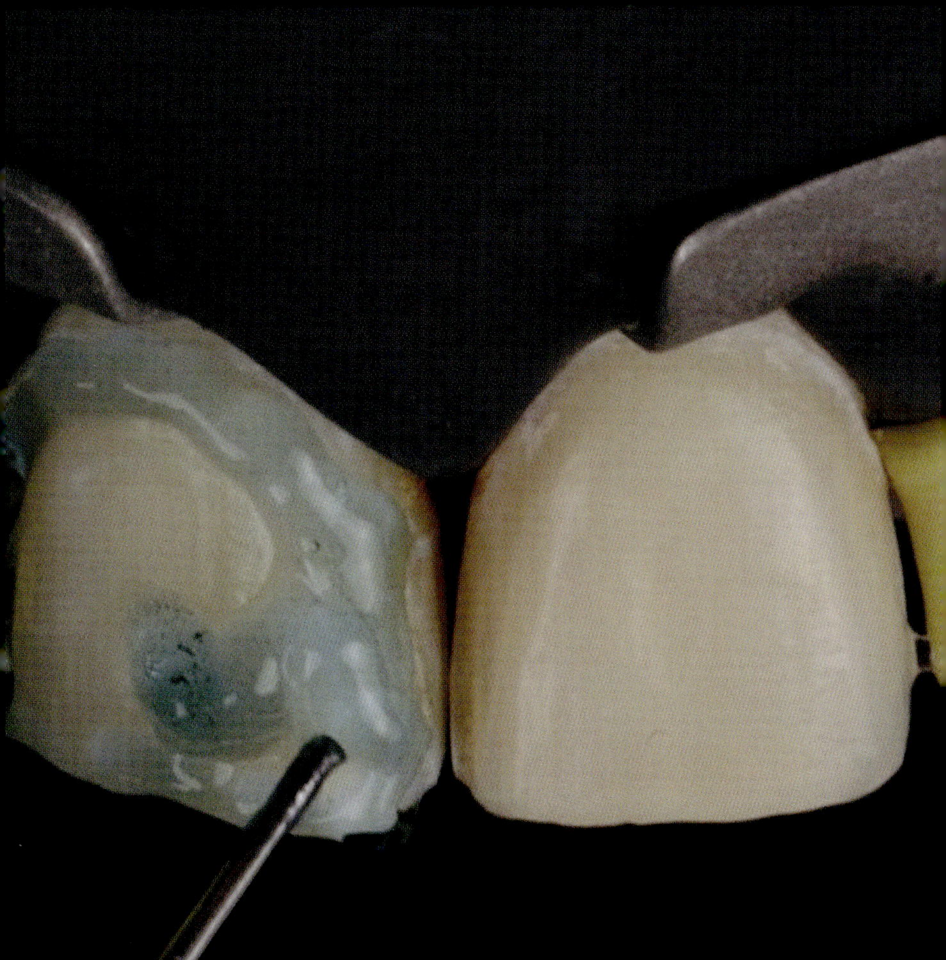

Phosphoric acid etching as per manufacturer instructions (15 to 30 s)

Rinse for a minimum of 15 s and **dry** thoroughly

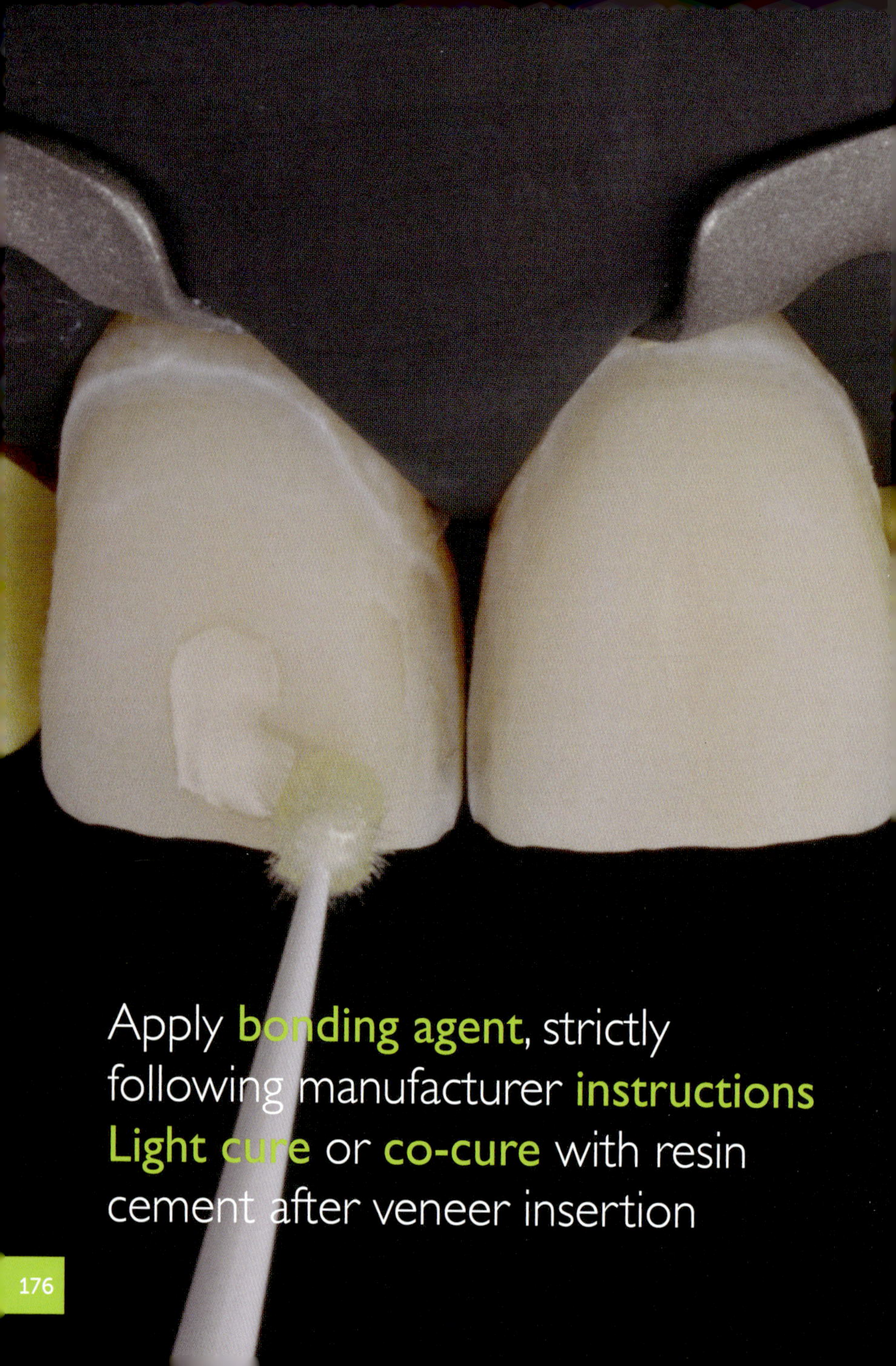

Apply **bonding agent**, strictly following manufacturer **instructions**
Light cure or **co-cure** with resin cement after veneer insertion

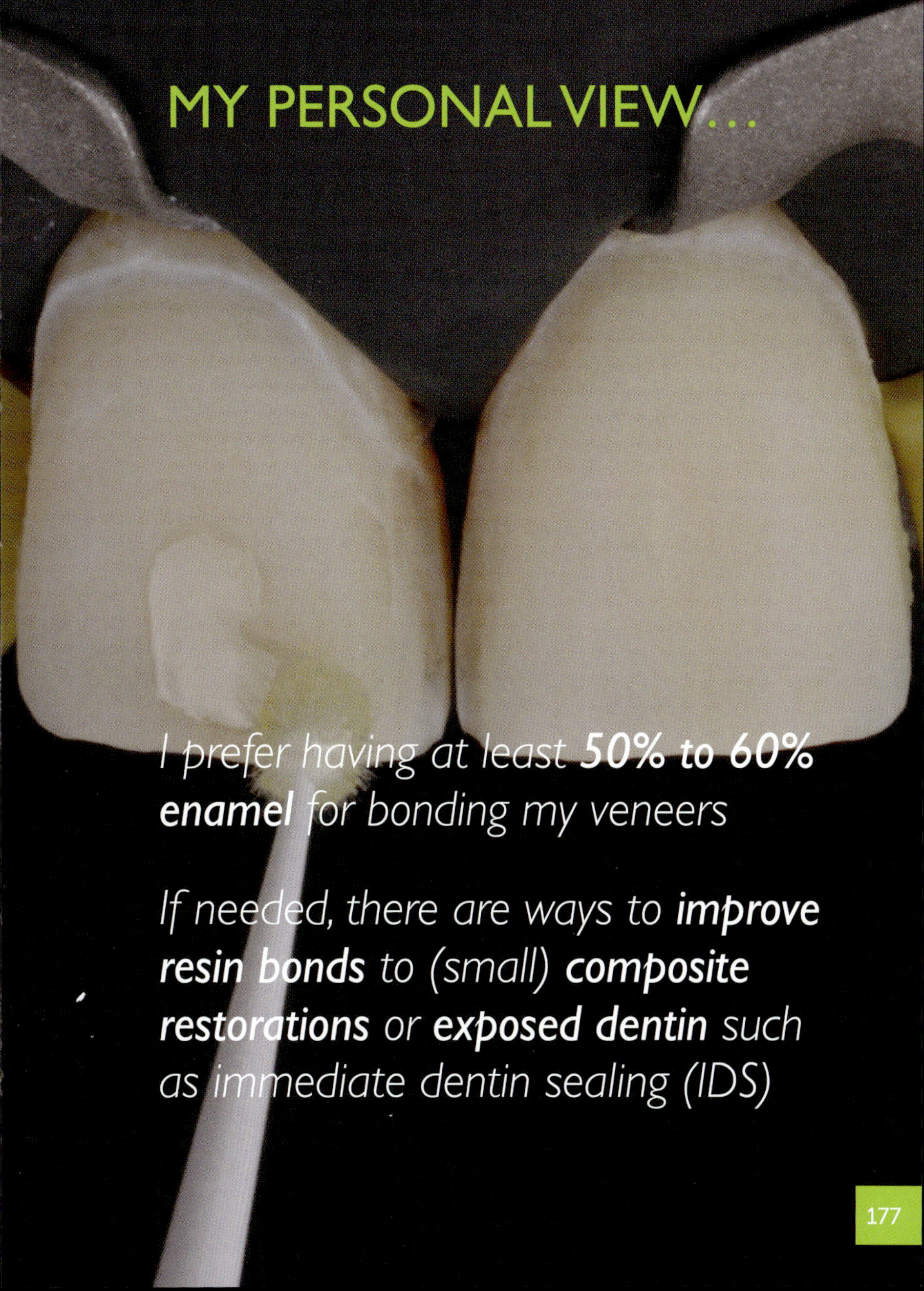

MY PERSONAL VIEW...

I prefer having at least ***50% to 60% enamel*** *for bonding my veneers*

If needed, there are ways to ***improve resin bonds*** *to (small)* ***composite restorations*** *or* ***exposed dentin*** *such as immediate dentin sealing (IDS)*

RESIN CEMENT

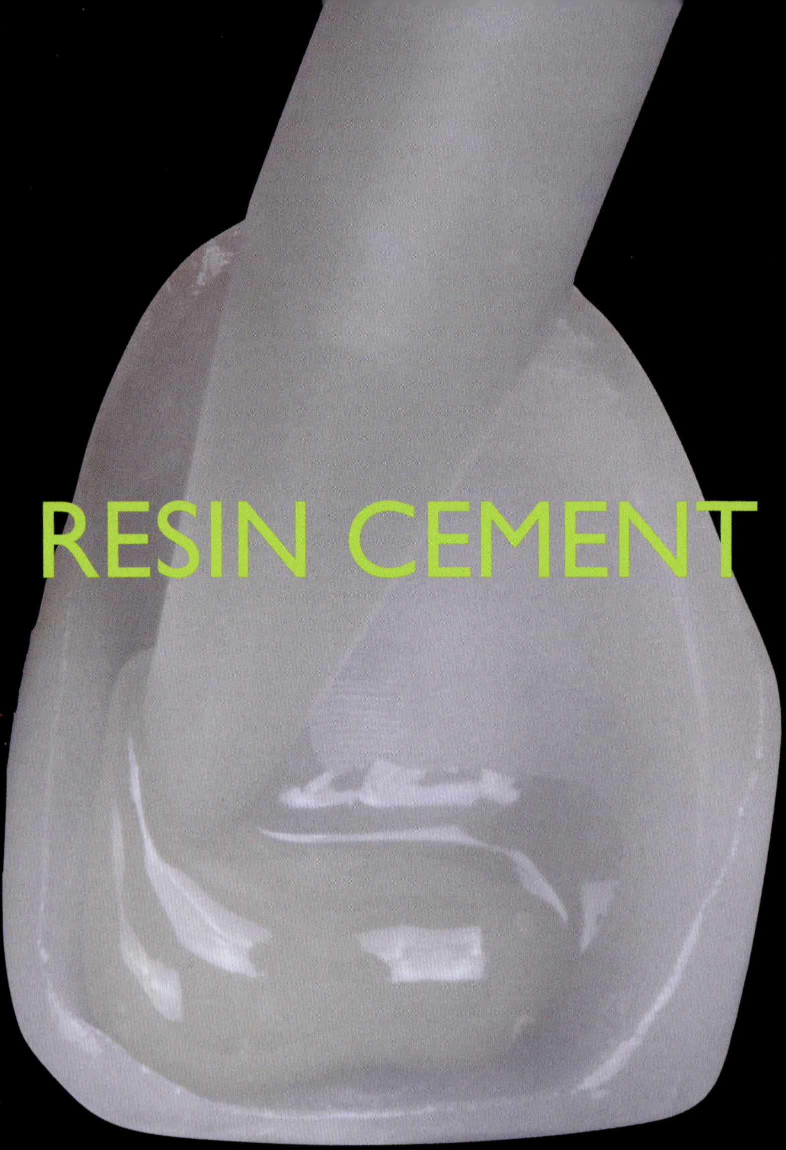

SELECTION

Dent Clin North Am 2022;66:603–625

Current protocols for resin-bonded dental ceramics

Blatz MB, Conejo J, Alammar A, Ayub J

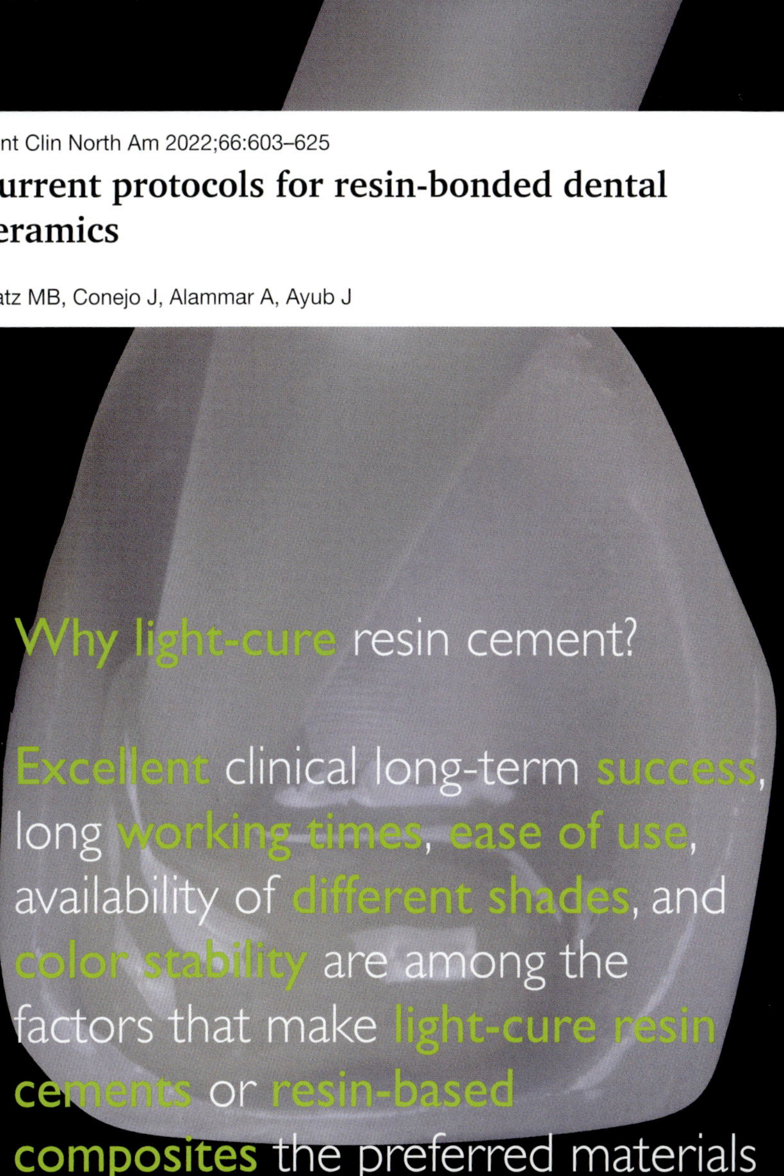

Why light-cure resin cement?

Excellent clinical long-term success, long working times, ease of use, availability of different shades, and color stability are among the factors that make light-cure resin cements or resin-based composites the preferred materials

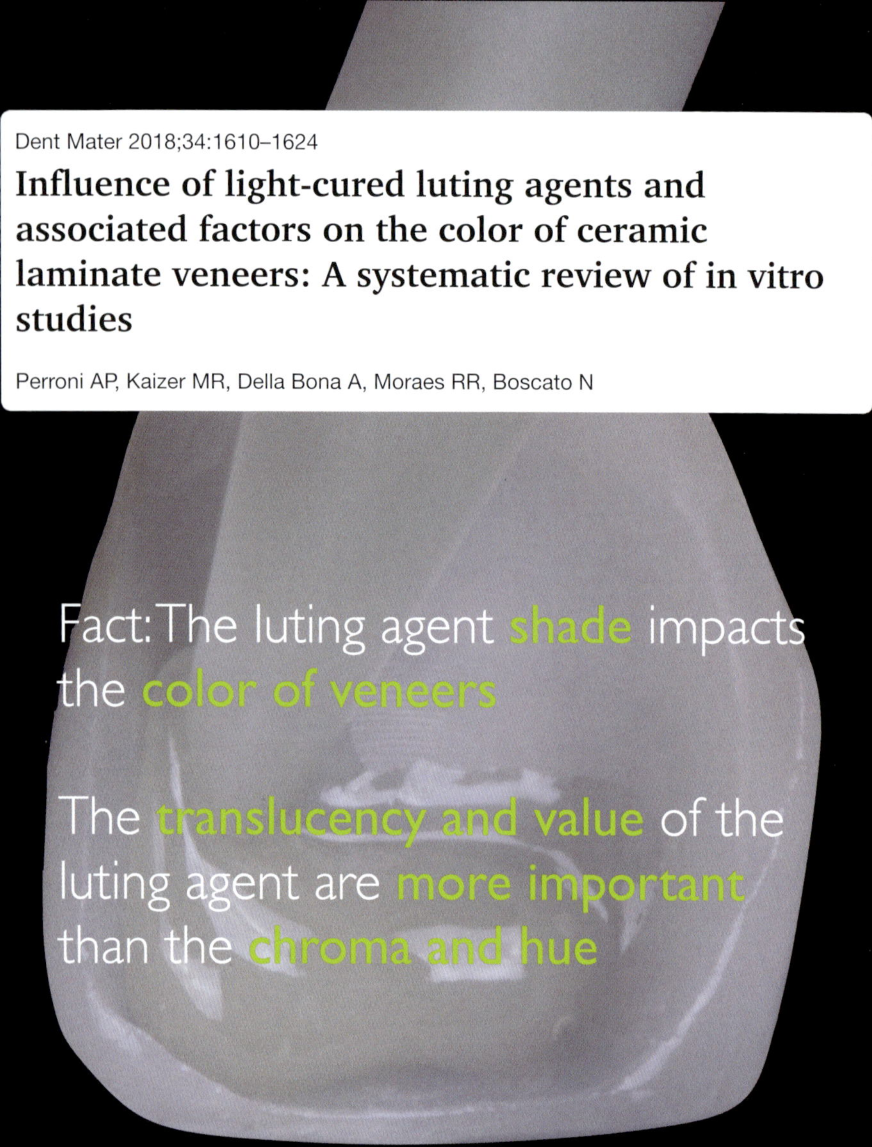

Dent Mater 2018;34:1610–1624

Influence of light-cured luting agents and associated factors on the color of ceramic laminate veneers: A systematic review of in vitro studies

Perroni AP, Kaizer MR, Della Bona A, Moraes RR, Boscato N

Fact: The luting agent shade impacts the color of veneers

The translucency and value of the luting agent are more important than the chroma and hue

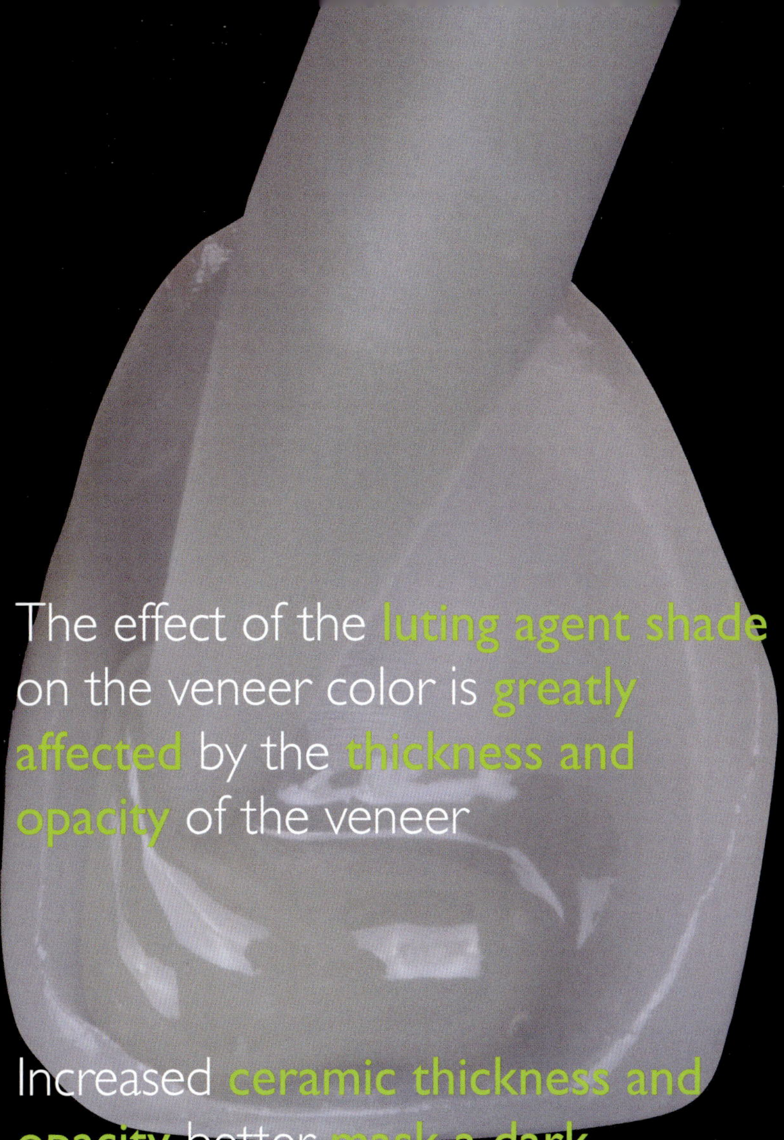

The effect of the **luting agent shade** on the veneer color is **greatly affected** by the **thickness and opacity** of the veneer

Increased **ceramic thickness and opacity** better **mask a dark background** and possible color changes due to aging

Perroni et al. Dent Mater 2018;34:1610–1624

MY PERSONAL VIEW…

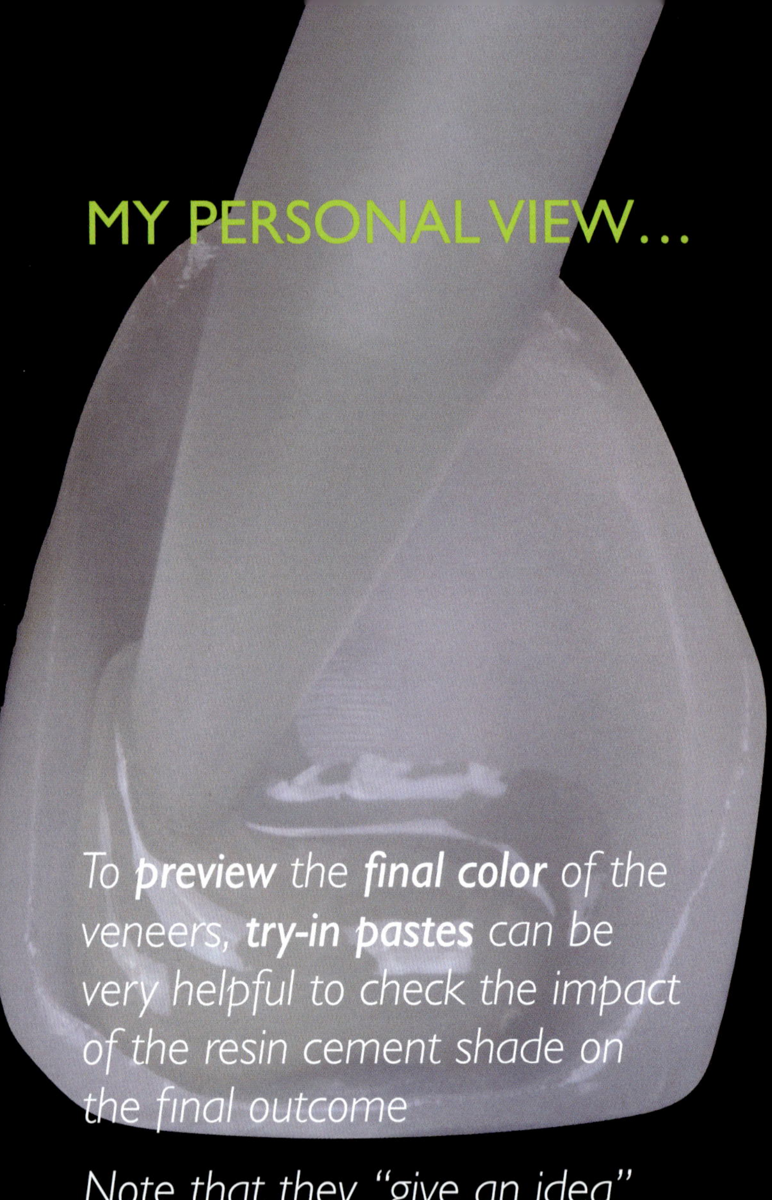

*To **preview** the **final color** of the veneers, **try-in pastes** can be very helpful to check the impact of the resin cement shade on the final outcome*

*Note that they "give an idea" but are **not 100%** accurate!*

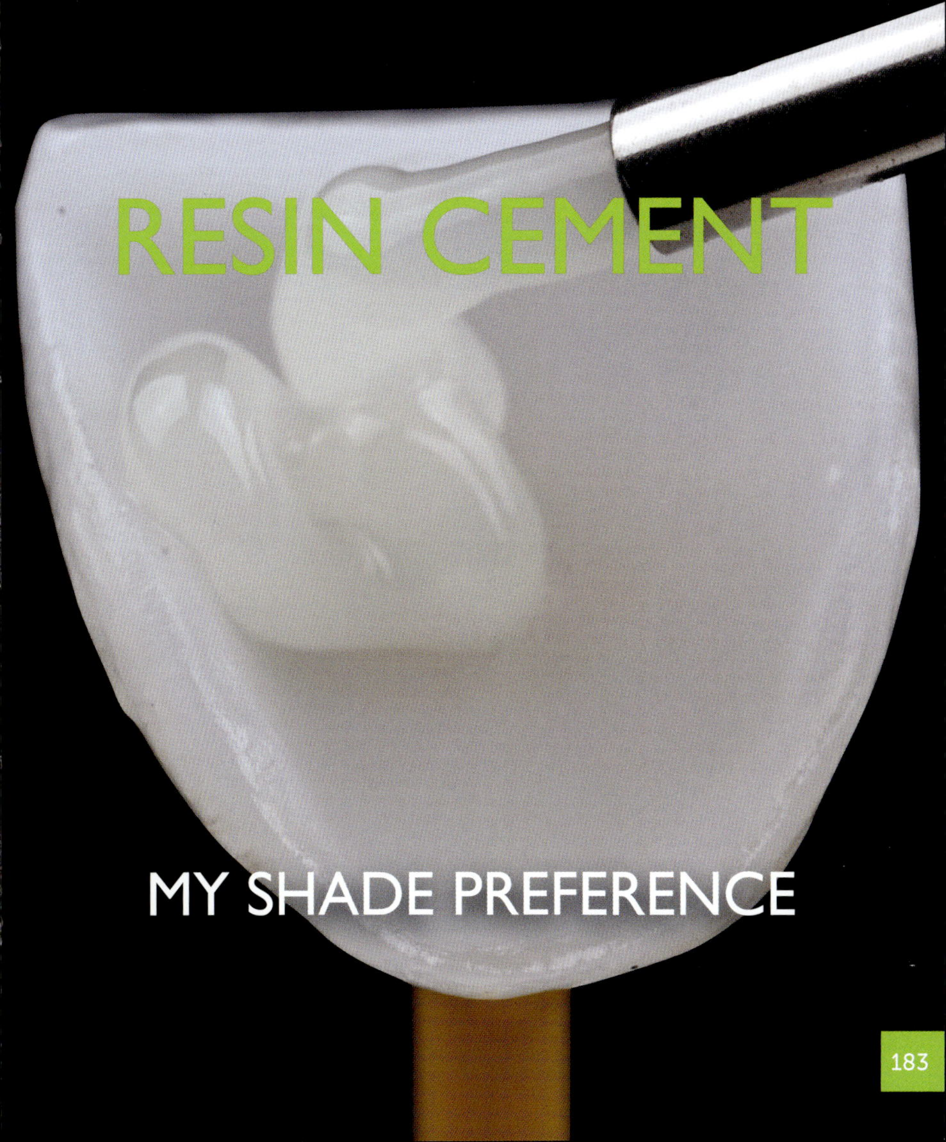

RESIN CEMENT

MY SHADE PREFERENCE

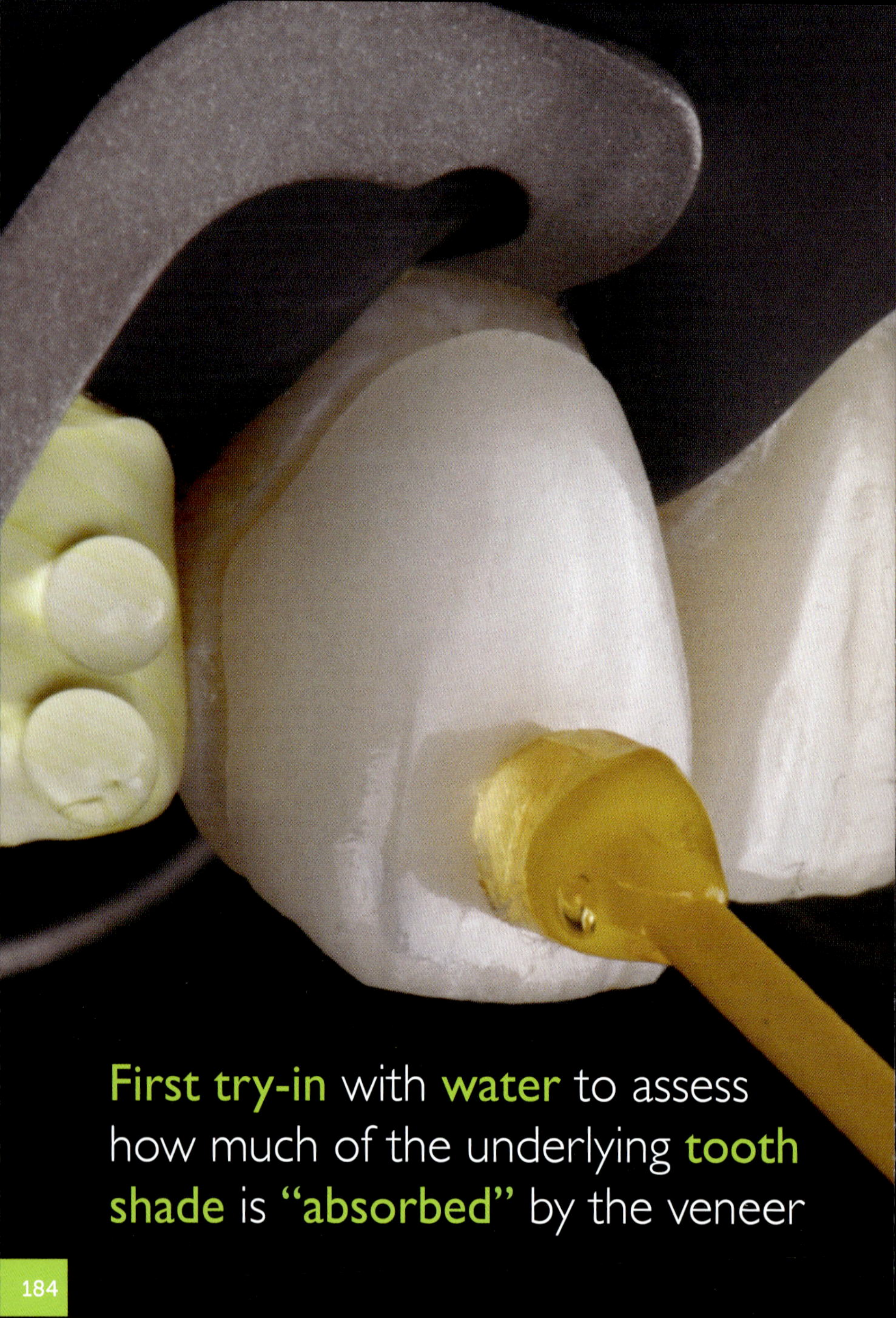

First try-in with water to assess how much of the underlying tooth shade is "absorbed" by the veneer

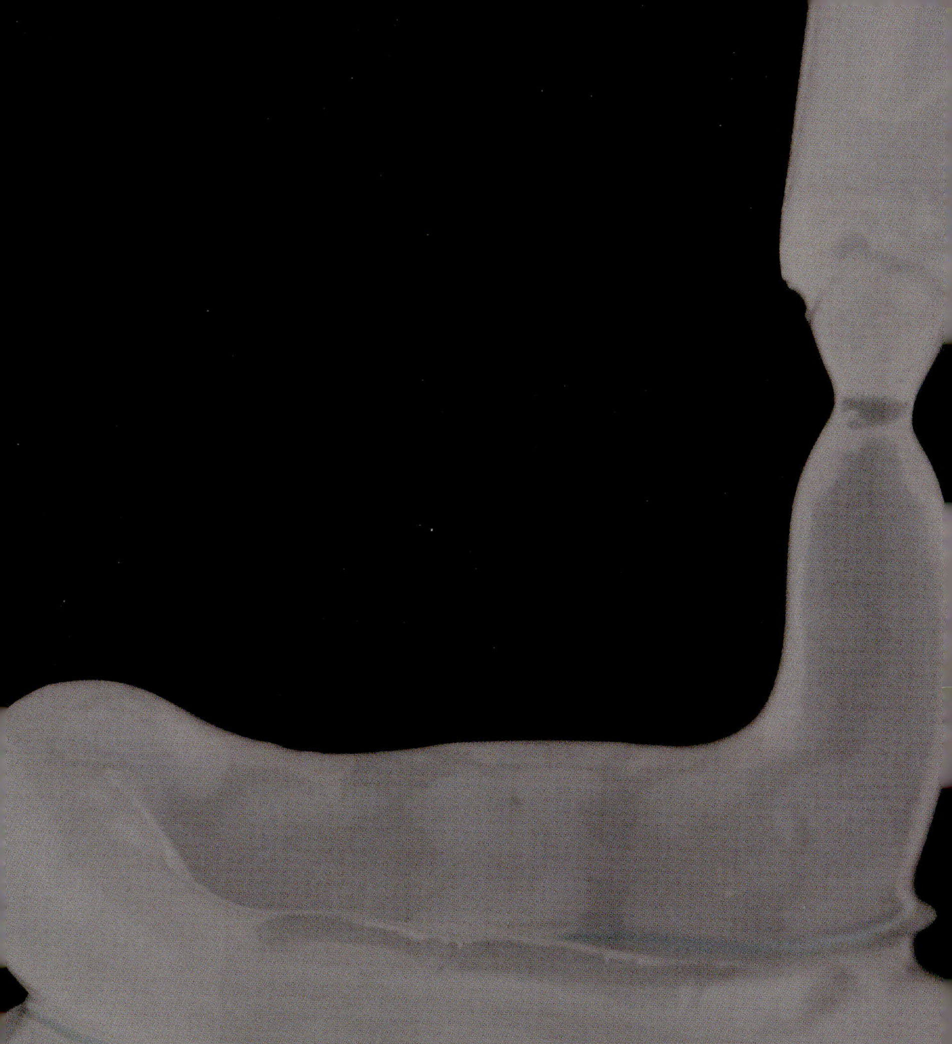

A **clear/transparent** resin cement **absorbs** the underlying **tooth shade** for a **natural appearance**

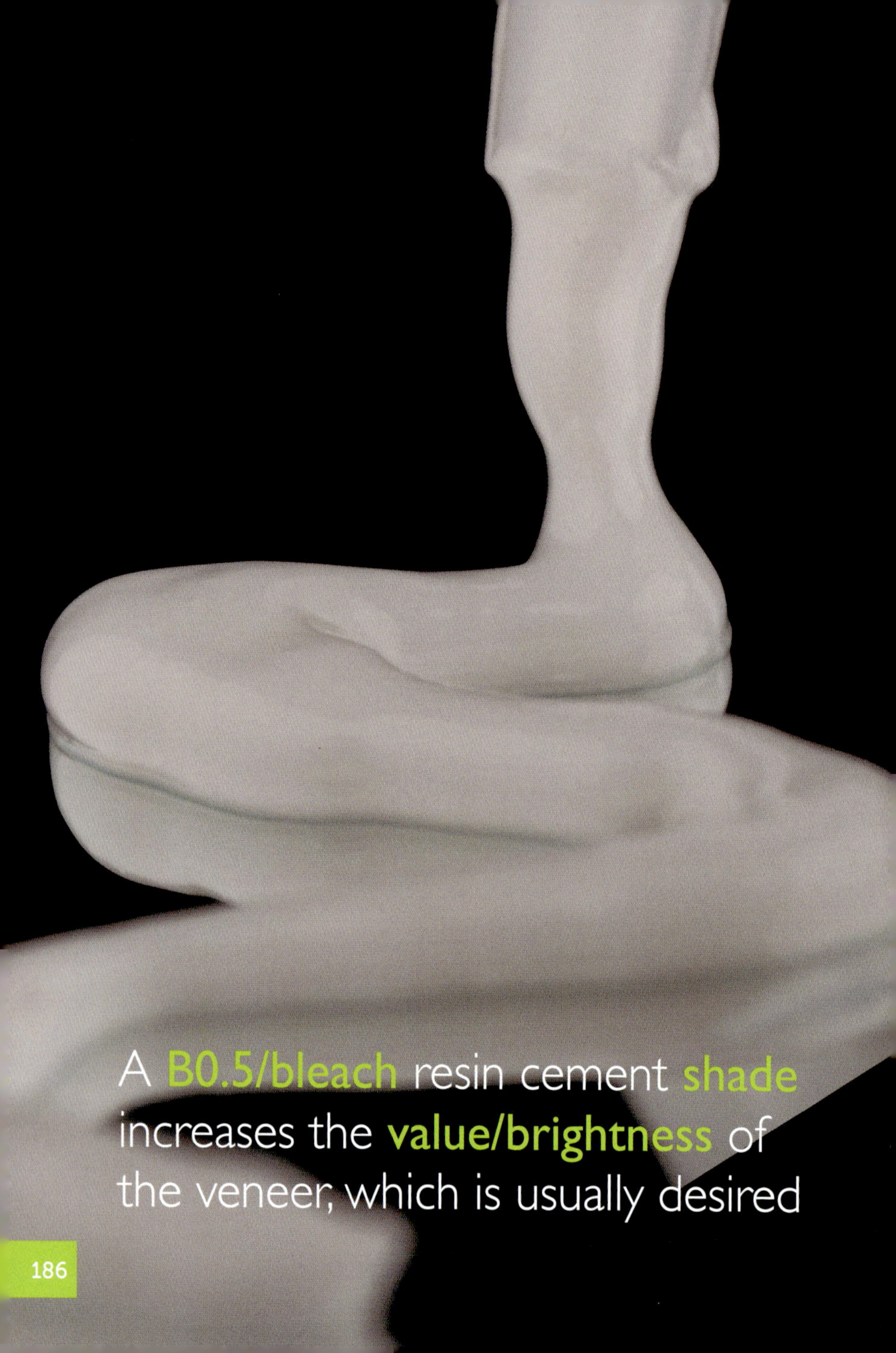

A **B0.5/bleach** resin cement **shade** increases the **value/brightness** of the veneer, which is usually desired

MY PREFERENCE

I mix **clear/transparent** with **B0.5/bleach shade** resin cement

Usually **60 : 40 ratio**
Thin veneers **80 : 20 ratio**

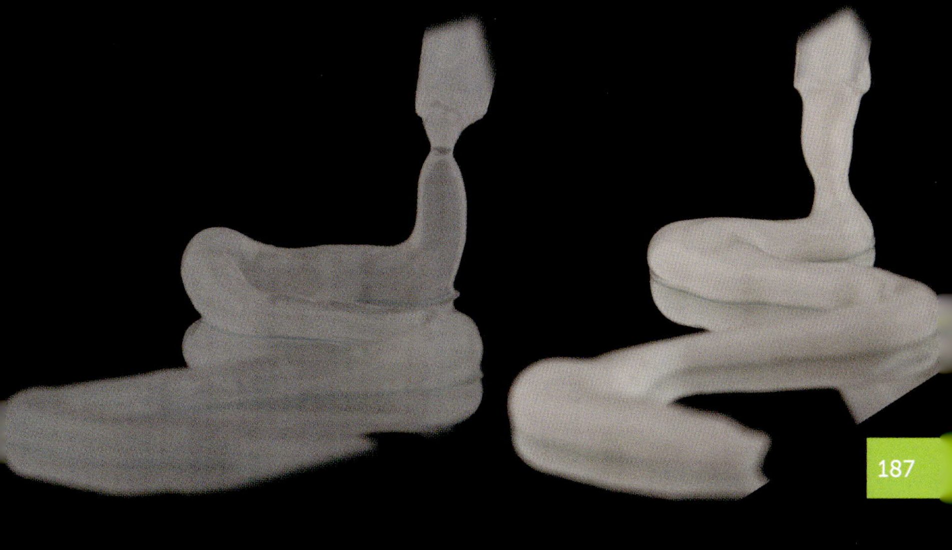

MY PREFERENCE

This mix **absorbs** some of the underlying **tooth** shade while **increasing the value** of the restoration

Adjust the mix **ratio** based on the supporting tooth **shade** and the thickness of the veneer

You may also find a **manufacturer** that offers your **preferred shade** and **translucency** mix in **one resin cement product**

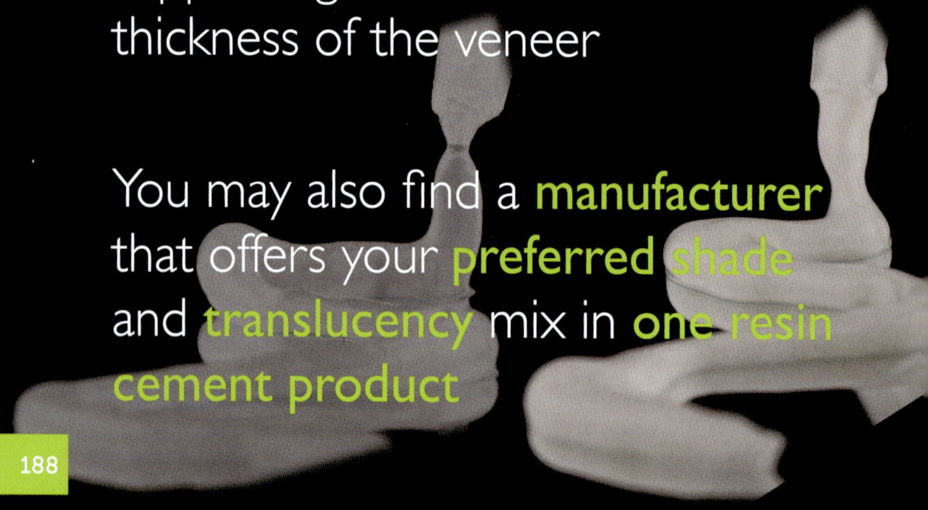

INSERT VENEER

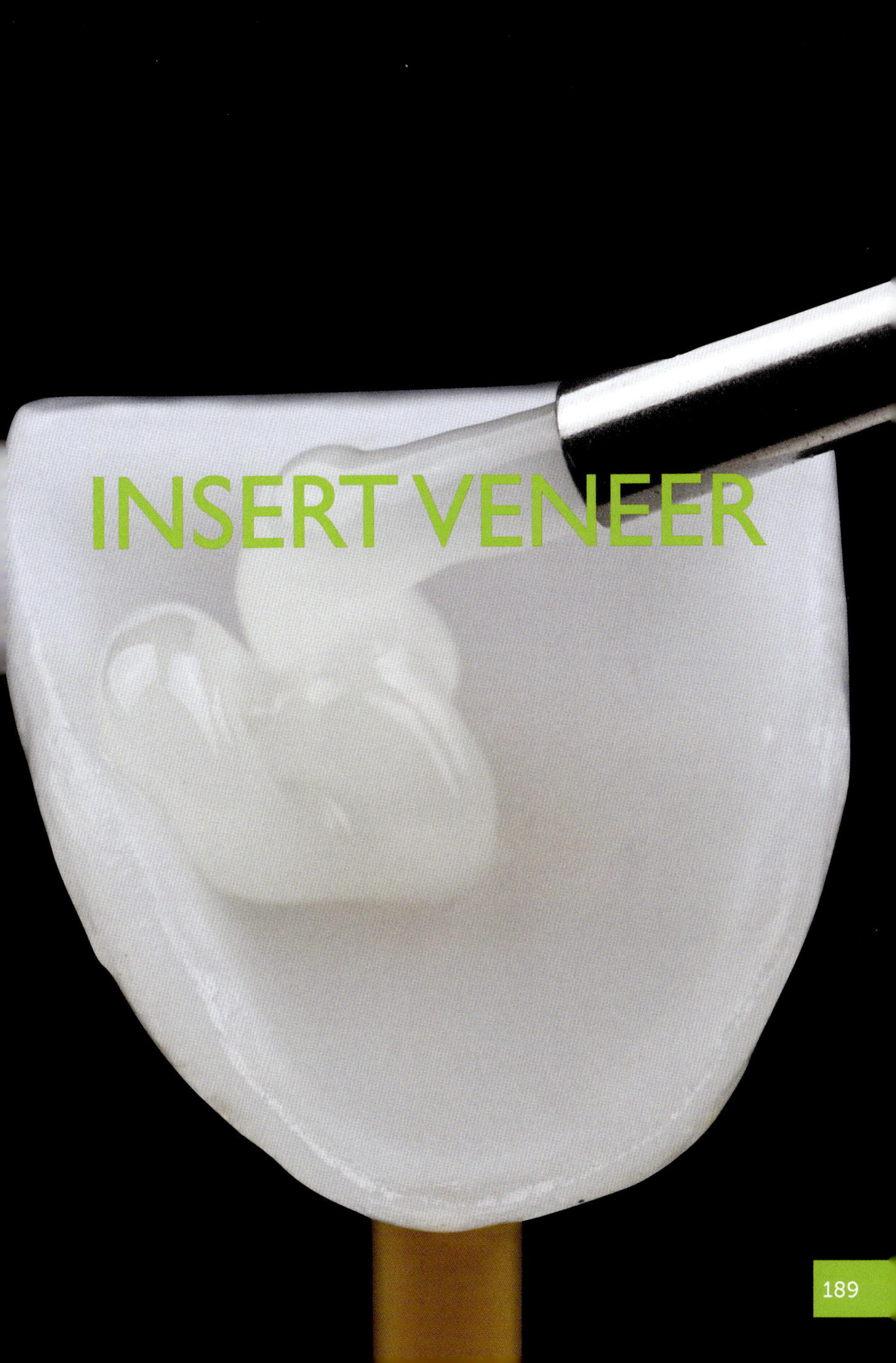

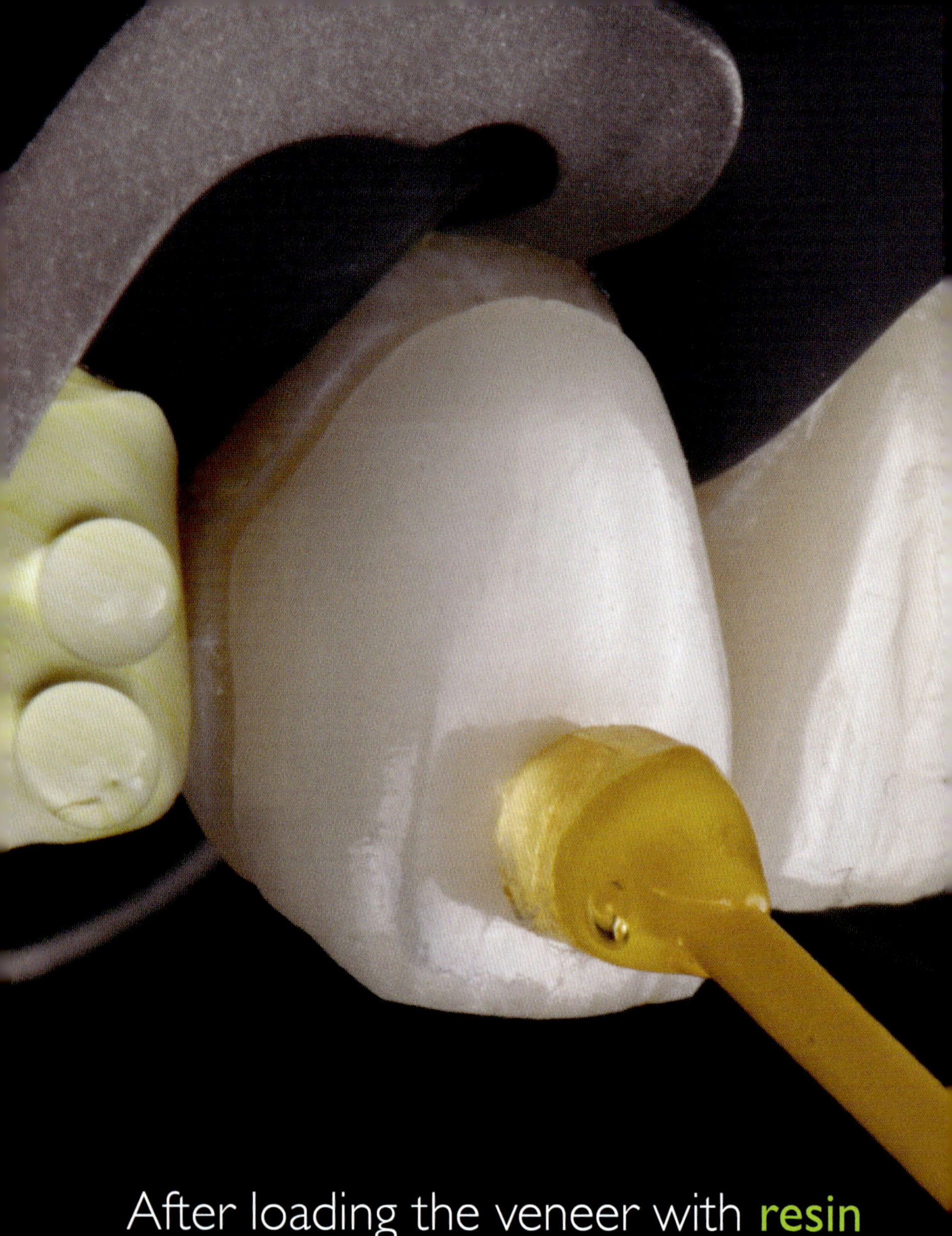

After loading the veneer with resin cement…

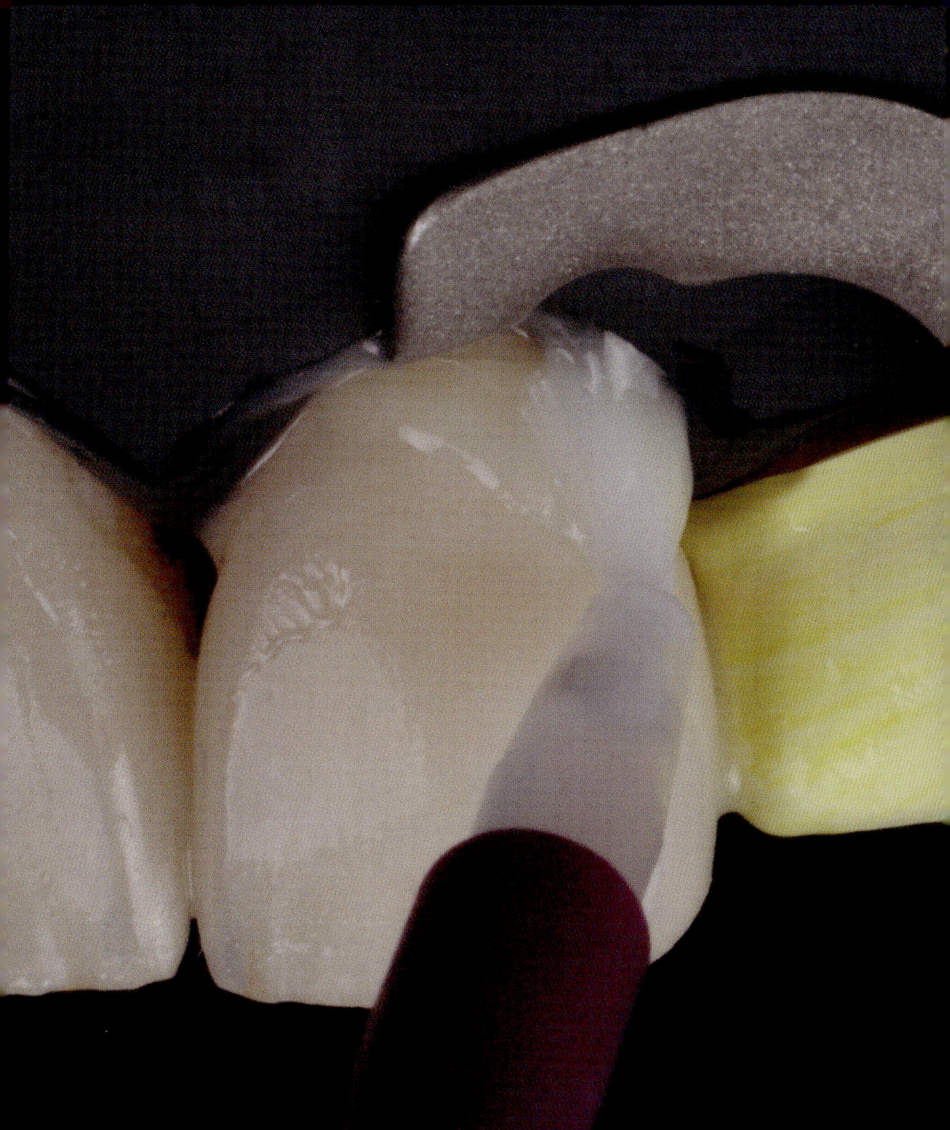

…**remove excess resin cement**, but do not "pull out" too much to keep tooth–veneer margins "filled"

LIGHT CURE

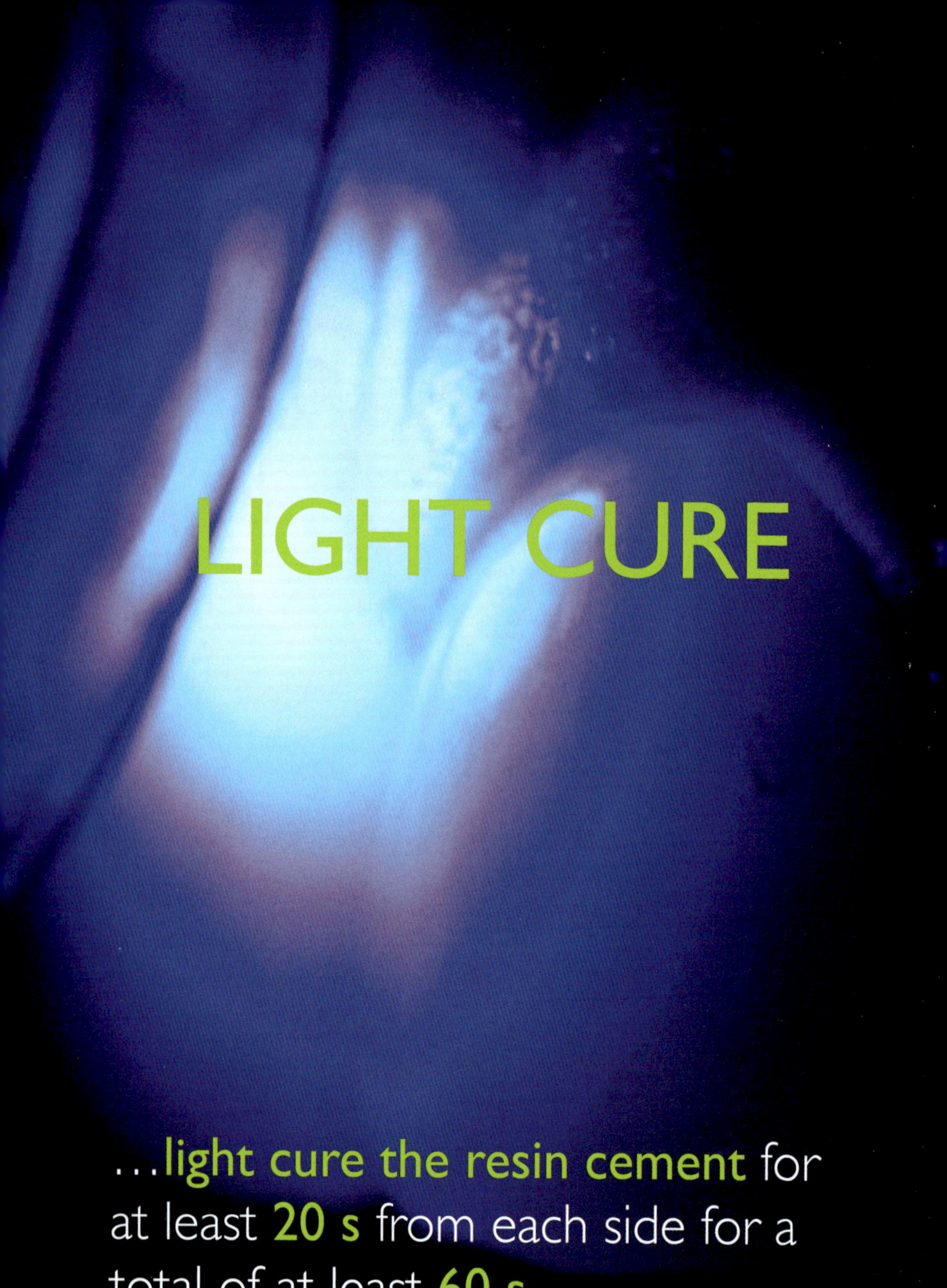

…**light cure the resin cement** for at least **20 s** from each side for a total of at least **60 s**

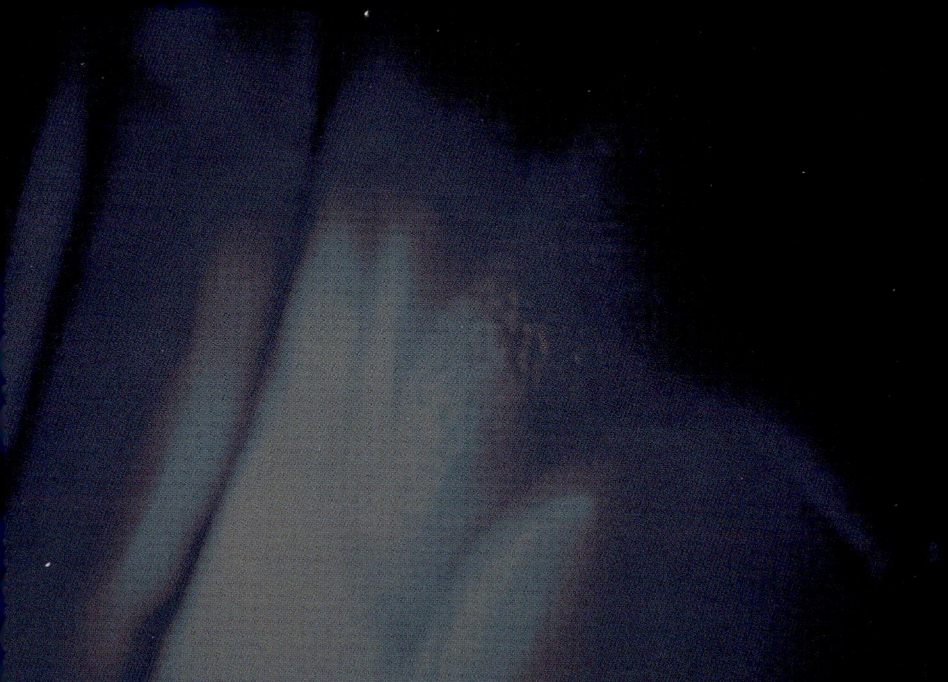

For easy cleaning, **TACK CURE** the composite **for 2 to 3 s before FULL CURING**, and **remove excess cement** while still "doughy"

...or use the **micro tip** of the curing light to first tack cure only in the **center** of the veneer, then remove excess composite before full curing

QUESTION

Should you **light cure** the **adhesive** on the tooth **first**, or **co-cure** the **adhesive** and the **resin cement** all at once?

Quintessence Int 2007;38:637–641

Precuring of self-etching bonding agents and its effect on bond strength of resin composite to dentin and enamel

Chapman JL, Burgess JO, Holst S, Sadan A, Blatz MB

Light curing self-etch adhesives **before** curing the **resin composite** produces **greater bond** strength to **dentin**

The curing technique had **no effect** on the **enamel** bond strength

Materials (Basel) 2021;14:7664

Effect of conventional adhesive application or co-curing technique on dentin bond strength

Vukelja J, Klarić Sever EK, Sever I, Jukić Krmek SJ, Tarle Z

The results showed a **significant difference** in dentin bond strength between conventional and co-curing methods

The **co-curing method** significantly **diminished bond** strength to **dentin**

MY PERSONAL VIEW…

*Bond strength is **better to dentin** when the bonding agent/ **adhesive** is **light cured** on the tooth before cementation*

*It does **not** seem to have a great effect when bonding to **enamel**; for example, when bonding **laminate veneers***

*Depending on the product, I typically **prefer** to **light cure** the **bonding agent separately** whenever I have good **control** over the **film thickness***

MY PERSONAL VIEW…

Most manufacturers recommend ***light curing*** *the bonding agent/****adhesive*** *on the tooth before composite/cement application*

Be careful:
Some *current* ***resin cement products*** *employ* ***"touch cure chemistry,"*** *which does* ***not*** *require* ***separate curing*** *when using* ***matching adhesive***

Follow manufacturer instructions *and stay* ***within one system***

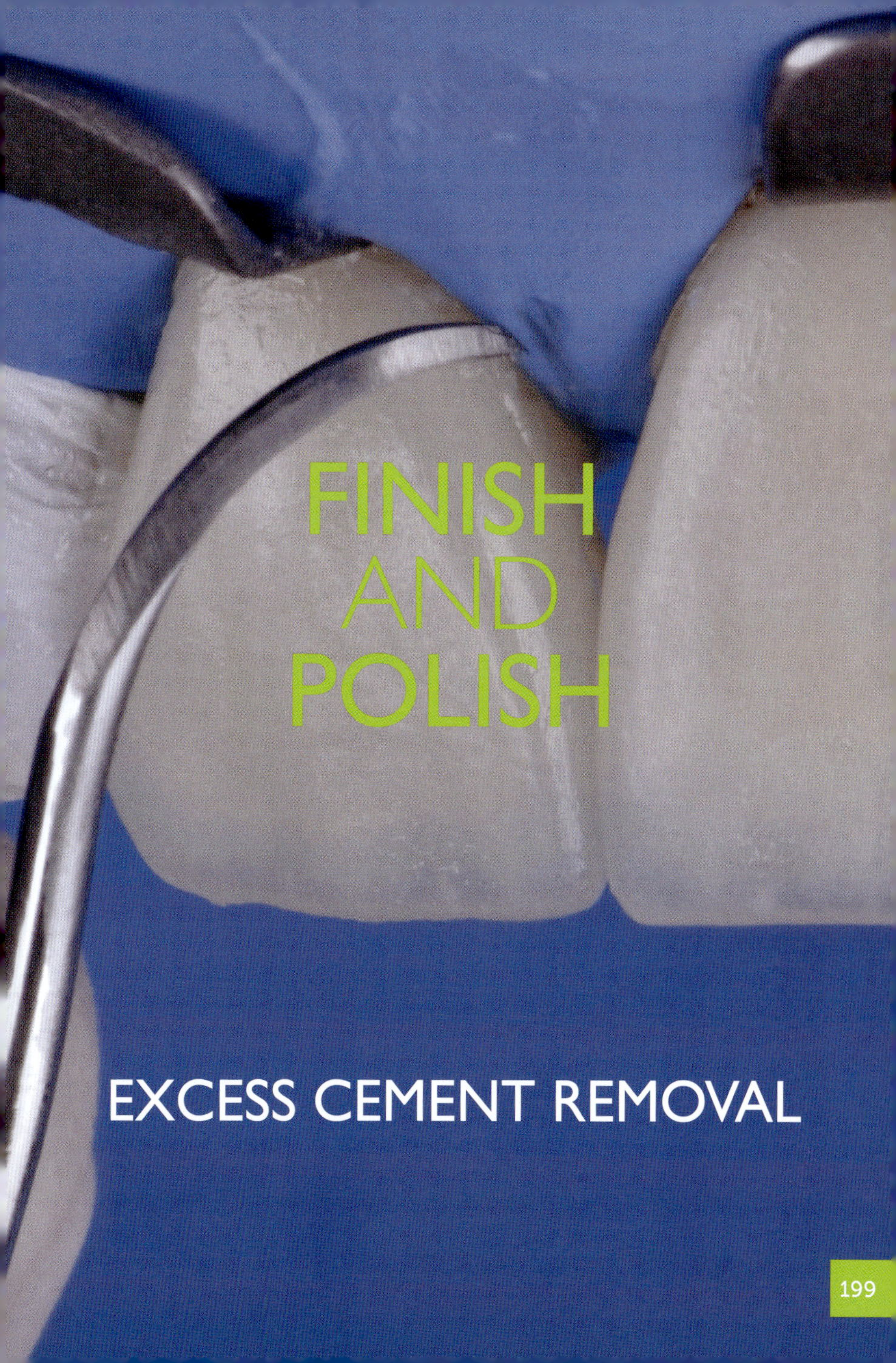

FINISH AND POLISH

EXCESS CEMENT REMOVAL

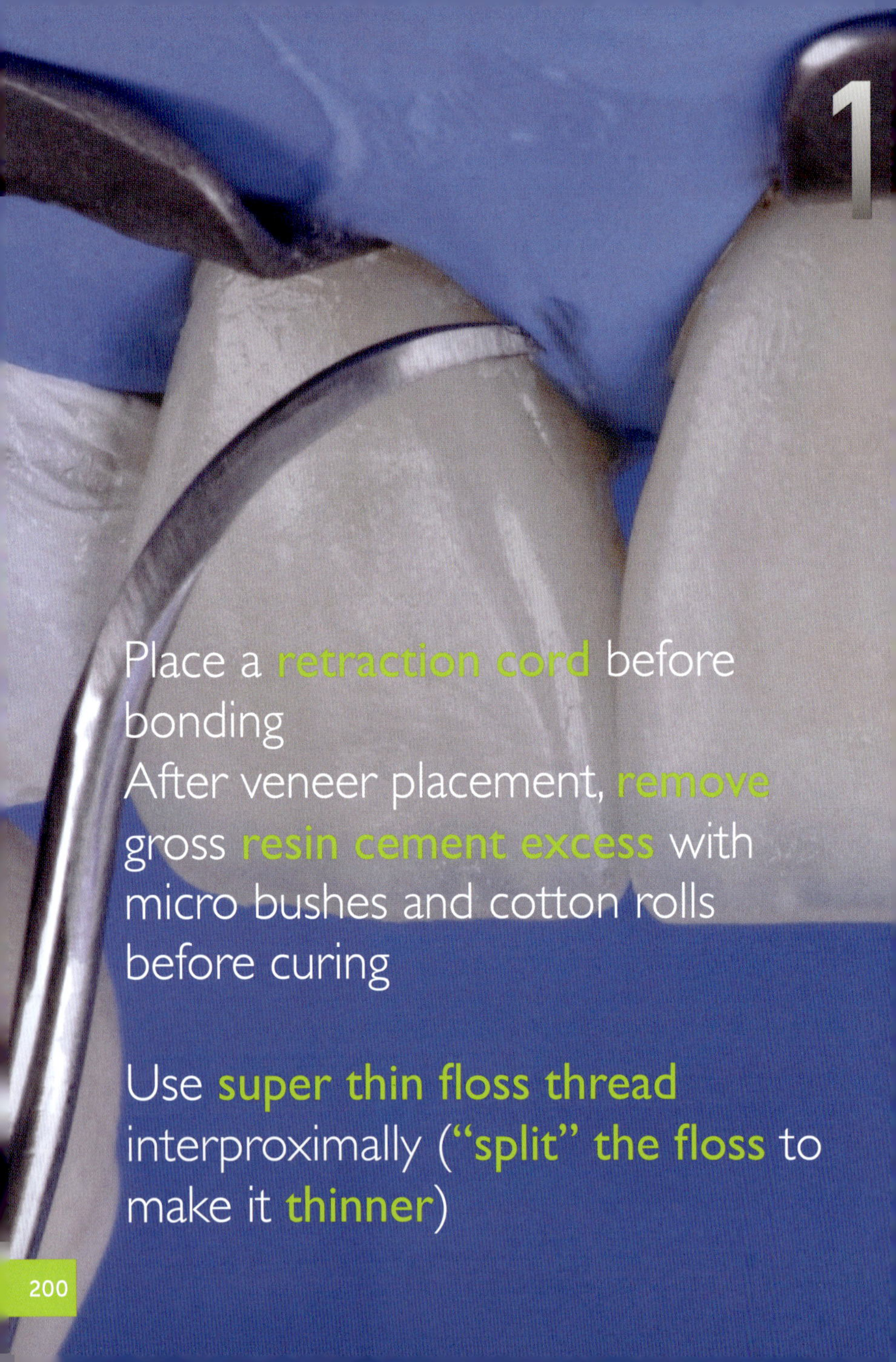

1

Place a retraction cord before bonding
After veneer placement, remove gross resin cement excess with micro bushes and cotton rolls before curing

Use **super thin floss thread** interproximally (**"split" the floss** to make it **thinner**)

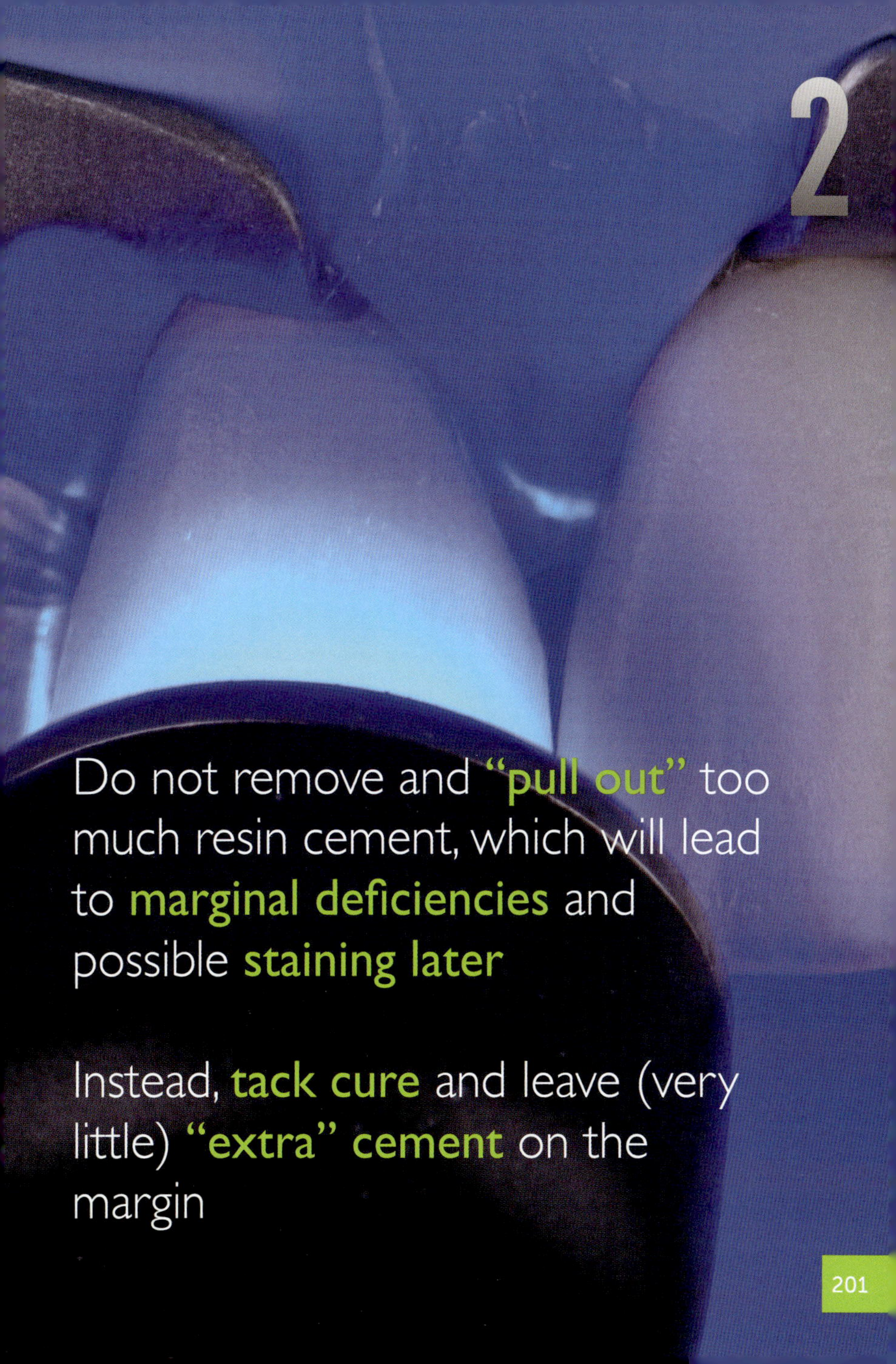

2

Do not remove and "**pull out**" too much resin cement, which will lead to **marginal deficiencies** and possible **staining later**

Instead, **tack cure** and leave (very little) **"extra" cement** on the margin

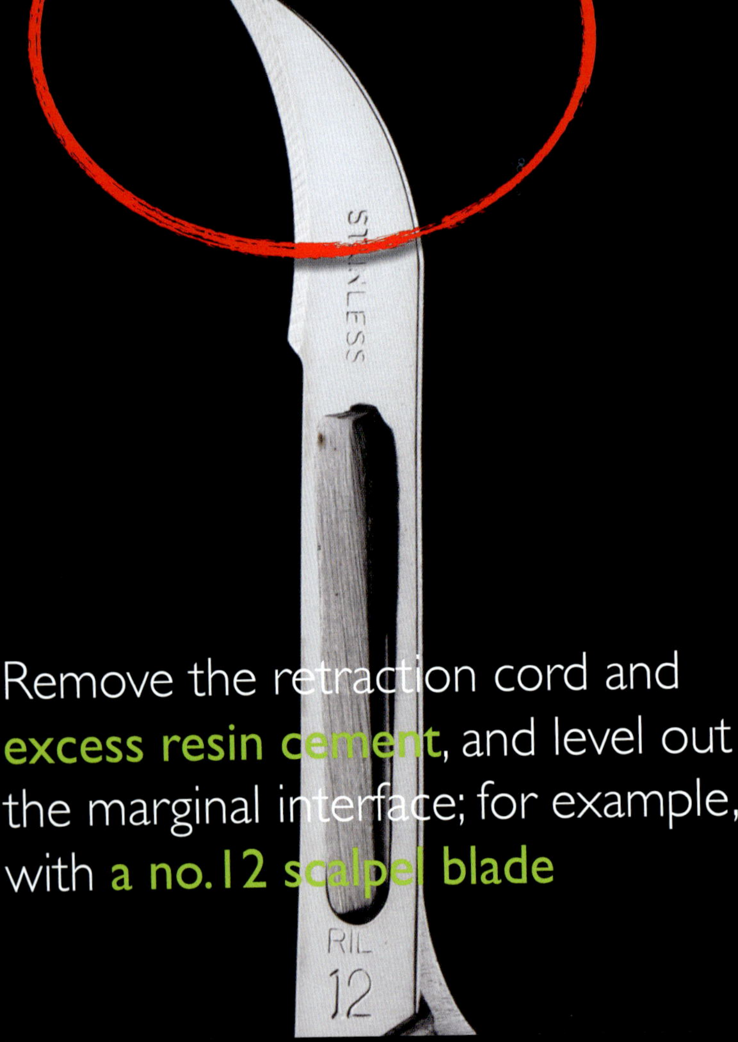
Remove the retraction cord and **excess resin cement**, and level out the marginal interface; for example, with **a no. 12 scalpel blade**
RIL
12

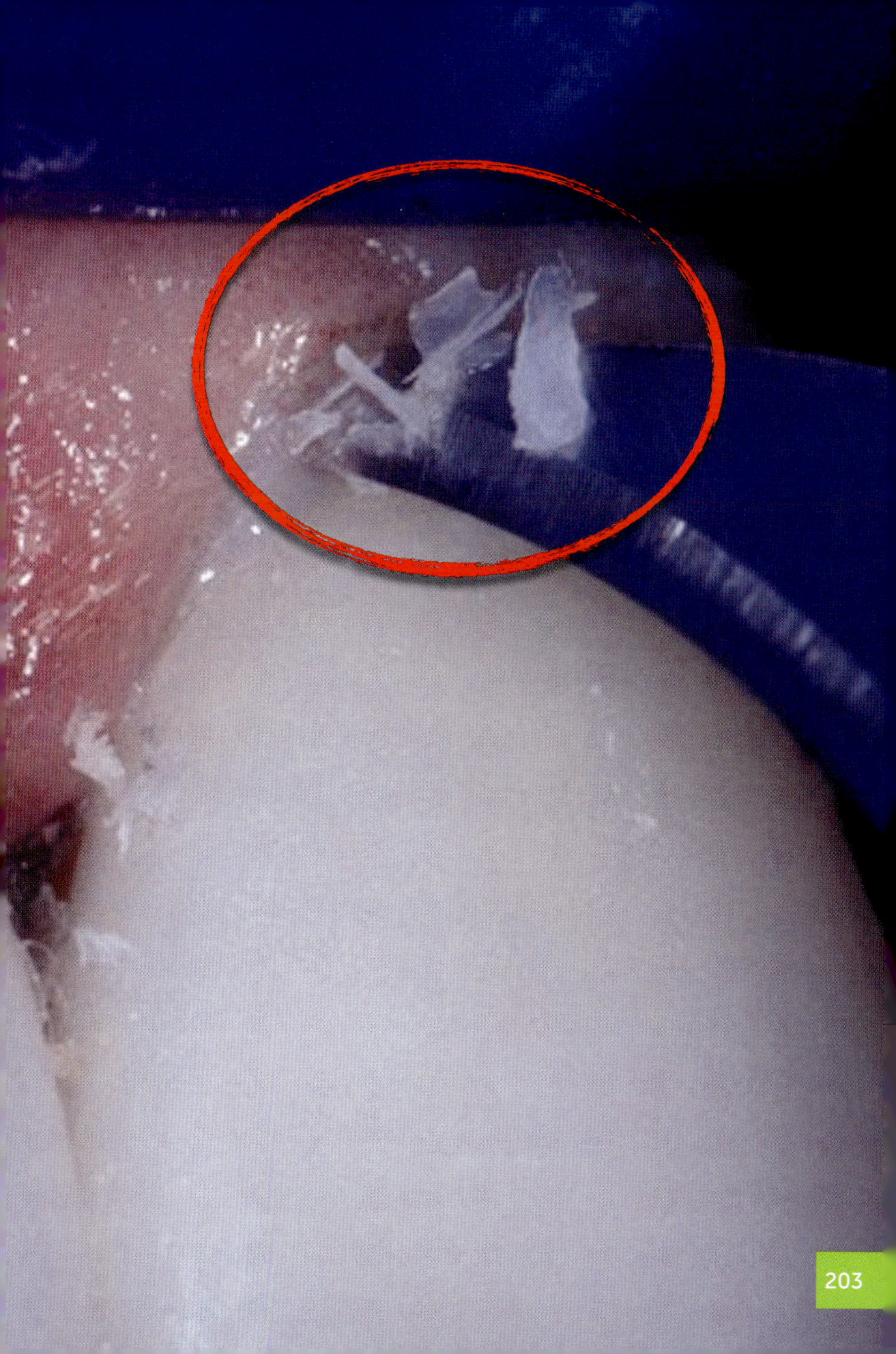

4

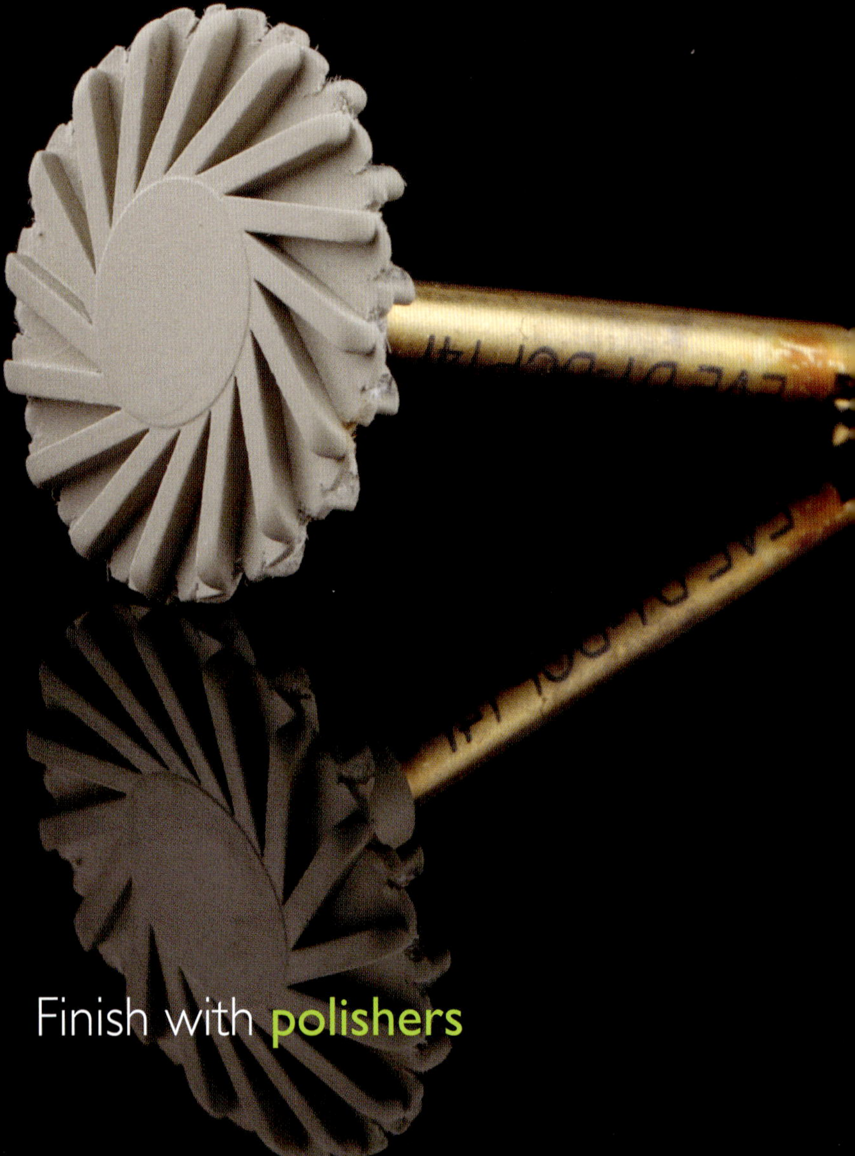

Finish with **polishers**

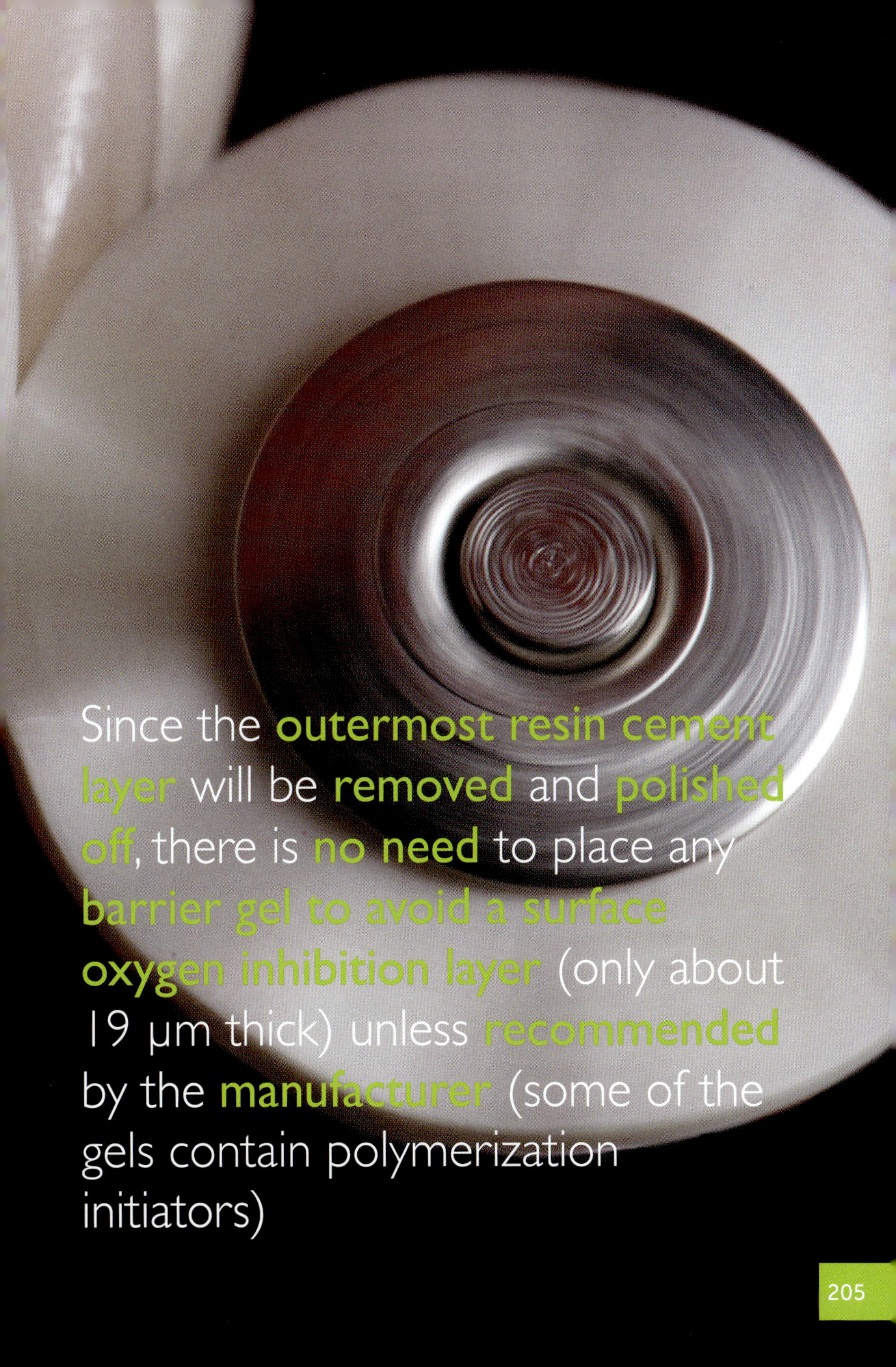

Since the **outermost resin cement layer** will be **removed** and **polished off**, there is **no need** to place any **barrier gel to avoid a surface oxygen inhibition layer** (only about 19 µm thick) unless **recommended** by the **manufacturer** (some of the gels contain polymerization initiators)

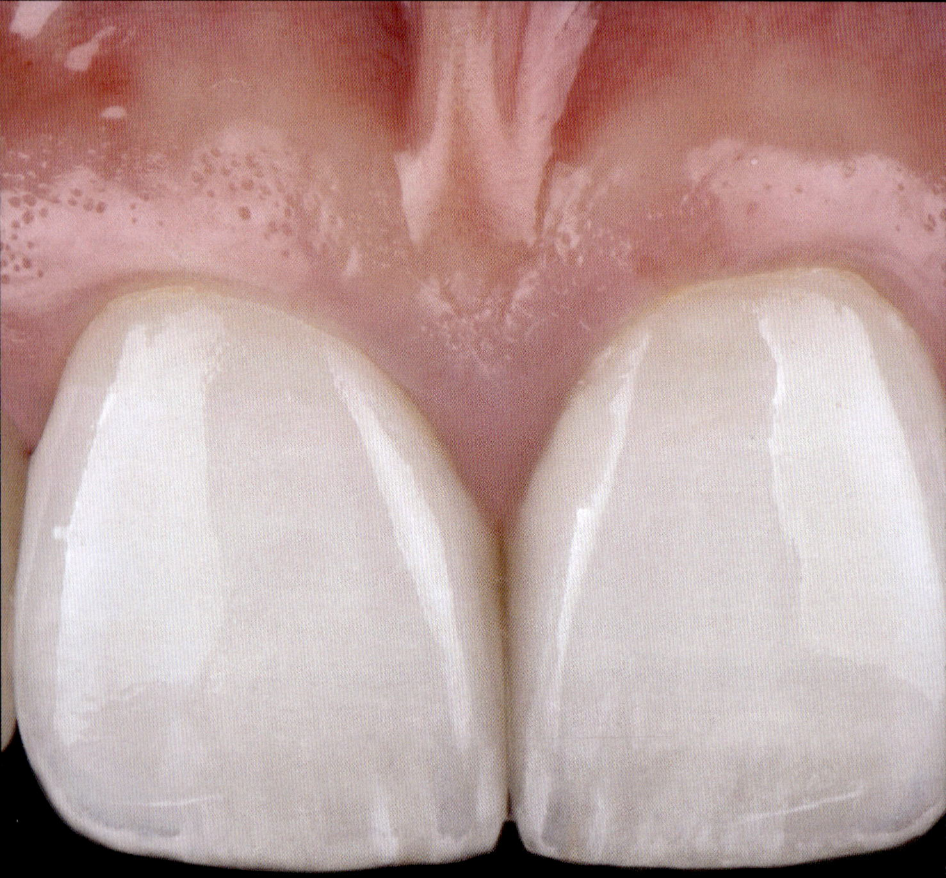

Schedule a **follow-up appointment** 1 to 2 weeks after bonding as well as **regular maintenance appointments**

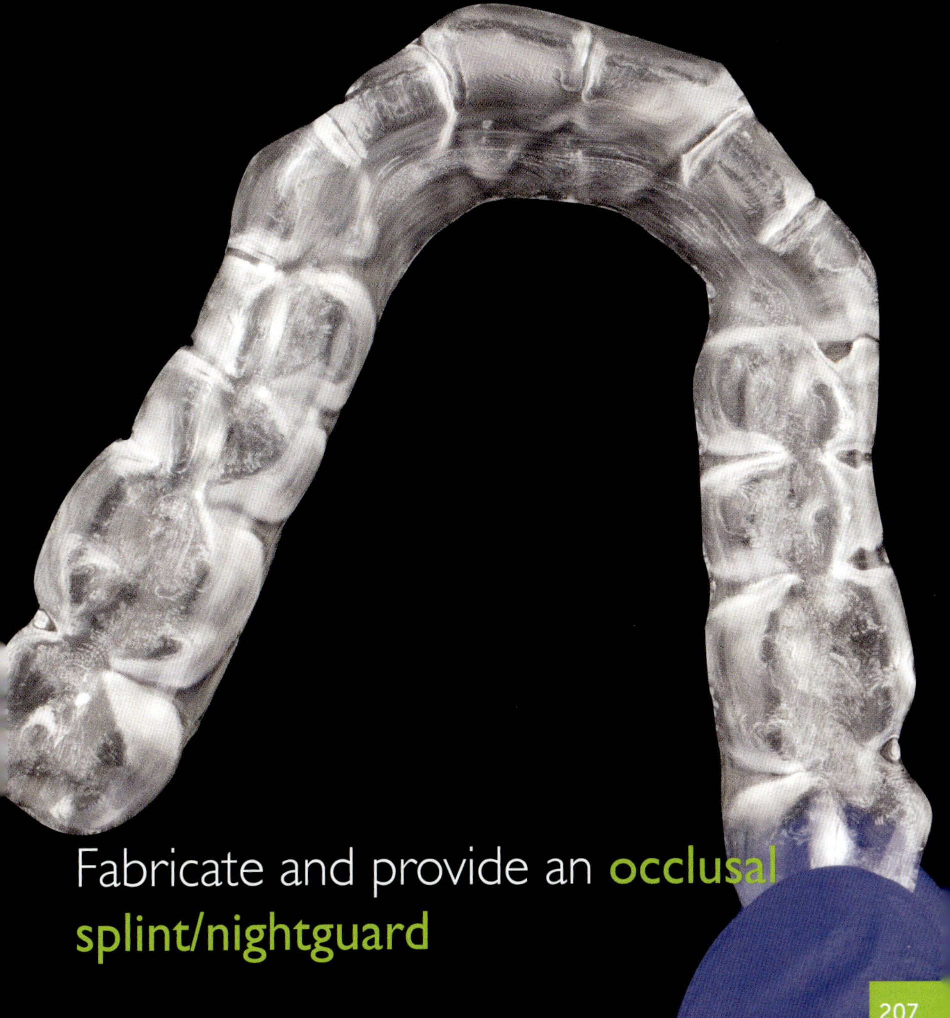

Fabricate and provide an occlusal splint/nightguard

Med Oral Patol Oral Cir Bucal 2014;19:e426–e432

Influence of bruxism on survival of porcelain laminate veneers

Granell-Ruiz M, Agustín-Panadero R, Fons-Font A, Román-Rodríguez JL, Solá-Ruíz MF

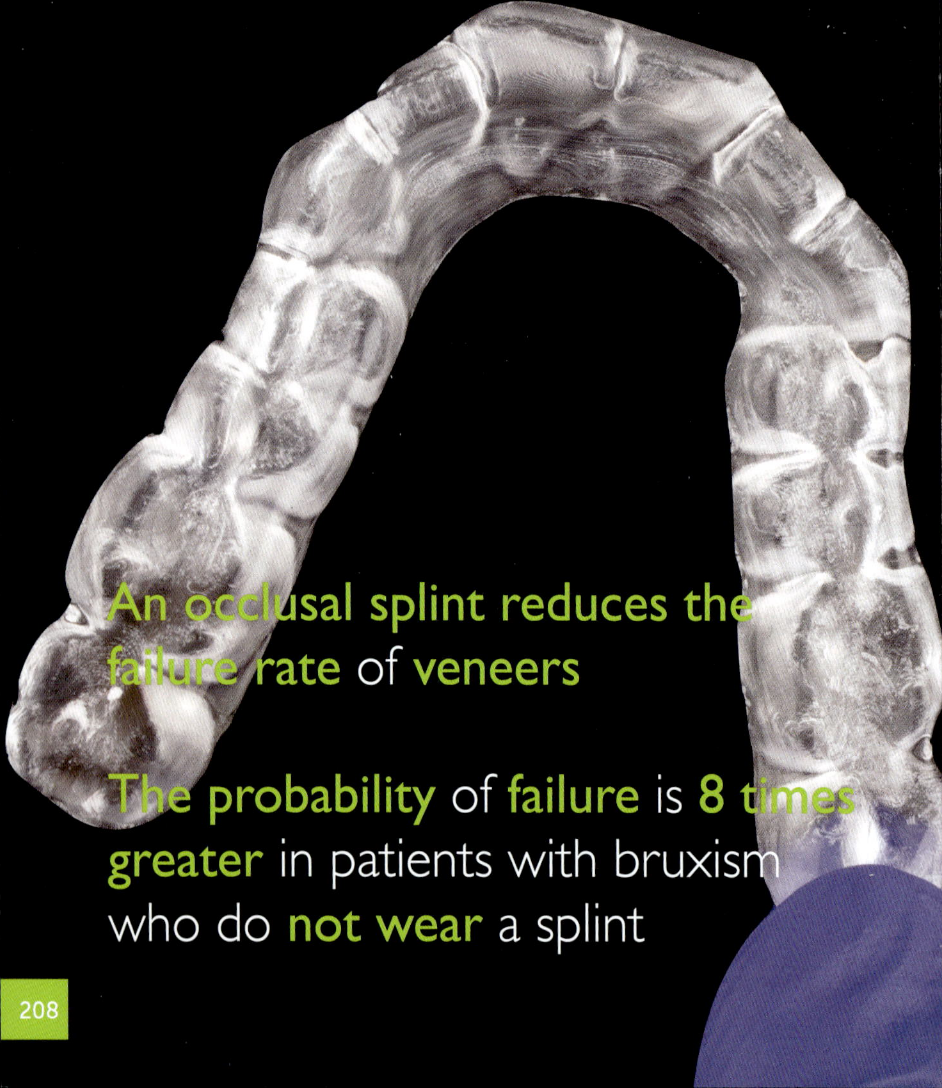

An occlusal splint reduces the failure rate of veneers

The probability of failure is 8 times greater in patients with bruxism who do not wear a splint

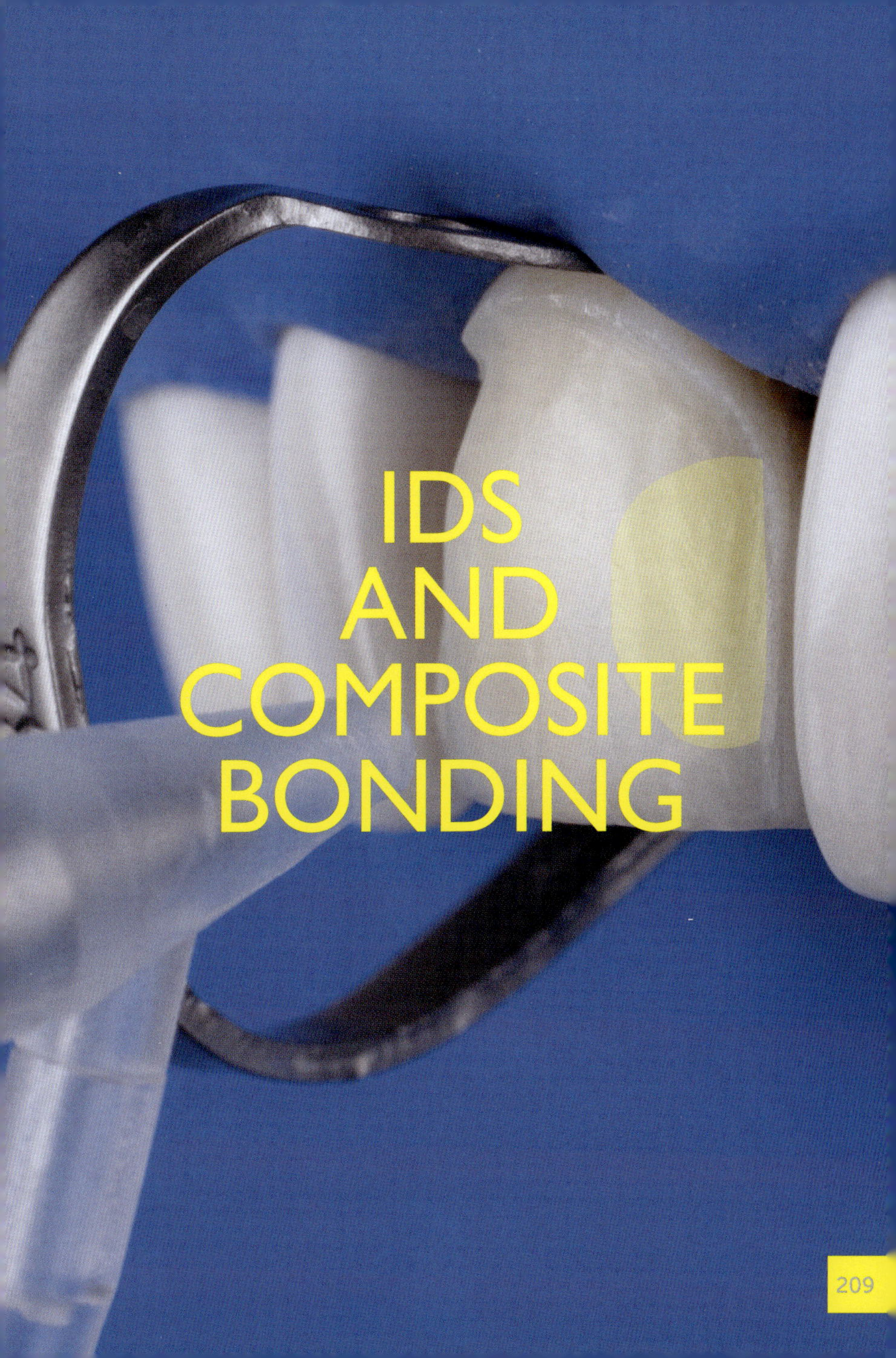

IDS AND COMPOSITE BONDING

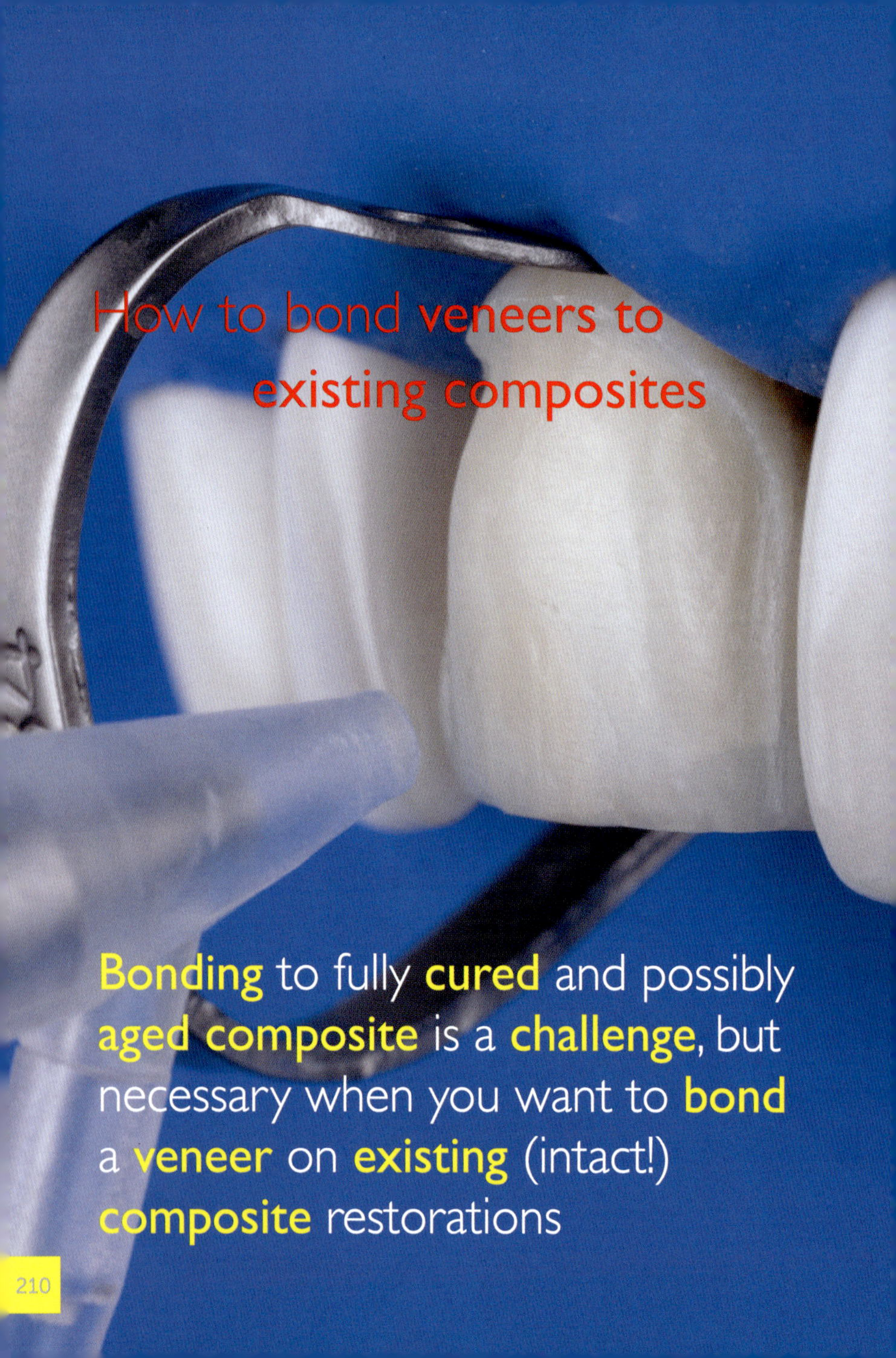

How to bond veneers to existing composites

Bonding to fully cured and possibly aged composite is a challenge, but necessary when you want to bond a veneer on existing (intact!) composite restorations

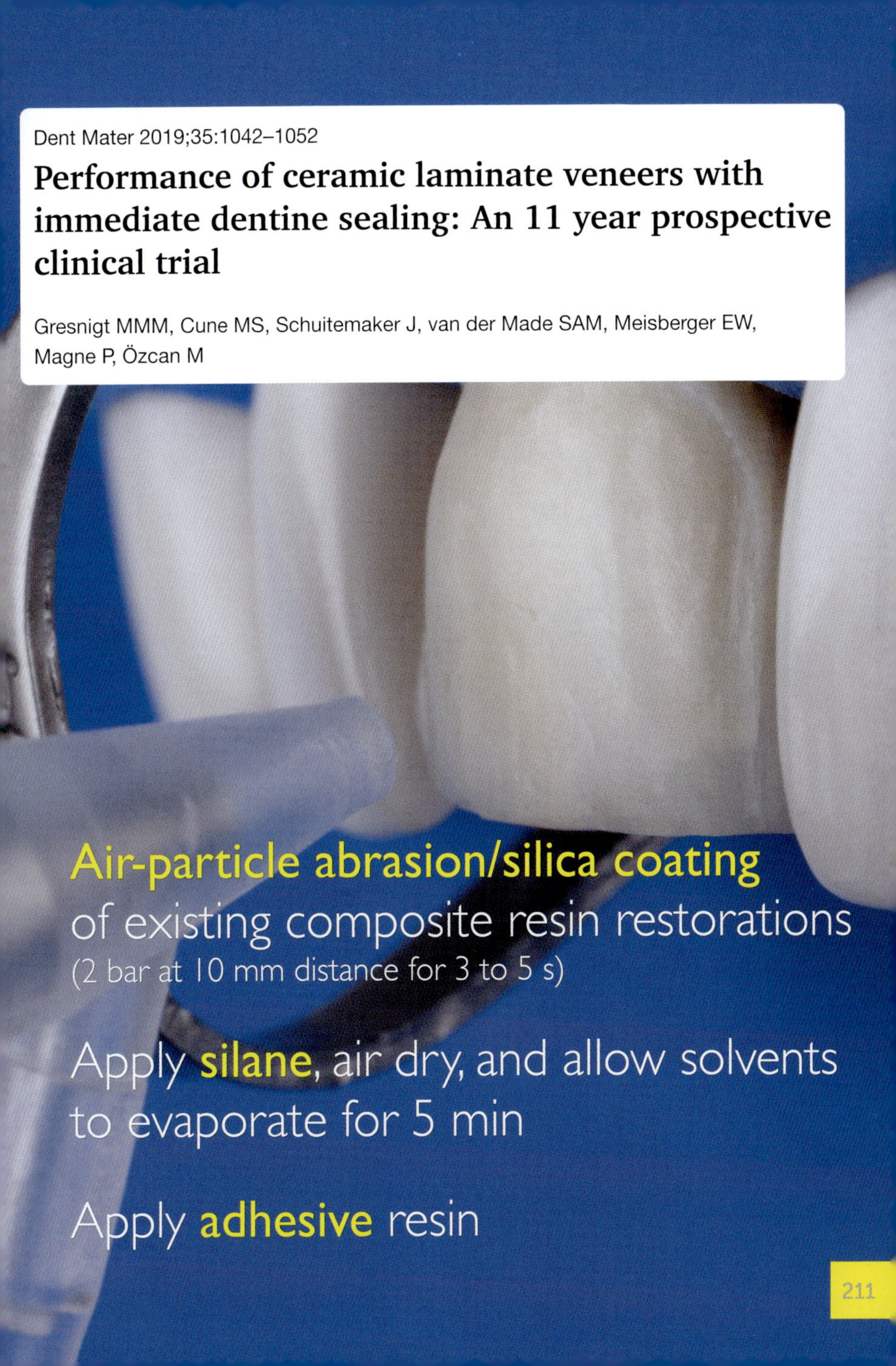

Dent Mater 2019;35:1042–1052

Performance of ceramic laminate veneers with immediate dentine sealing: An 11 year prospective clinical trial

Gresnigt MMM, Cune MS, Schuitemaker J, van der Made SAM, Meisberger EW, Magne P, Özcan M

Air-particle abrasion/silica coating of existing composite resin restorations
(2 bar at 10 mm distance for 3 to 5 s)

Apply **silane**, air dry, and allow solvents to evaporate for 5 min

Apply **adhesive** resin

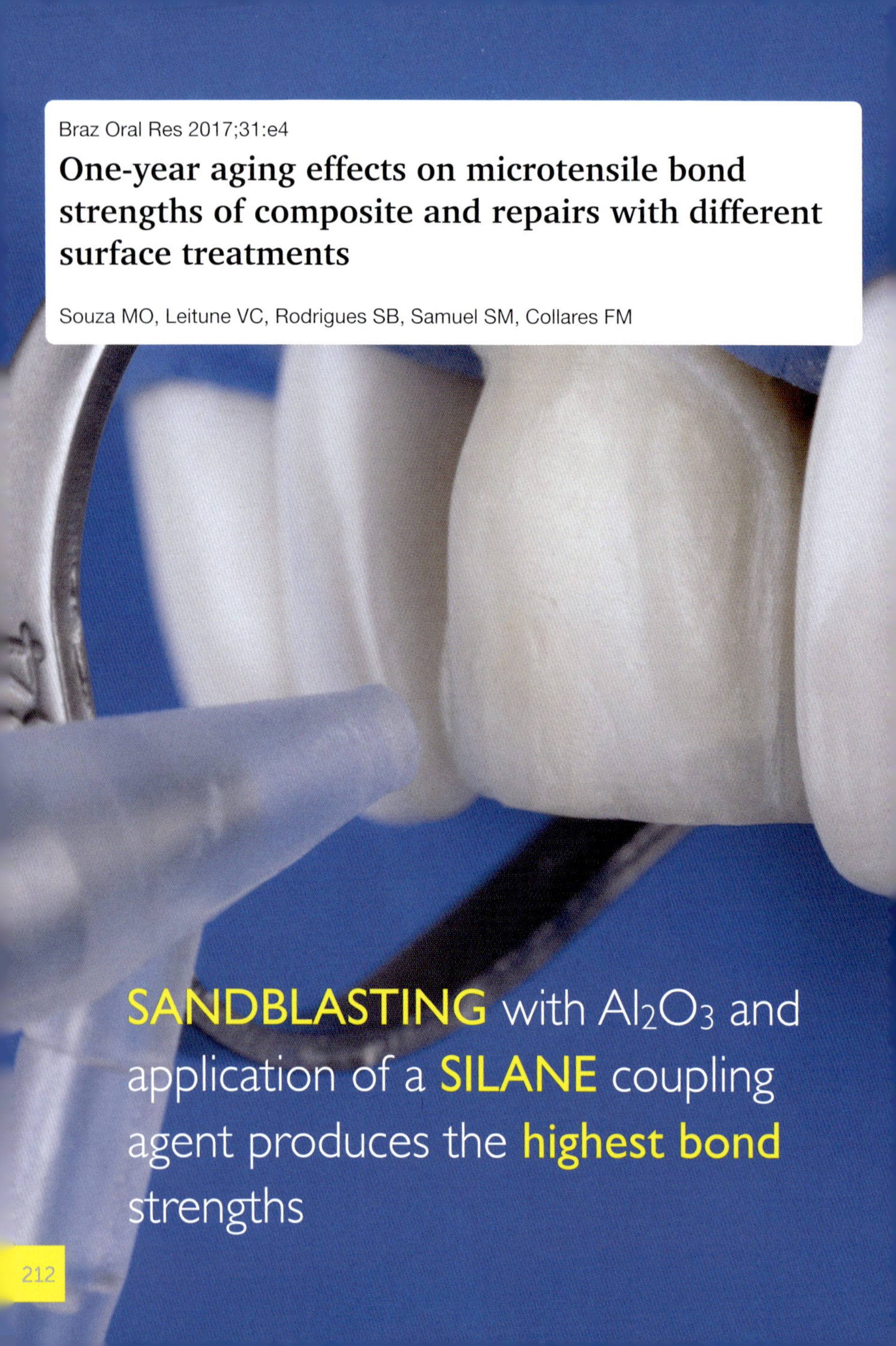

Braz Oral Res 2017;31:e4

One-year aging effects on microtensile bond strengths of composite and repairs with different surface treatments

Souza MO, Leitune VC, Rodrigues SB, Samuel SM, Collares FM

SANDBLASTING with Al_2O_3 and application of a **SILANE** coupling agent produces the **highest bond** strengths

Polymers (Basel) 2020;12:950

Silane effect of universal adhesive on the composite-composite repair bond strength after different surface pretreatments

Michelotti G, Niedzwiecki M, Bidjan D, Dieckmann P, Deari S, Attin T, Tauböck TT

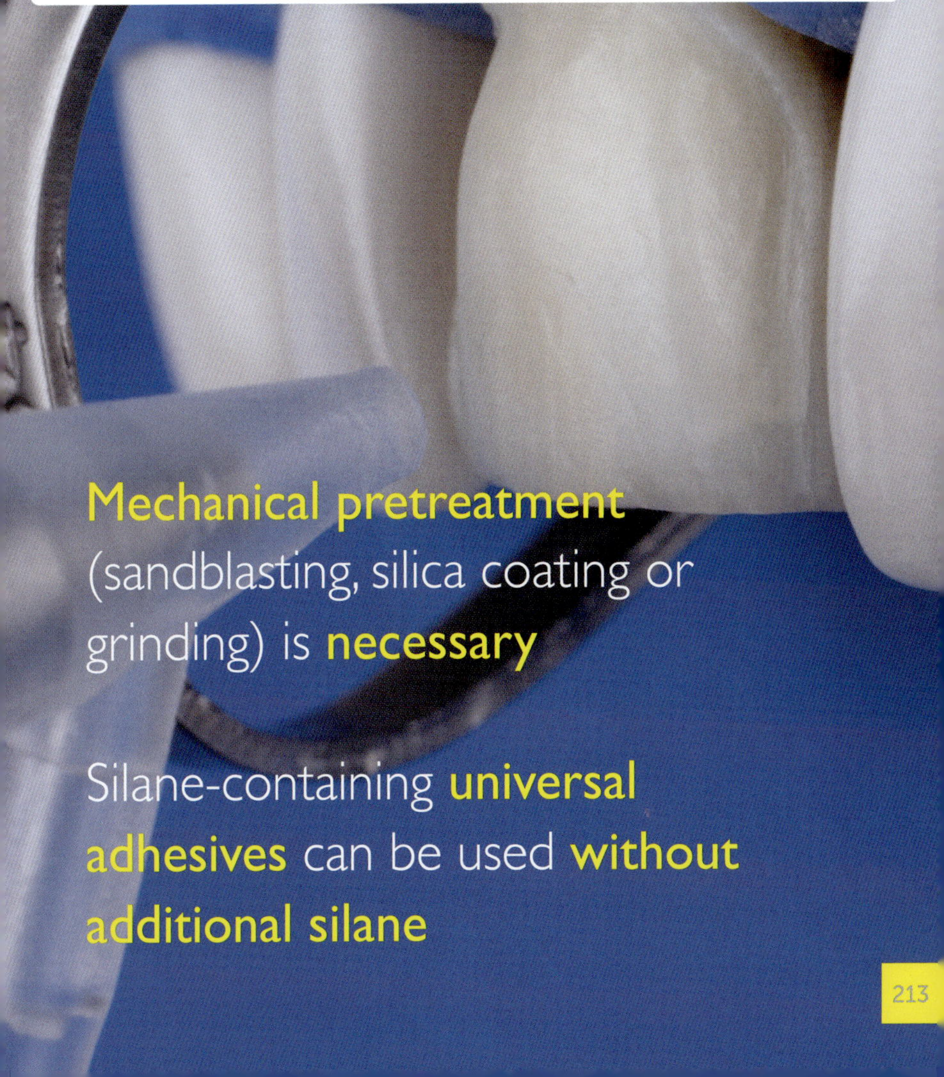

Mechanical pretreatment (sandblasting, silica coating or grinding) is **necessary**

Silane-containing **universal adhesives** can be used **without additional silane**

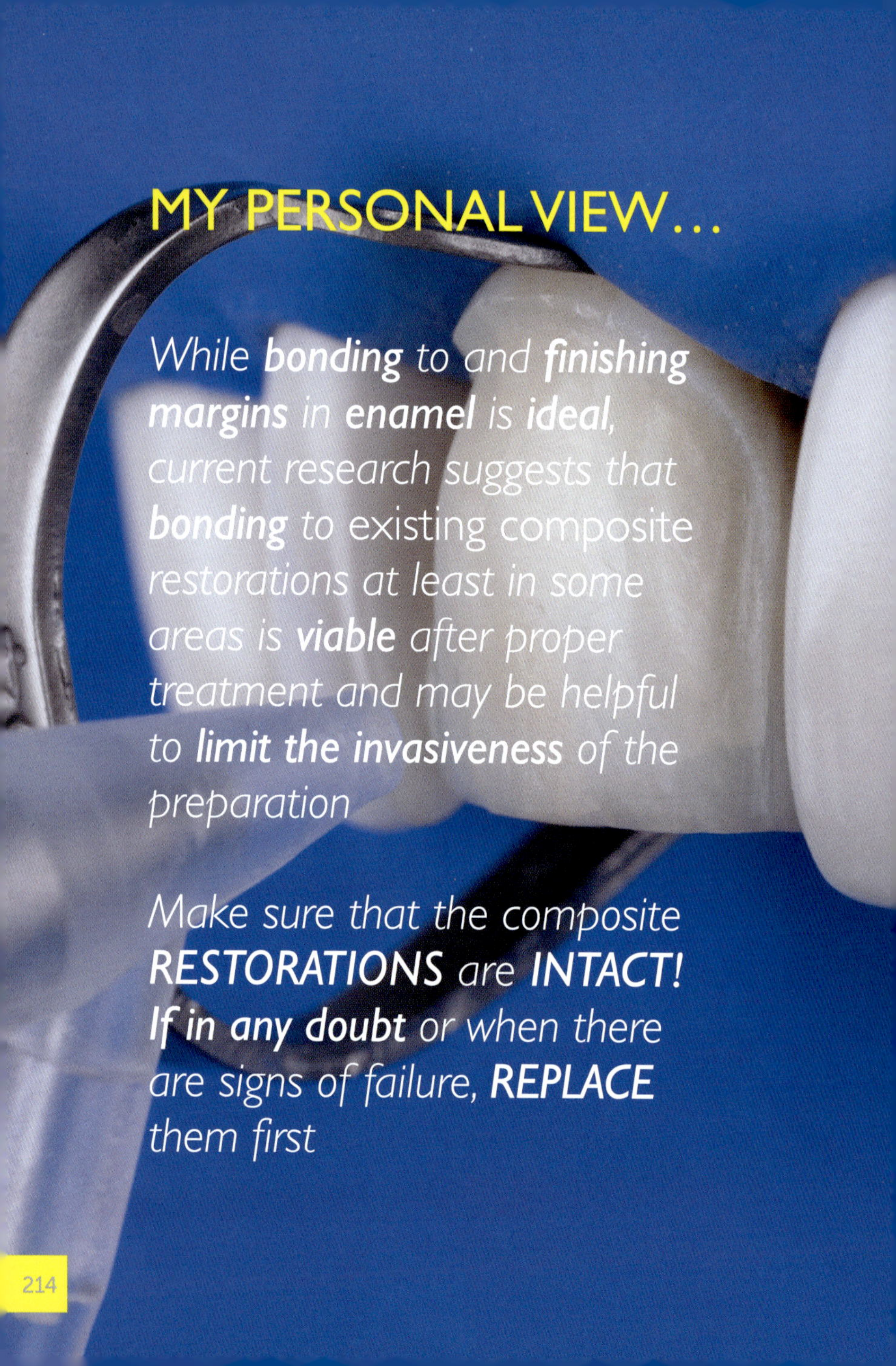

MY PERSONAL VIEW...

While ***bonding*** *to and* ***finishing margins*** *in* ***enamel*** *is* ***ideal****, current research suggests that* **bonding** to existing composite *restorations at least in some areas is* ***viable*** *after proper treatment and may be helpful to* ***limit the invasiveness*** *of the preparation*

Make sure that the composite **RESTORATIONS** *are* **INTACT!** ***If in any doubt*** *or when there are signs of failure,* **REPLACE** *them first*

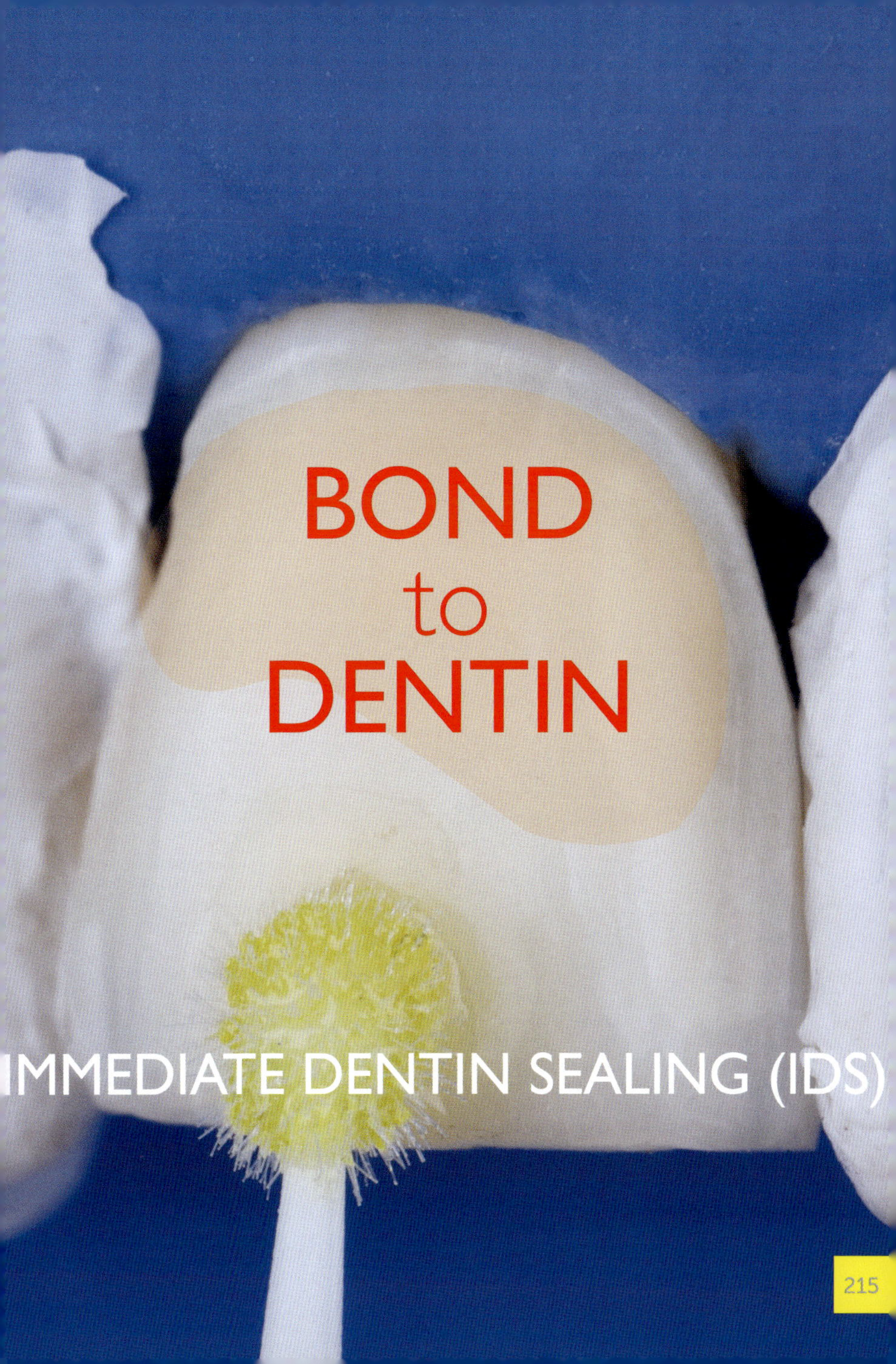
BOND
to
DENTIN
IMMEDIATE DENTIN SEALING (IDS)

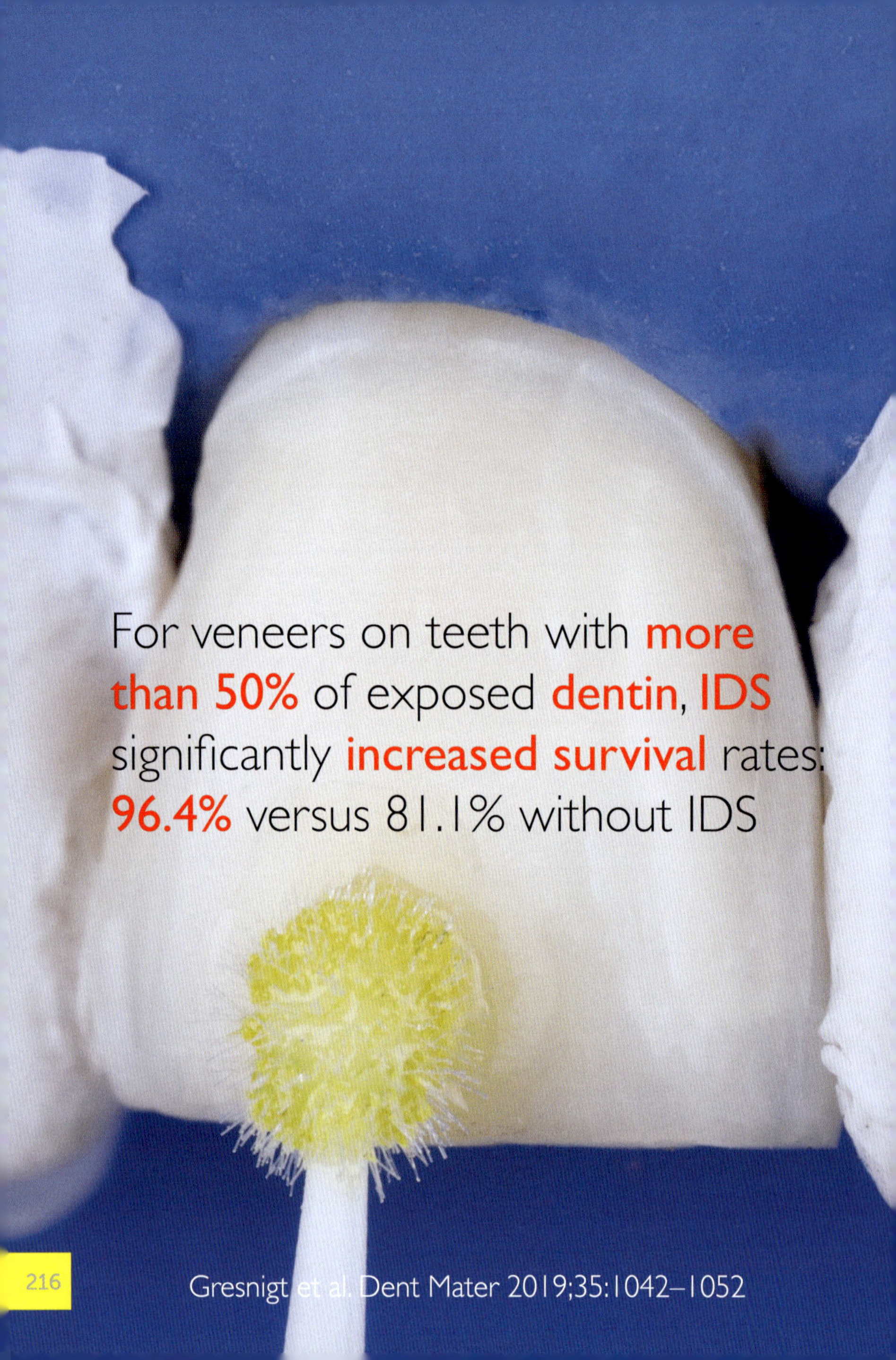

For veneers on teeth with **more than 50%** of exposed **dentin, IDS** significantly **increased survival** rates: **96.4%** versus 81.1% without IDS

Gresnigt et al. Dent Mater 2019;35:1042–1052

Gels 2022;8:175

Immediate dentin sealing for adhesive cementation of indirect restorations: A systematic review and meta-analysis

Hardan L, Devoto W, Bourgi R, Cuevas-Suárez CE, Lukomska-Szymanska M, Fernández-Barrera MÁ, Cornejo-Ríos E, Monteiro P, Zarow M, Jakubowicz N, Mancino D, Haikel Y, Kharouf N

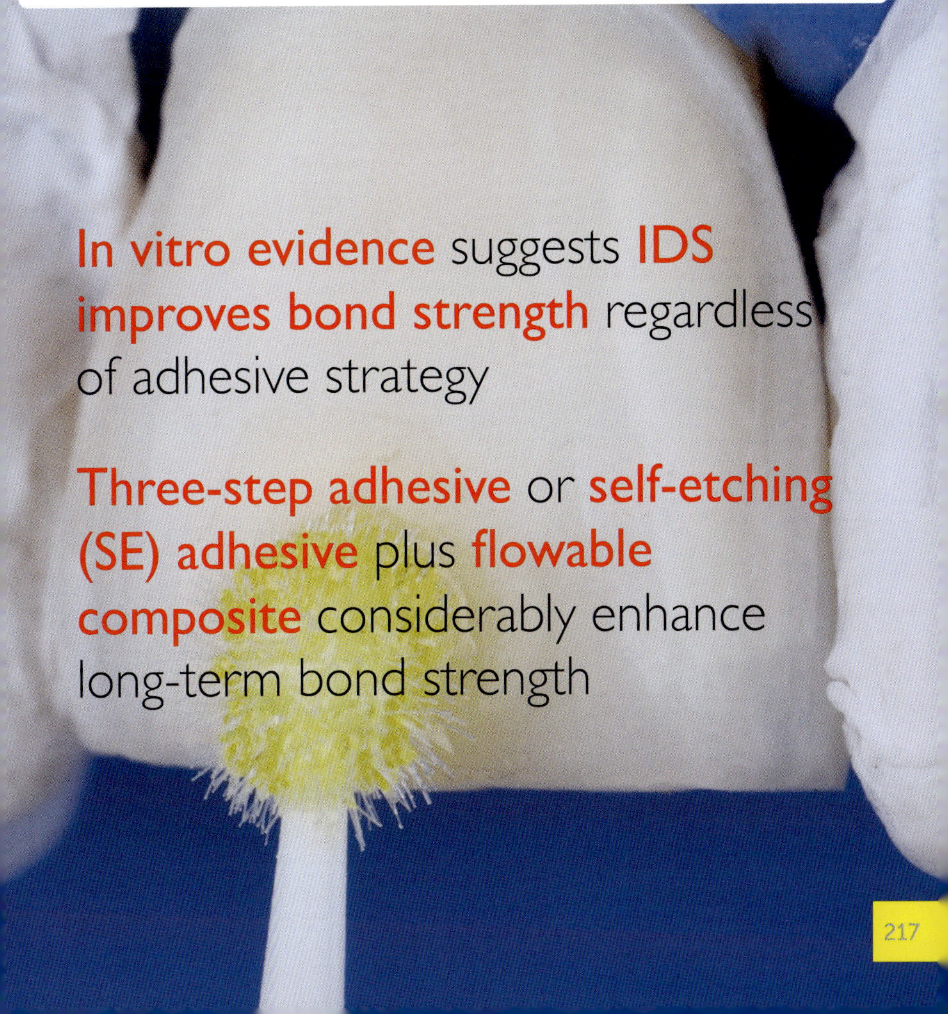

In vitro evidence suggests **IDS improves bond strength** regardless of adhesive strategy

Three-step adhesive or **self-etching (SE) adhesive** plus **flowable composite** considerably enhance long-term bond strength

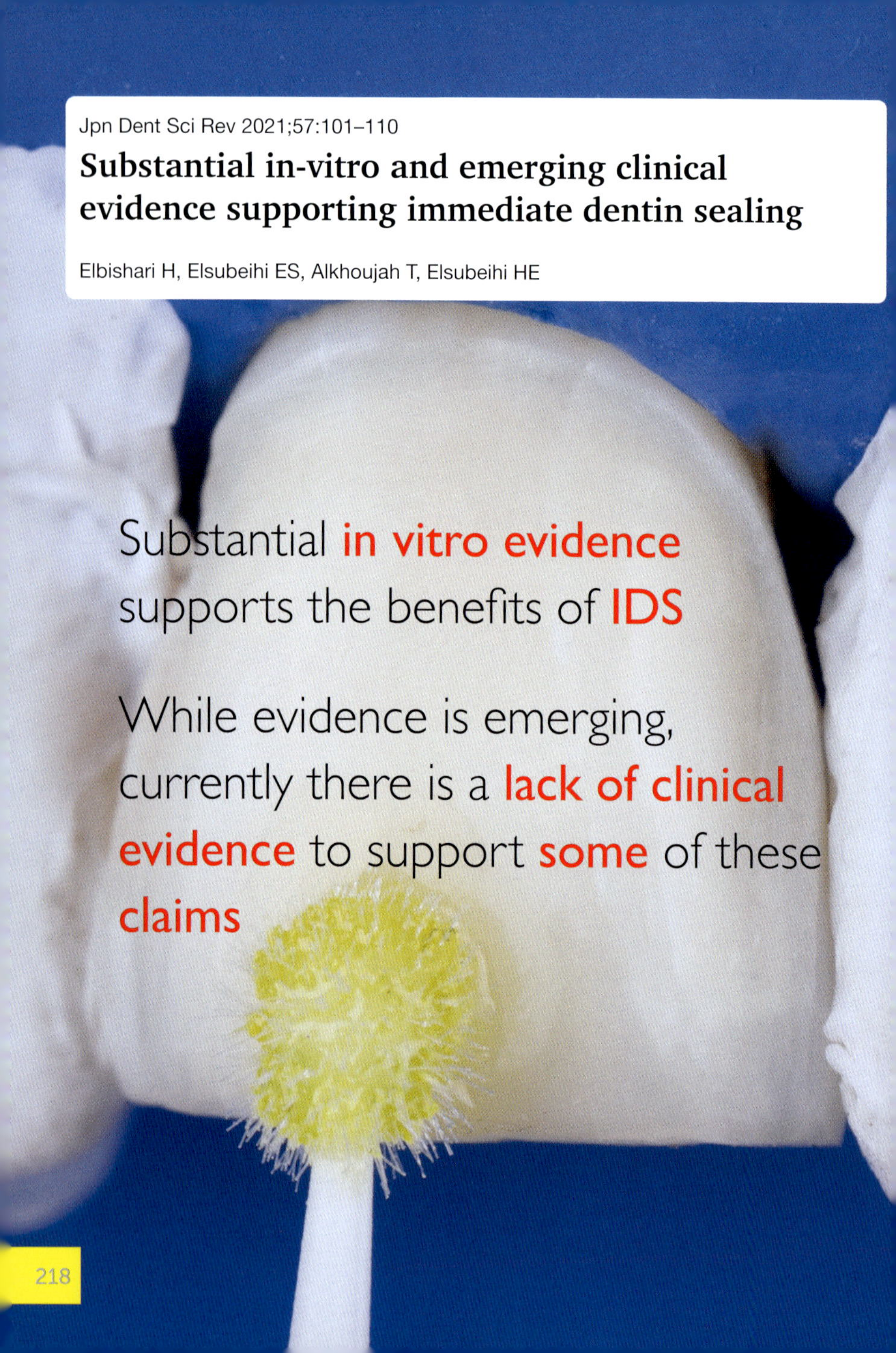

Jpn Dent Sci Rev 2021;57:101–110

Substantial in-vitro and emerging clinical evidence supporting immediate dentin sealing

Elbishari H, Elsubeihi ES, Alkhoujah T, Elsubeihi HE

Substantial **in vitro evidence** supports the benefits of **IDS**

While evidence is emerging, currently there is a **lack of clinical evidence** to support **some** of these **claims**

Clin Cosmet Investig Dent 2021;13:233–256

Immediate dentin sealing: A literature review

Samartzi TK, Papalexopoulos D, Sarafianou A, Kourtis S

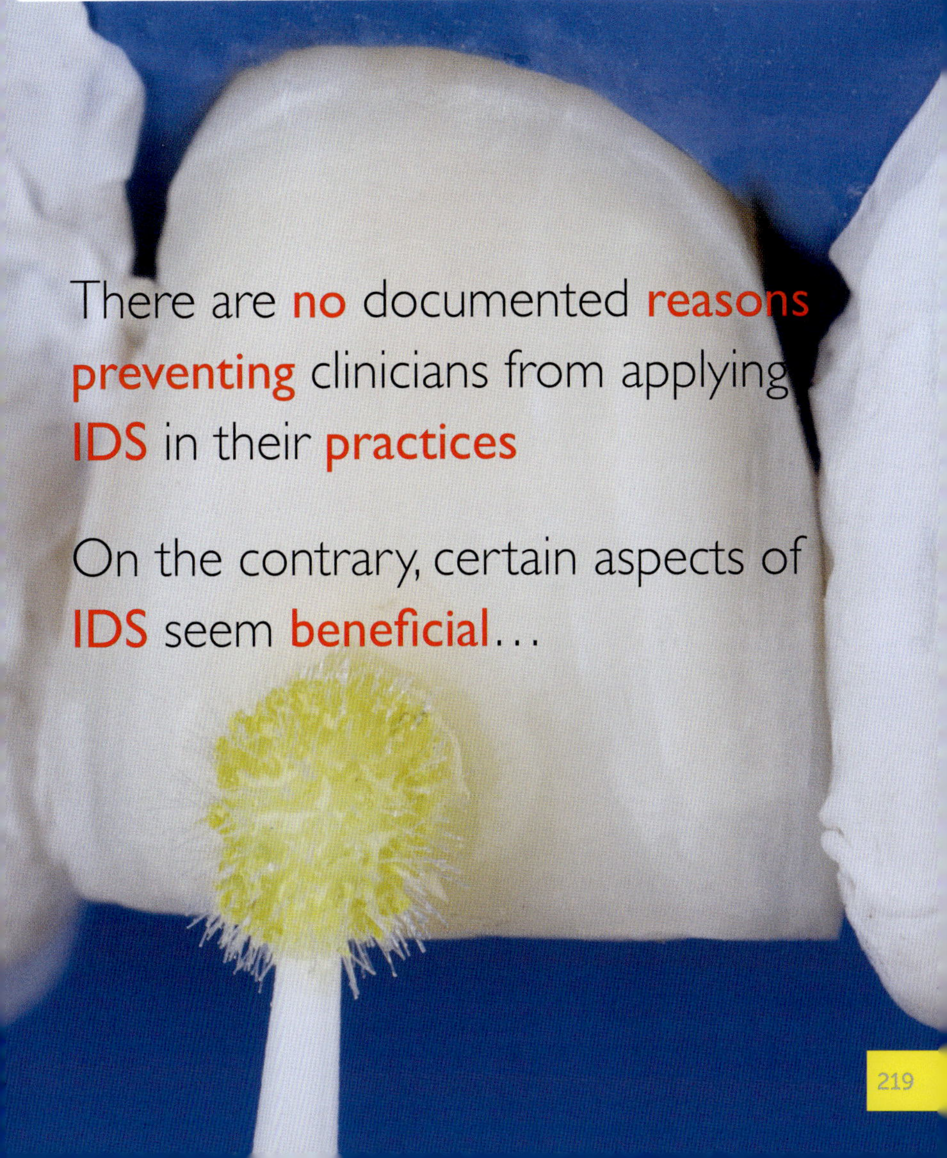

Biomimetics (Basel) 2024;9:182

Effect of immediate dentin sealing on the bonding performance of indirect restorations: A systematic review

Ozer F, Eken ZB, Hao J, Tuloglu N, Blatz MB

IDS improves the bond strength of indirect restorations to dentin and reduces the negative effects of temporary materials on the bond durability of final indirect restorations

Filled dentin bonding agents or combinations with flowable compostie resin are preferred to protect the IDS layer from conditioning procedures

MY PERSONAL VIEW...

Laboratory studies confirm the ***benefits of IDS*** *or the* ***"resin coating technique"*** *with* ***more clinical support needed****, although this support is* ***emerging*** *in the literature*

Remember that ***every technique*** *is only* ***as good as its clinical execution****, so* ***familiarize*** *yourself with* ***IDS*** *should you choose to apply it*

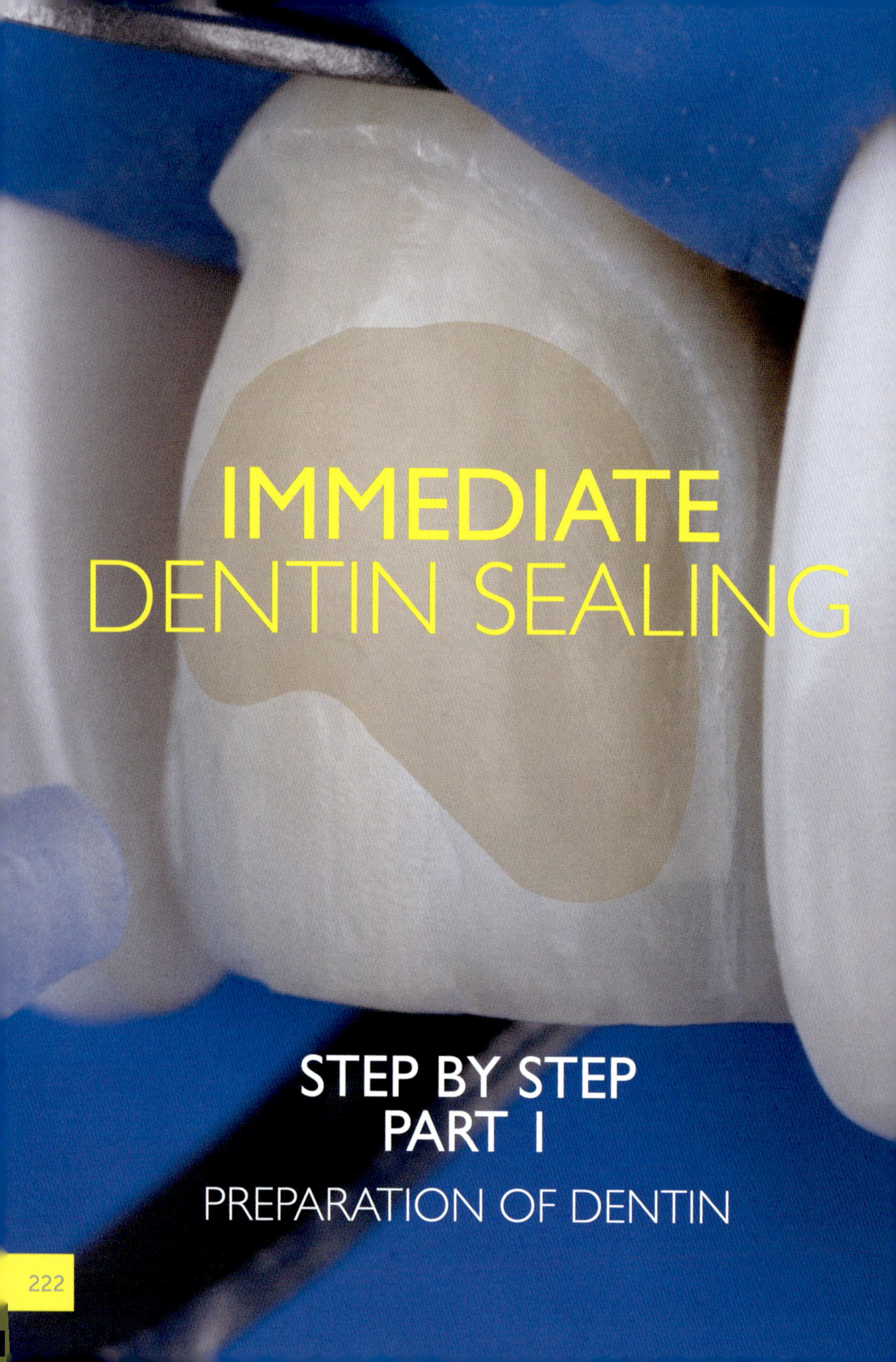

IMMEDIATE DENTIN SEALING

STEP BY STEP PART I

PREPARATION OF DENTIN

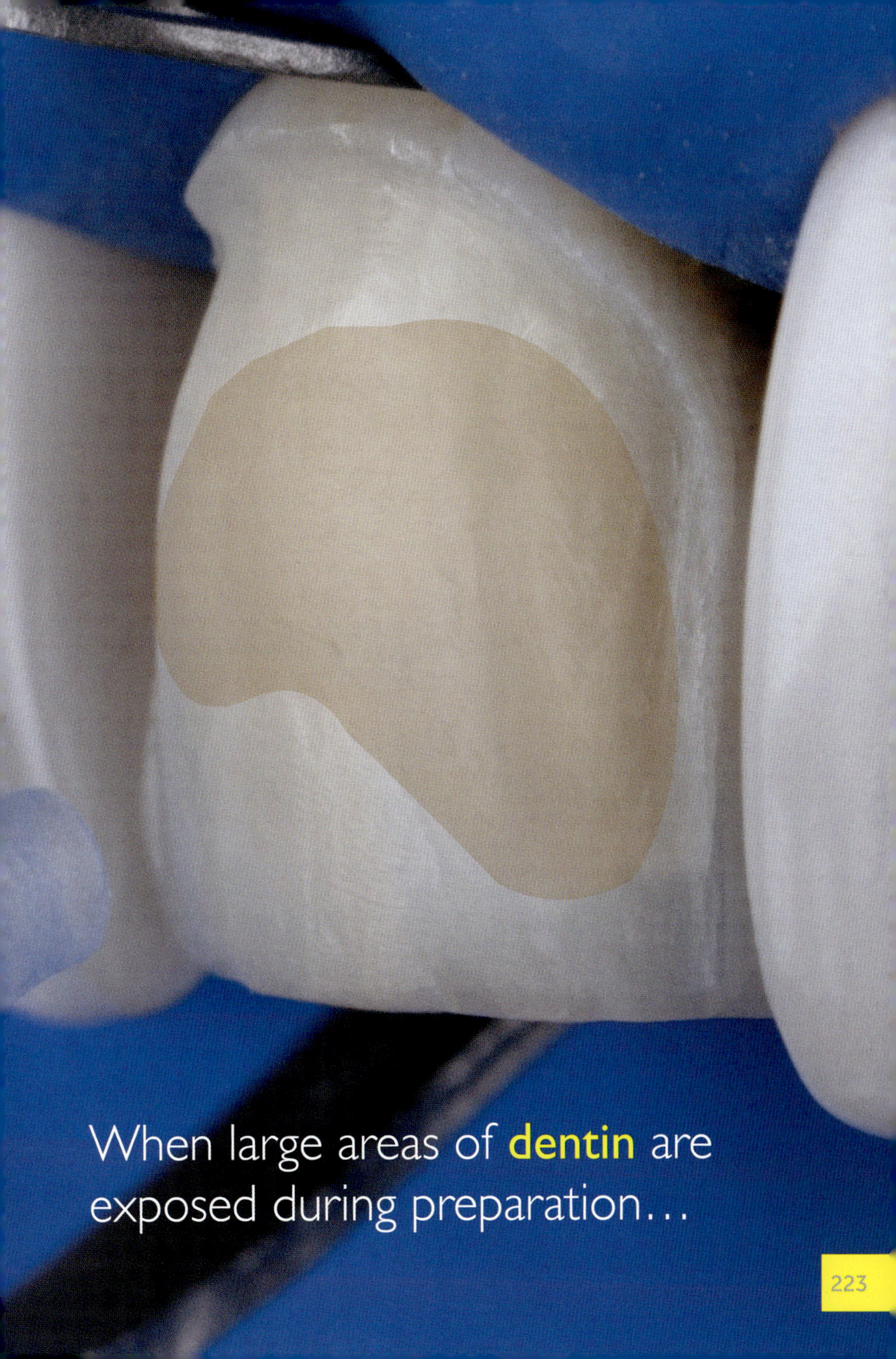

When large areas of **dentin** are exposed during preparation…

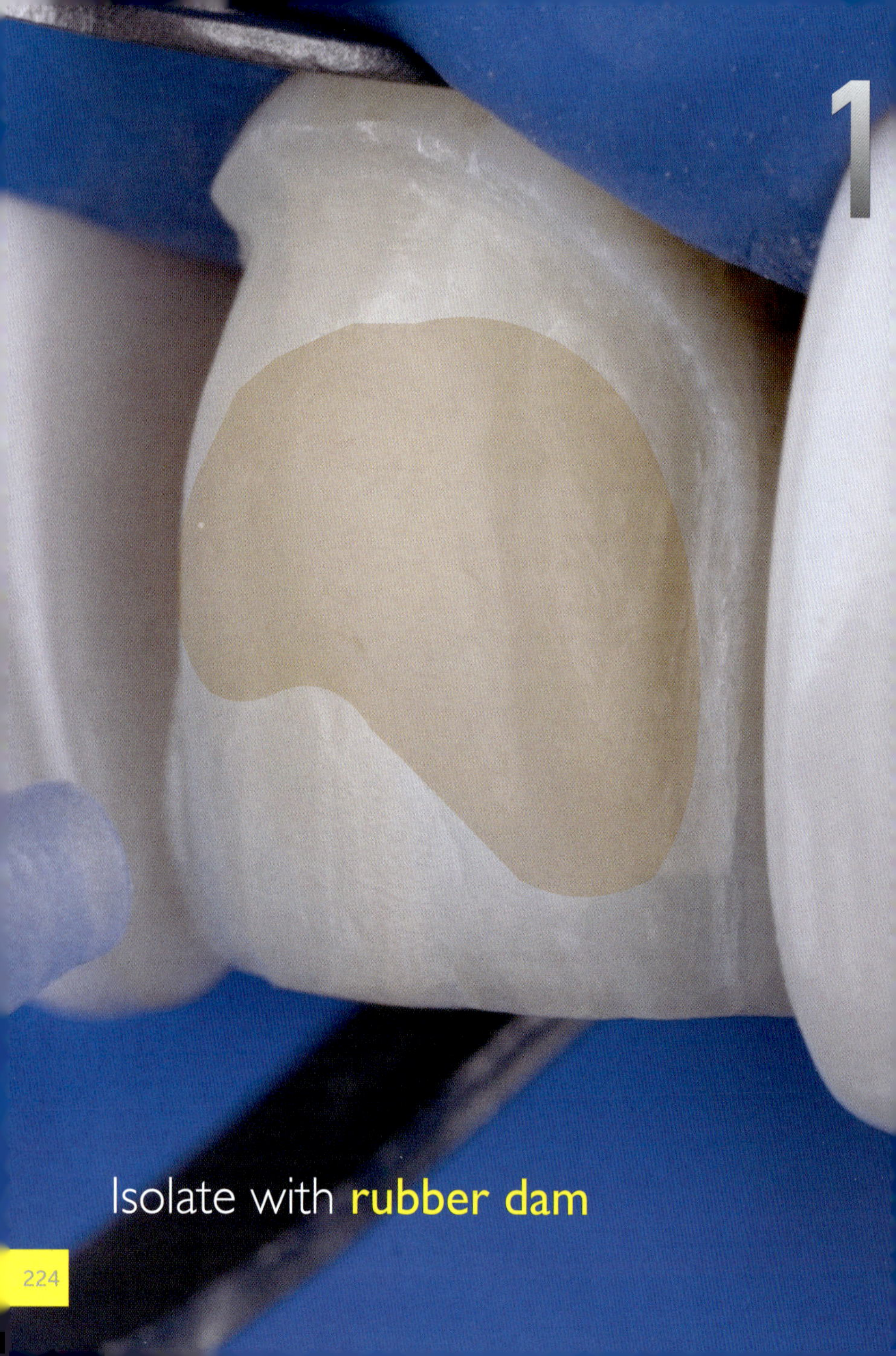

1

Isolate with **rubber dam**

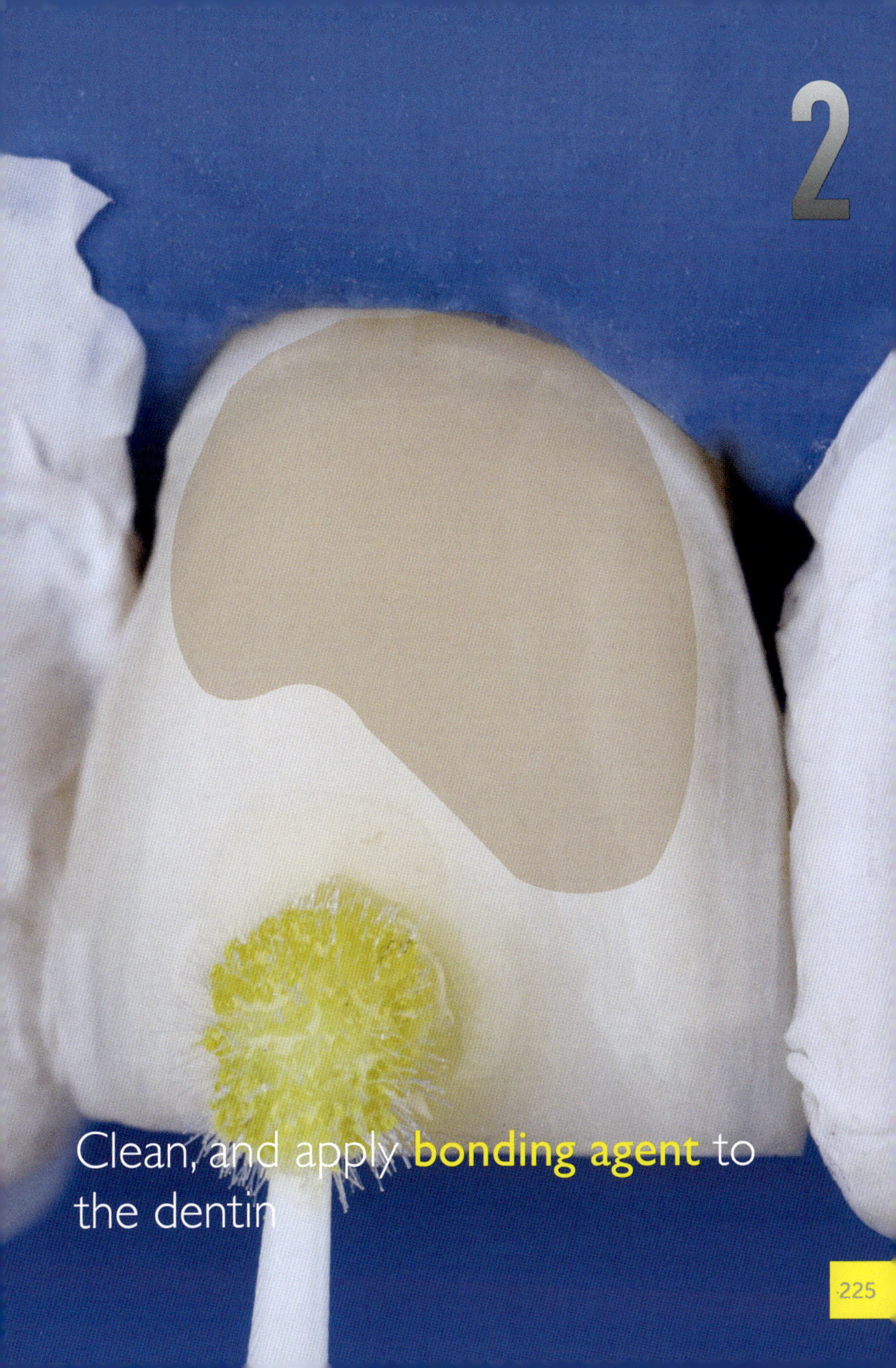

2

Clean, and apply **bonding agent** to the dentin

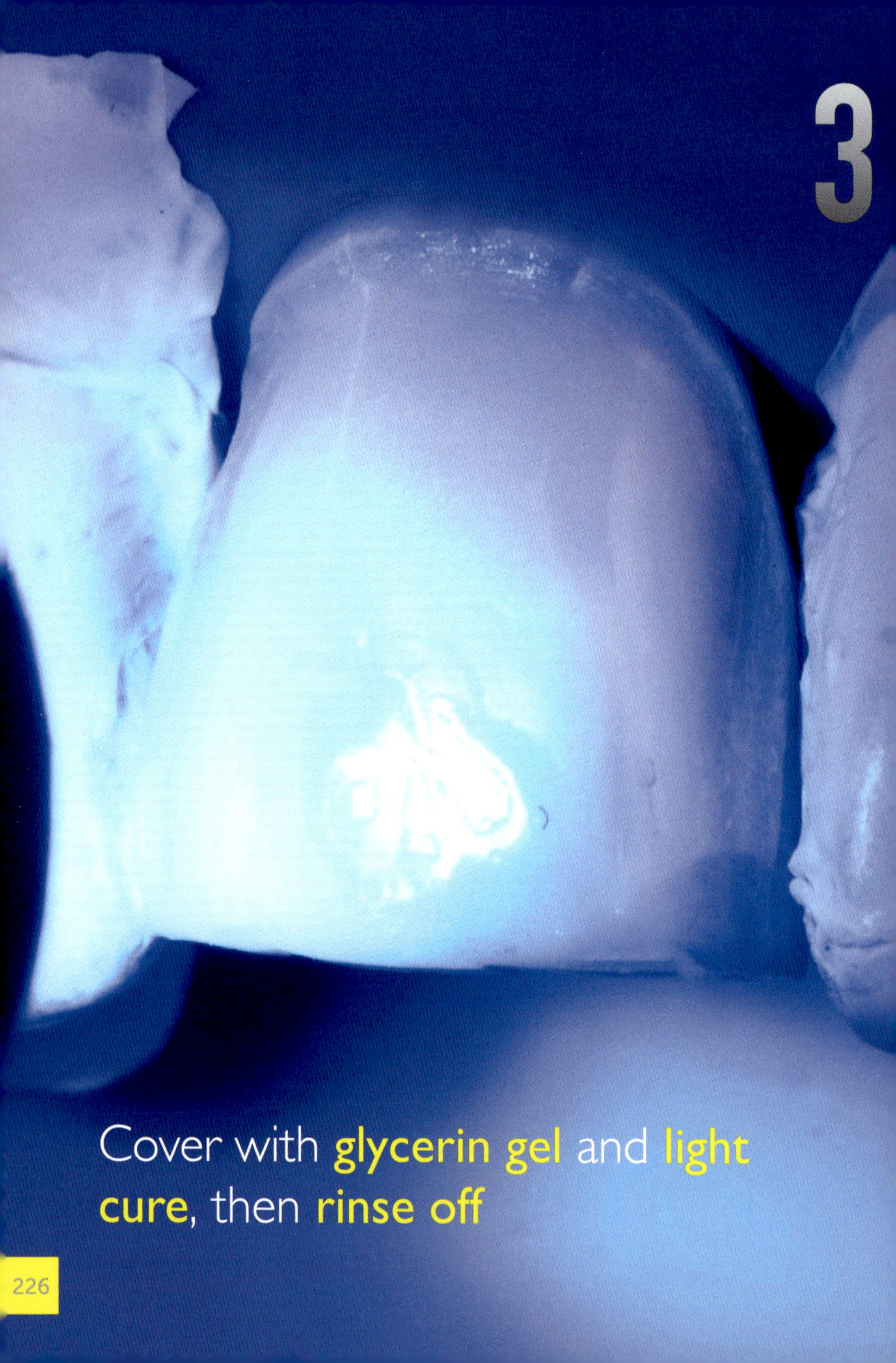

3

Cover with **glycerin gel** and **light cure**, then **rinse off**

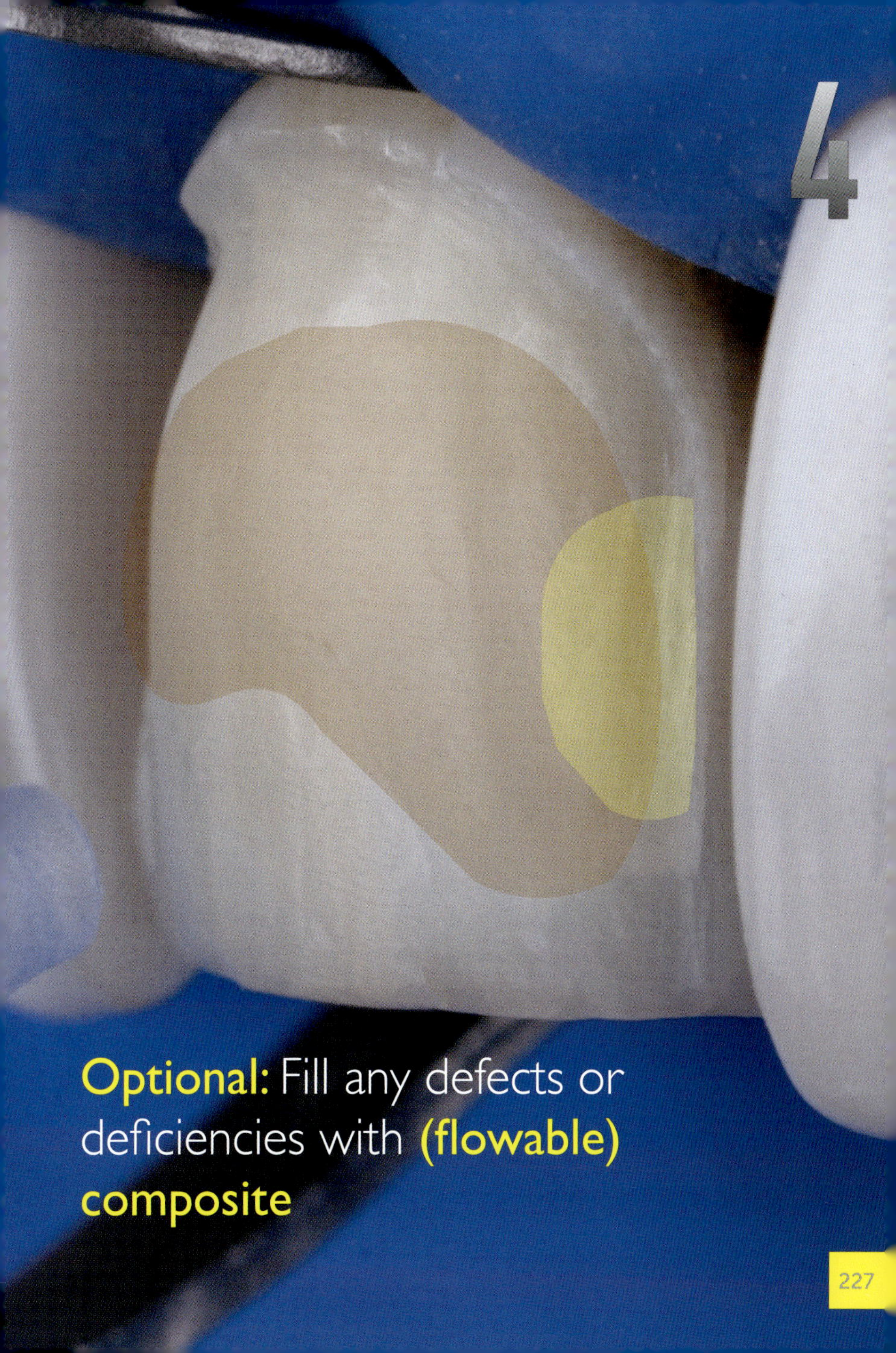

4

Optional: Fill any defects or deficiencies with **(flowable) composite**

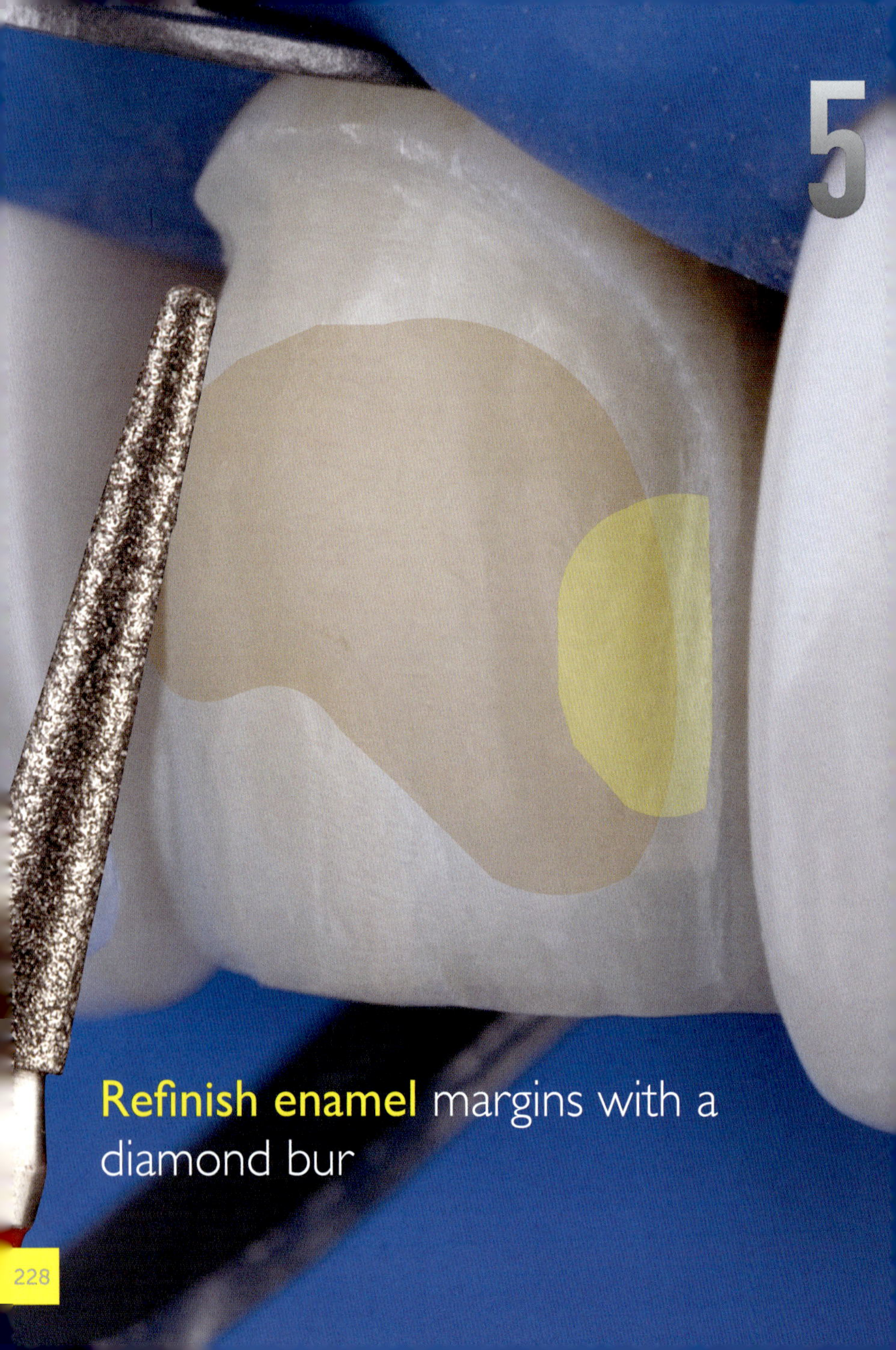

5

Refinish enamel margins with a diamond bur

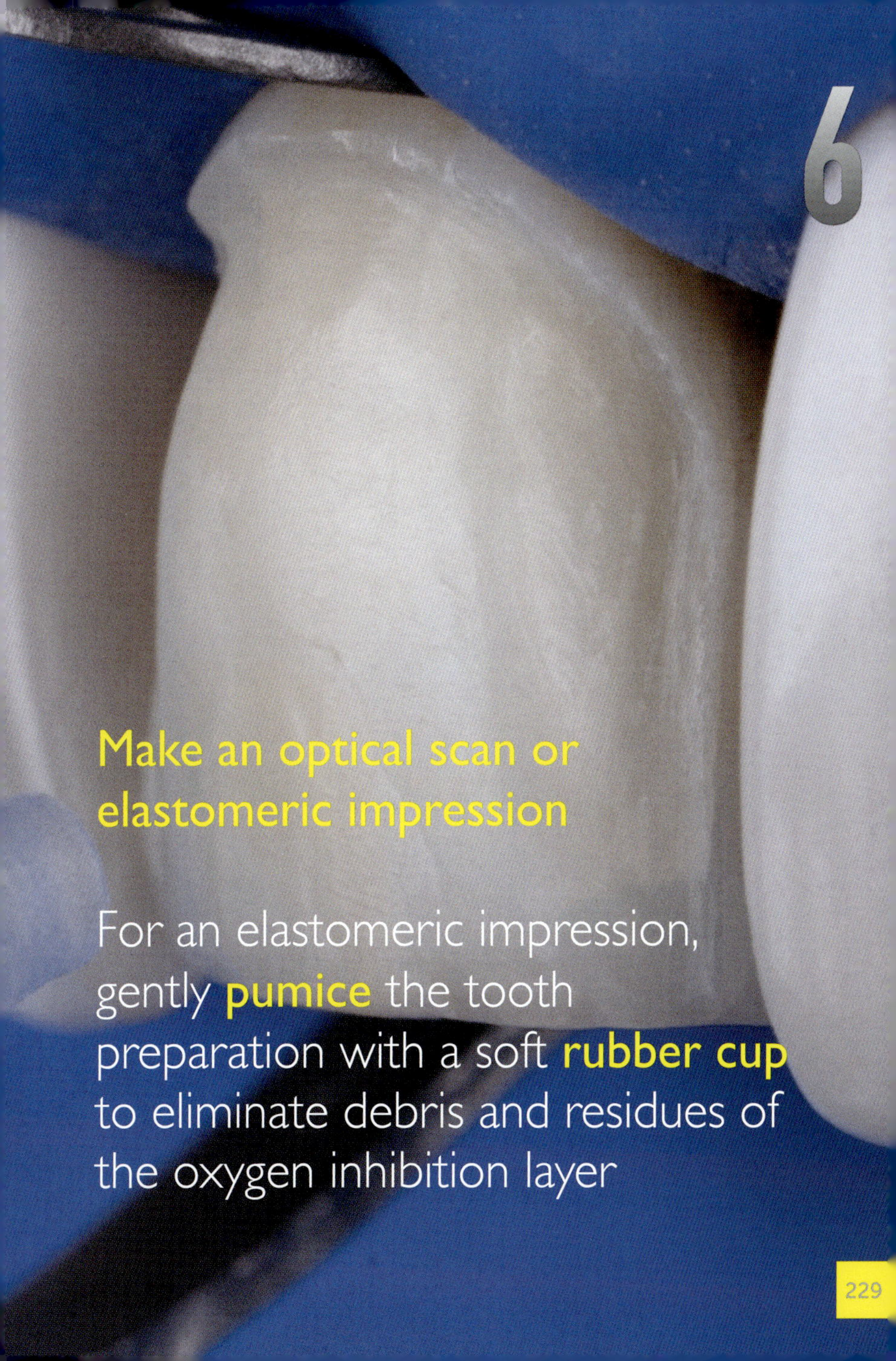

6

Make an optical scan or elastomeric impression

For an elastomeric impression, gently **pumice** the tooth preparation with a soft **rubber cup** to eliminate debris and residues of the oxygen inhibition layer

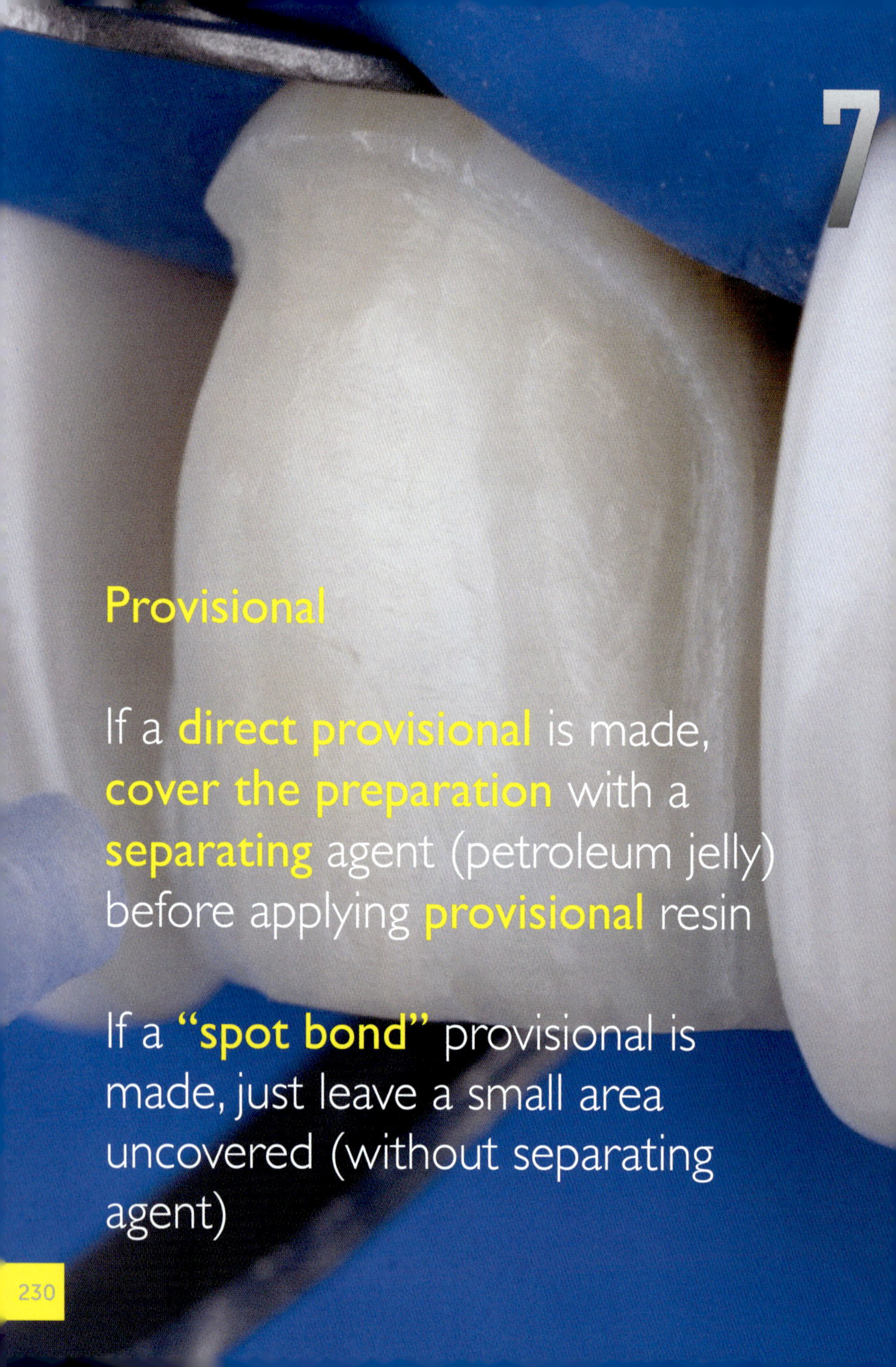

Provisional

If a **direct provisional** is made, **cover the preparation** with a **separating** agent (petroleum jelly) before applying **provisional** resin

If a **"spot bond"** provisional is made, just leave a small area uncovered (without separating agent)

IDS PREPARATION OF DENTIN

CHEAT SHEET

1. Isolate with rubber dam
2. Clean and apply bonding agent to the dentin
3. Cover with glycerin gel and light cure, then rinse off
4. Optional: Fill any defects or deficiencies with (flowable) composite
5. Refinish enamel margins with a diamond bur
6. Make an optical scan or elastomeric impression
   For an elastomeric impression, gently pumice the tooth preparation

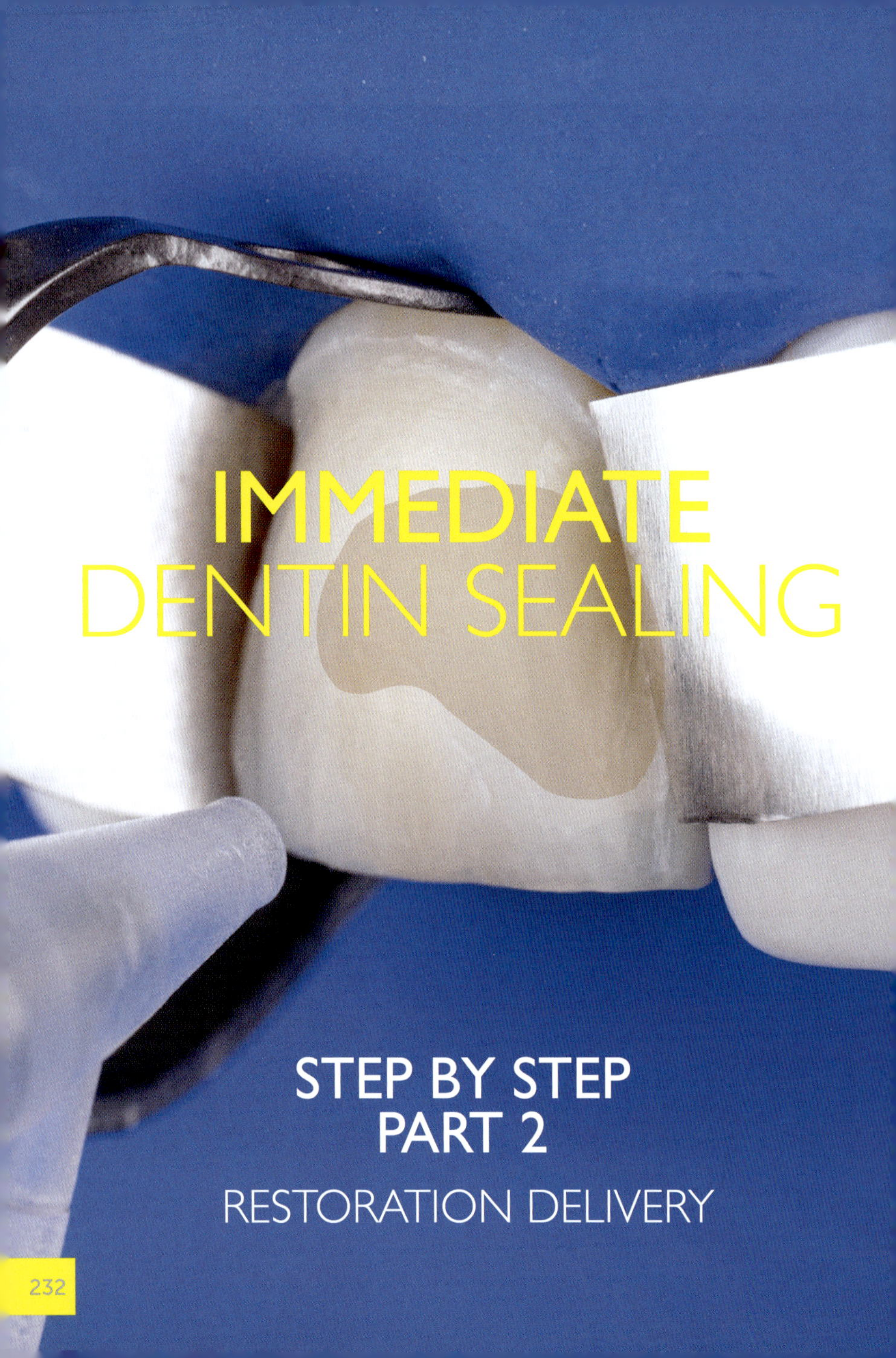

IMMEDIATE DENTIN SEALING

STEP BY STEP PART 2

RESTORATION DELIVERY

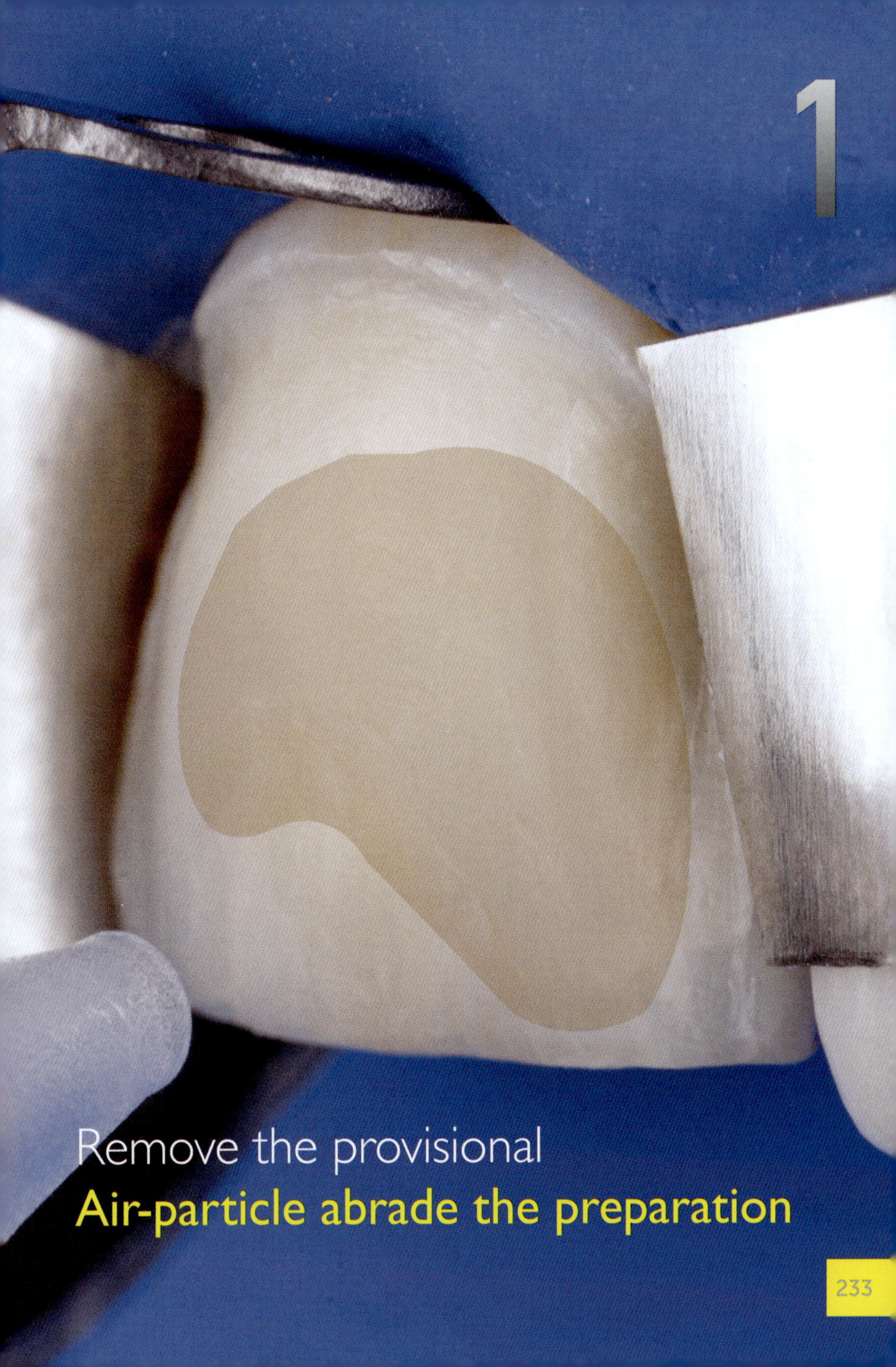

1

Remove the provisional

Air-particle abrade the preparation

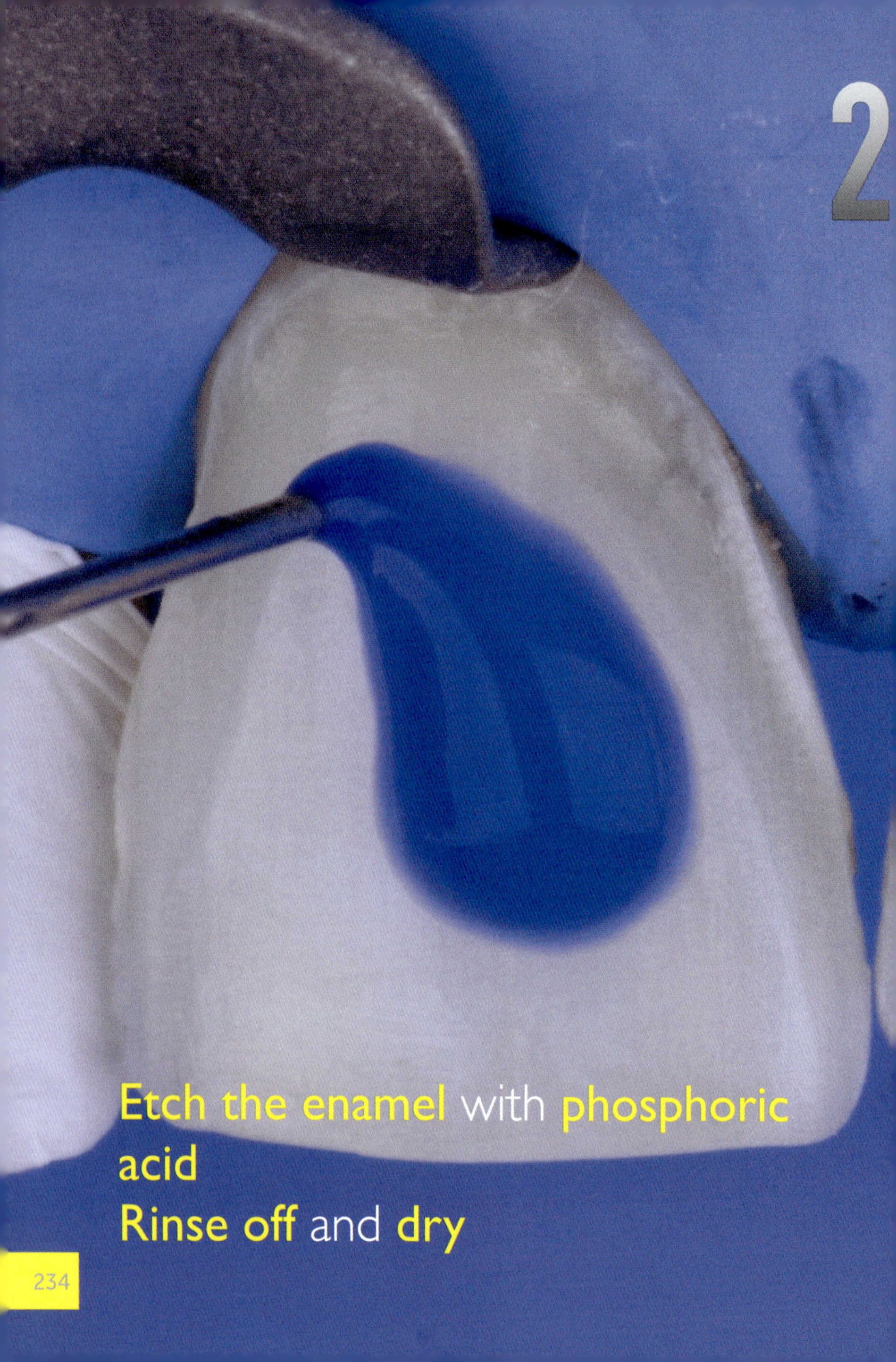

2

Etch the enamel with phosphoric acid
Rinse off and dry

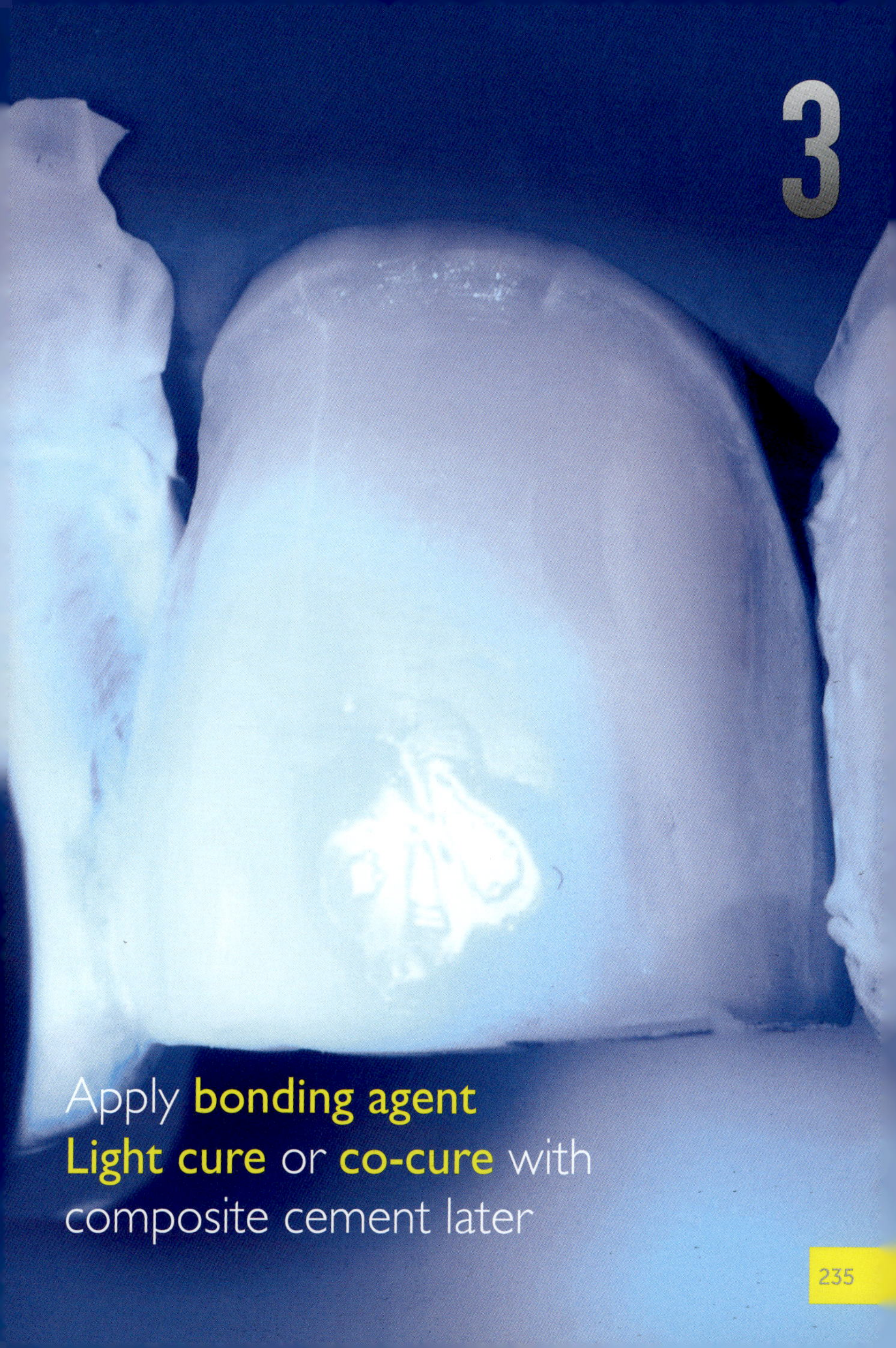

3

Apply **bonding agent**
Light cure or **co-cure** with composite cement later

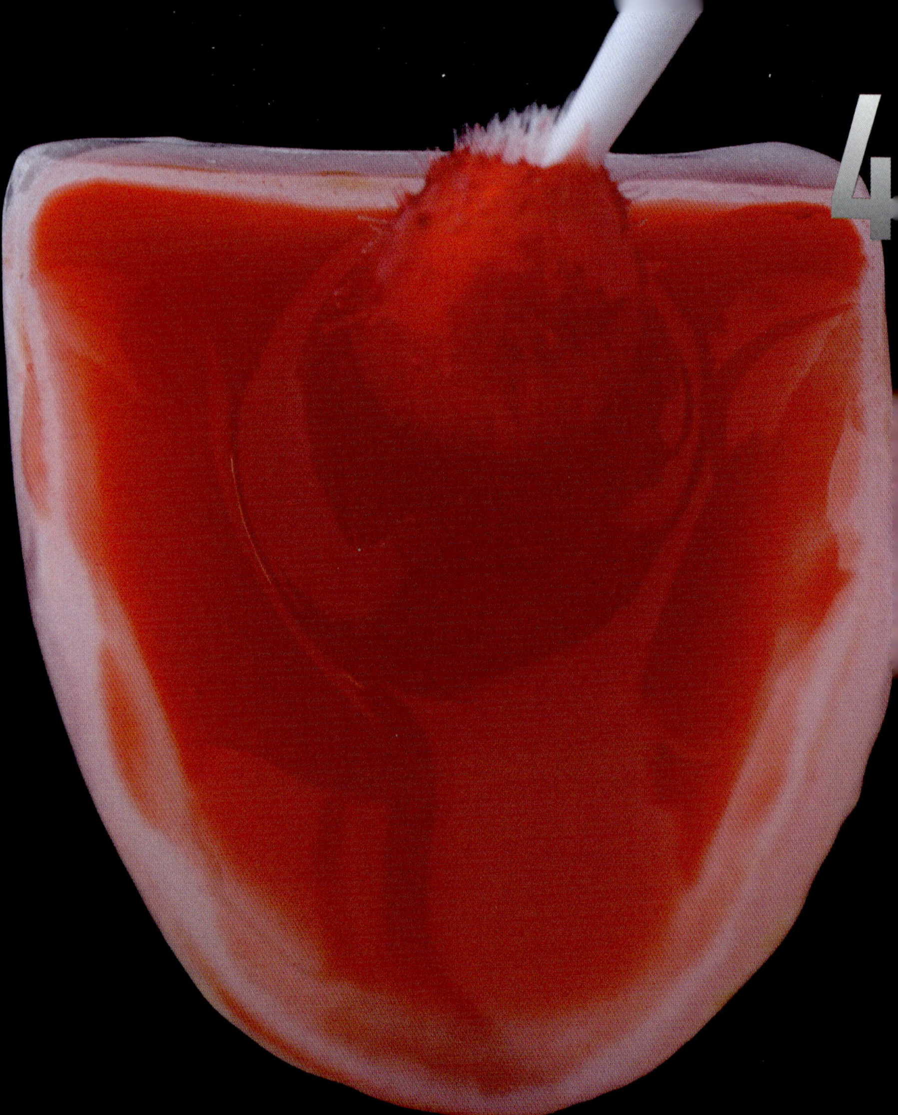

Properly pretreat the **restoration**: **Hydrofluoric acid (HF) etching** for silica ceramics

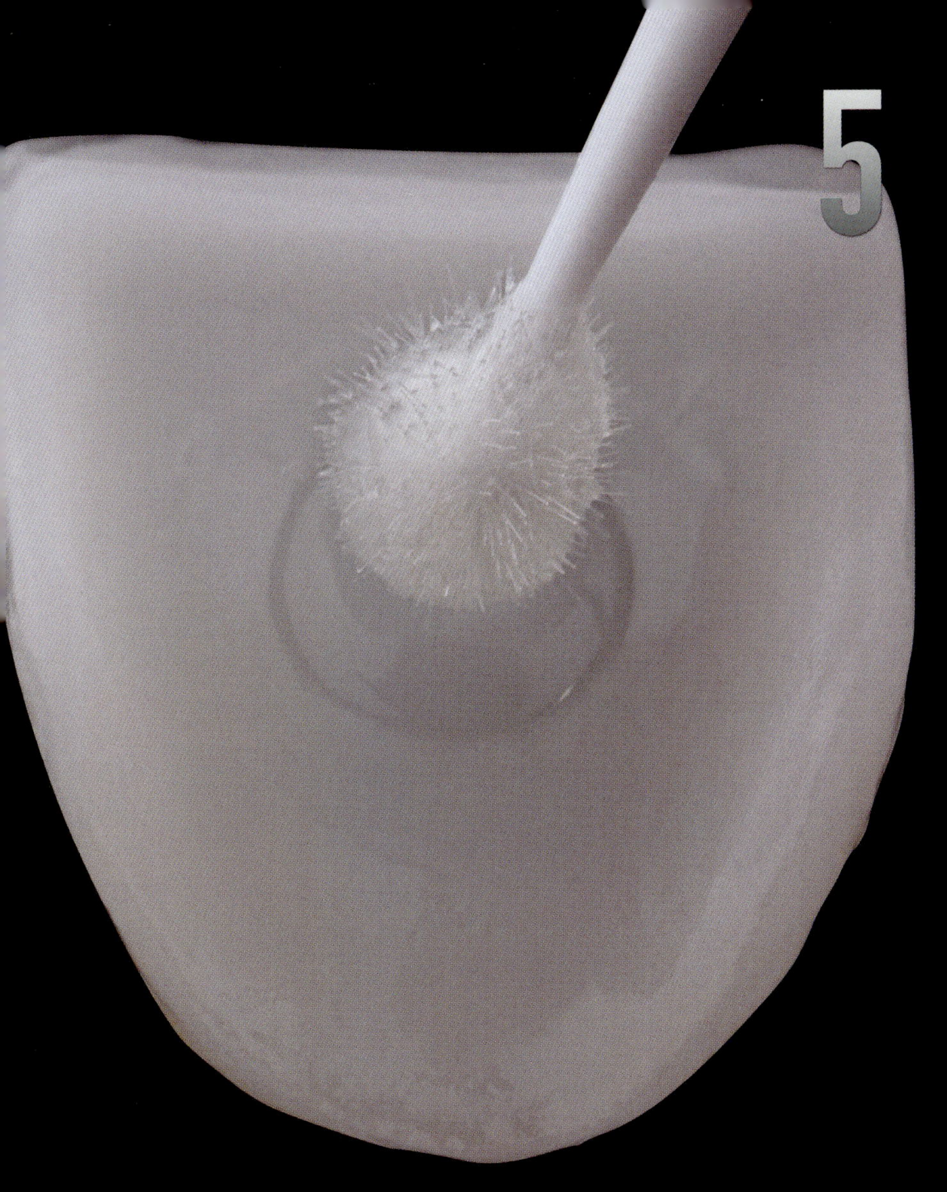

5

Clean in an ultrasonic bath, dry, and apply **silane coupling agent**

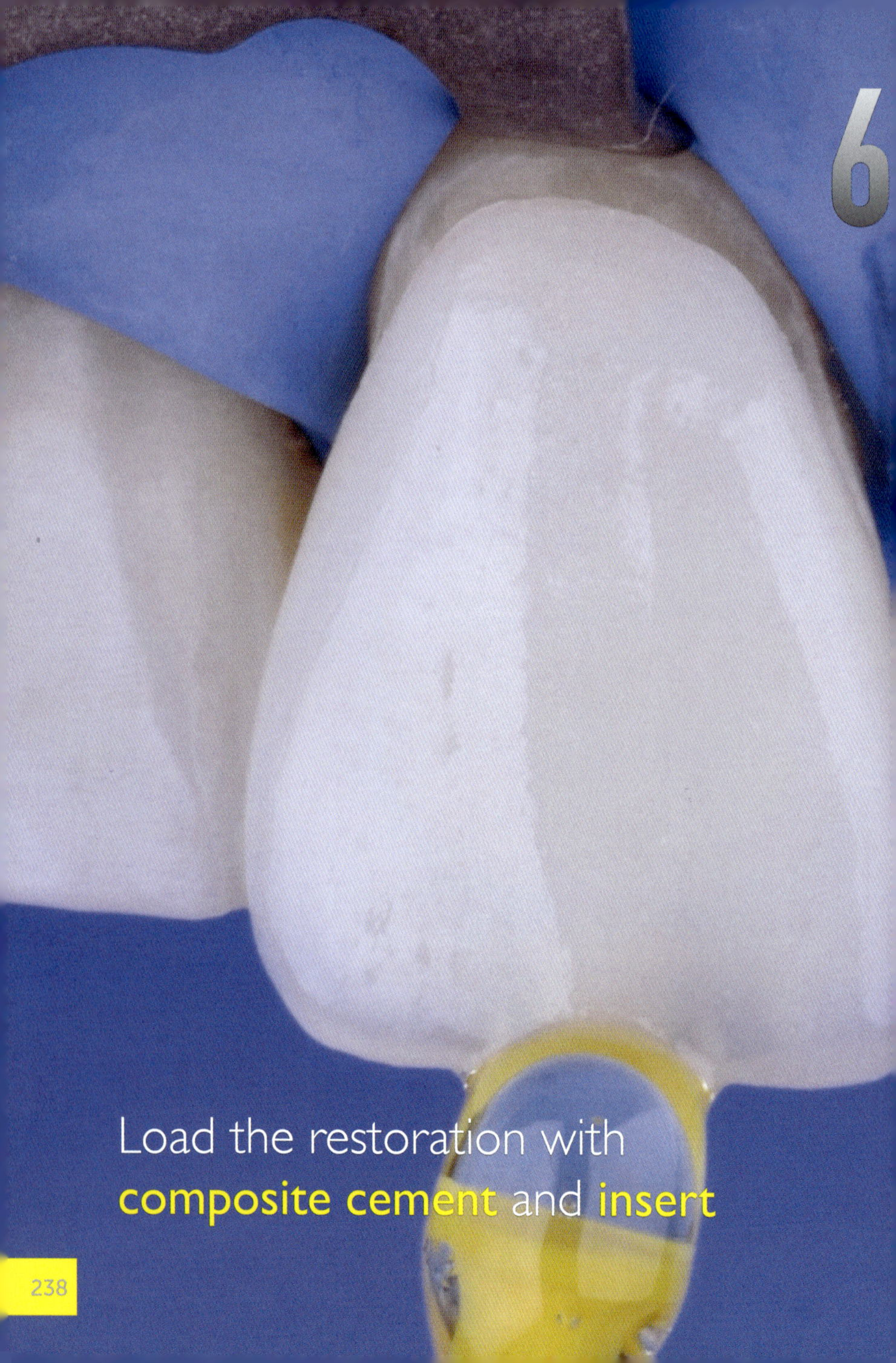
6
Load the restoration with
composite cement and insert

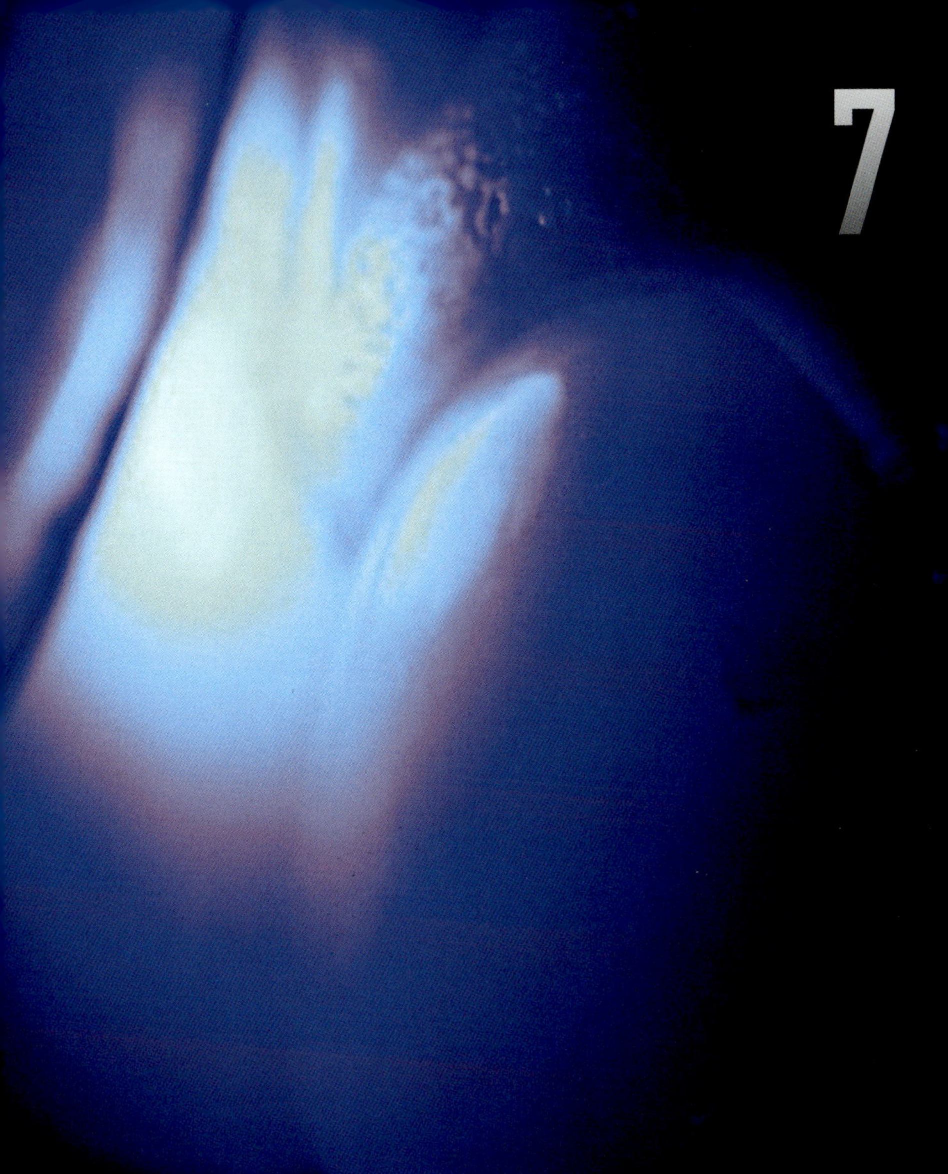

7

Remove excess and **light cure**

Finish and **polish**

IDS RESTORATION DELIVERY

CHEAT SHEET

1. Remove the provisional
   Air-particle abrade the preparation
2. Etch the enamel with phosphoric acid
   Rinse off and dry
3. Apply bonding agent
   Light cure or co-cure later
4. Properly pretreat the restoration: HF etching for silica ceramics
5. Clean in an ultrasonic bath, dry, and apply silane coupling agent
6. Load the restoration with composite cement and insert
7. Remove excess and light cure
   Finish and polish

MATERIAL SELECTION

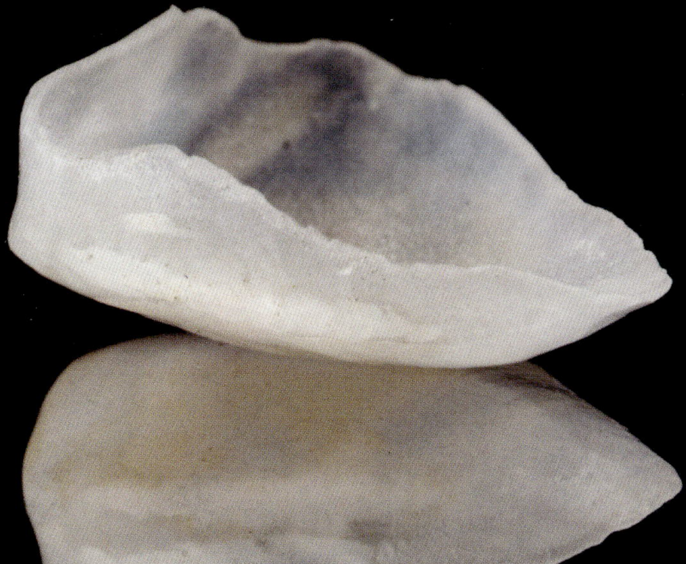

Material options for bonded laminate veneers include most **indirect esthetic materials**, fabricated either conventionally or with CAD/CAM technologies:

Feldspathic porcelain
Silica-based ceramics
Hybrid ceramics
Composites
Zirconia

Their selection depends on **functional** and **esthetic needs**

Note that each material requires **specific bonding protocols** for long-term success

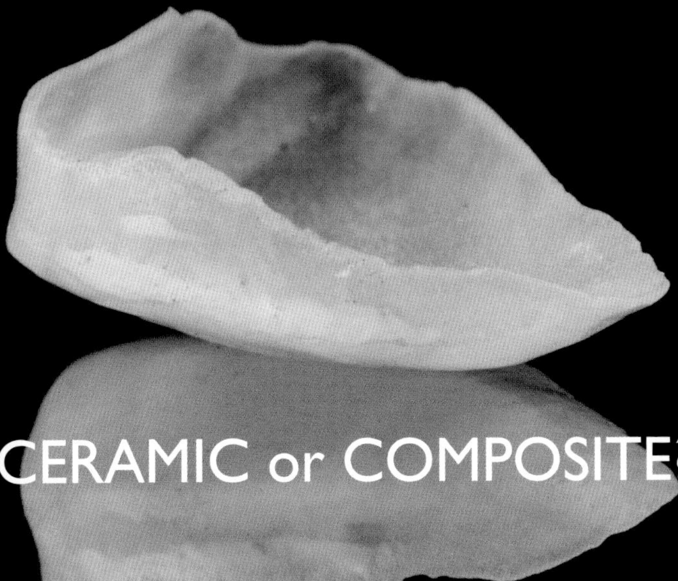

CERAMIC or COMPOSITE?

J Dent 2019;86:102–109

Randomized clinical trial on indirect resin composite and ceramic laminate veneers: Up to 10-year findings

Gresnight MMM, Cune MS, Jansen K, van der Made SAM, Özcan M

Ceramic veneers on maxillary anterior teeth performed **significantly better** than **composite indirect** veneers after a **decade**, both in terms of **survival** and **quality** of surviving restorations

Int J Prosthodont 2019;32:59–65

Comparison of failure and complication risks of porcelain laminate and indirect resin veneer restorations: A meta-analysis

Liu M, Gai K, Chen J, Jiang L

Porcelain laminate veneers have a better prognosis than indirect resin-based composite veneers

Resin-based composite veneers could still be an option in specific cases

Note the recommended **bonding protocols**, which are **significantly different** from the ones applied to **ceramic** materials

J Esthet Restor Dent 2014;26:382–393

Resin bond to indirect composite and new ceramic/polymer materials: a review of the literature

Spitznagel FA, Horvath SD, Guess PC, Blatz MB

1. **Clean** composite veneers in an **ultrasonic cleaning** bath for 2 to 5 min (alcohol) and dry
2. **Air-particle abrasion** (for example, 60-μm alumina particles at 2 bar for 10 s)
3. Apply **silane coupling** agent or **universal bonding agent** containing silane (additional adhesive is not necessary unless recommended by the manufacturer)
4. Insert the restoration with **resin-based composite** cement

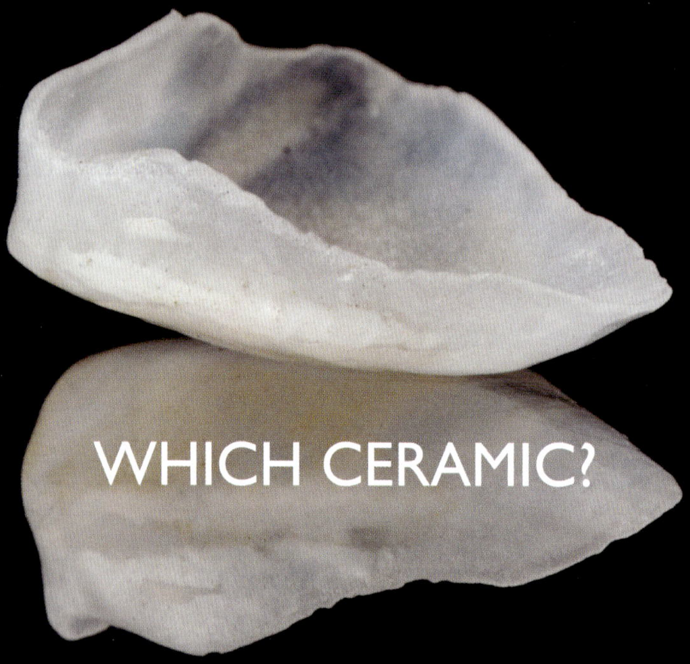

WHICH CERAMIC?

CERAMIC SELECTION

FRACTURE STRENGTH

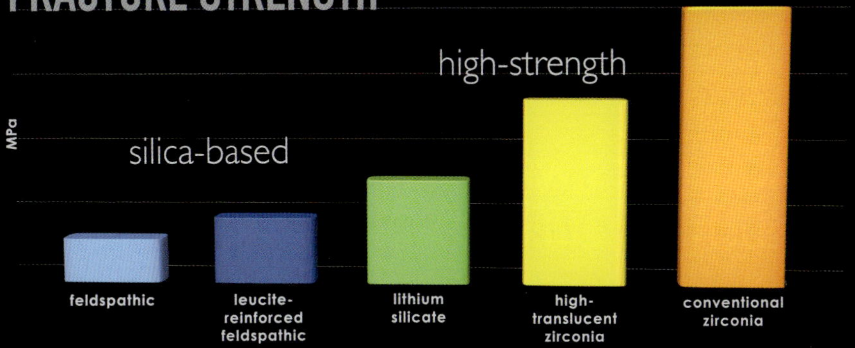

TRANSLUCENCY

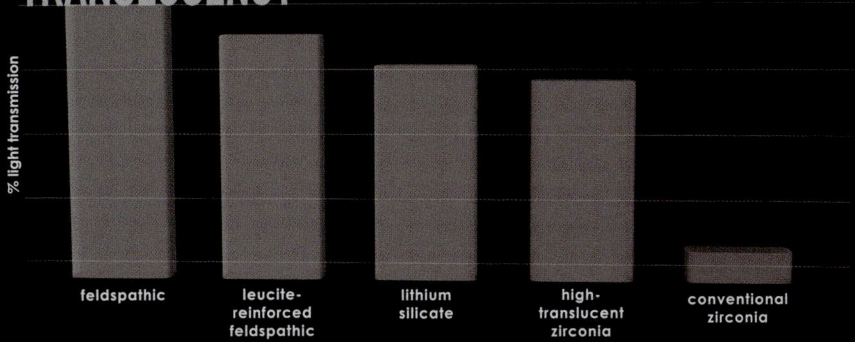

FRACTURE STRENGTH AND TRANSLUCENCY

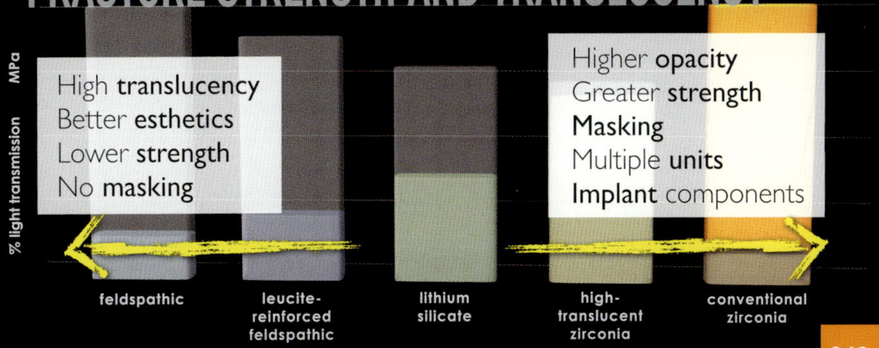

CERAMIC SELECTION

Ceramics with **higher translucency** such as **feldspathic porcelains** and **silica-based ceramics** are typically preferred for bonded laminate veneers

However, **greater shade changes** may require **more opaque** ceramics and/or greater **material thickness**

Lithium silicate ceramics provide some flexibility and can be fabricated either through **CAD/CAM** or the **pressing technique**

Evid Based Dent 2013;14:15–16

Review suggests high survival rates for veneers at five and ten years

Watt E, Conway DI

When bonded to an **enamel substrate**, feldspathic porcelain **veneers** have a very high **10-year survival** rate of 96%

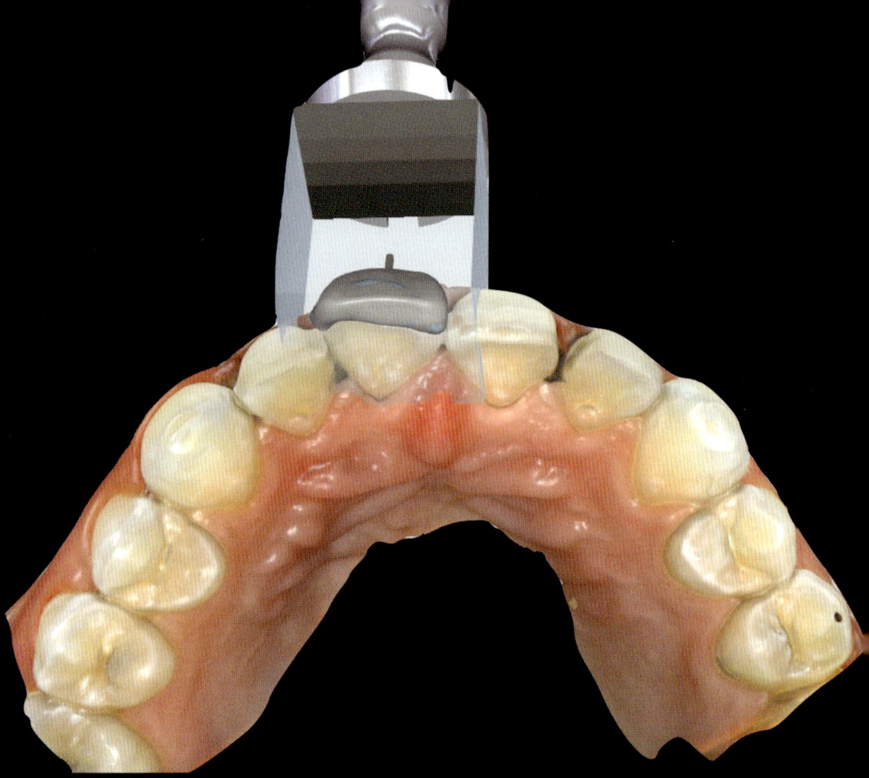

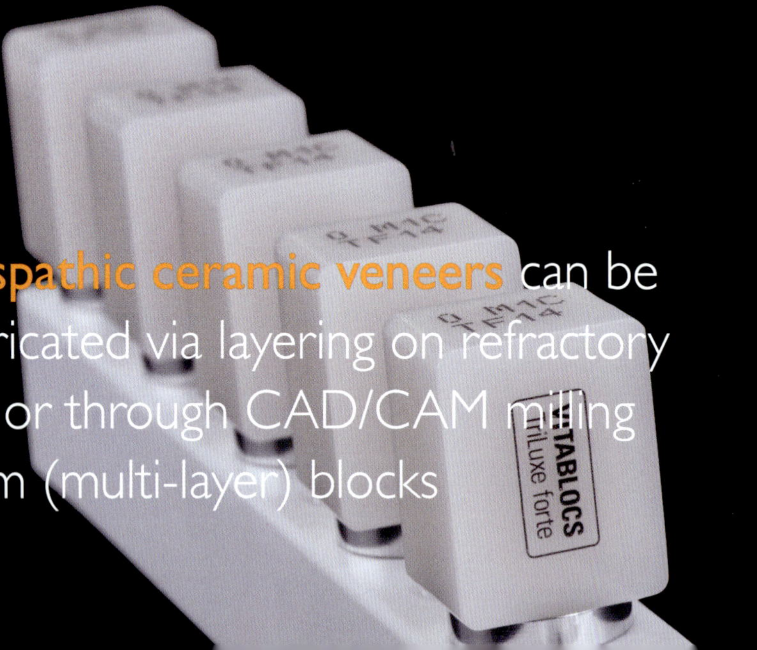

Felspathic ceramic veneers can be fabricated via layering on refractory die or through CAD/CAM milling from (multi-layer) blocks

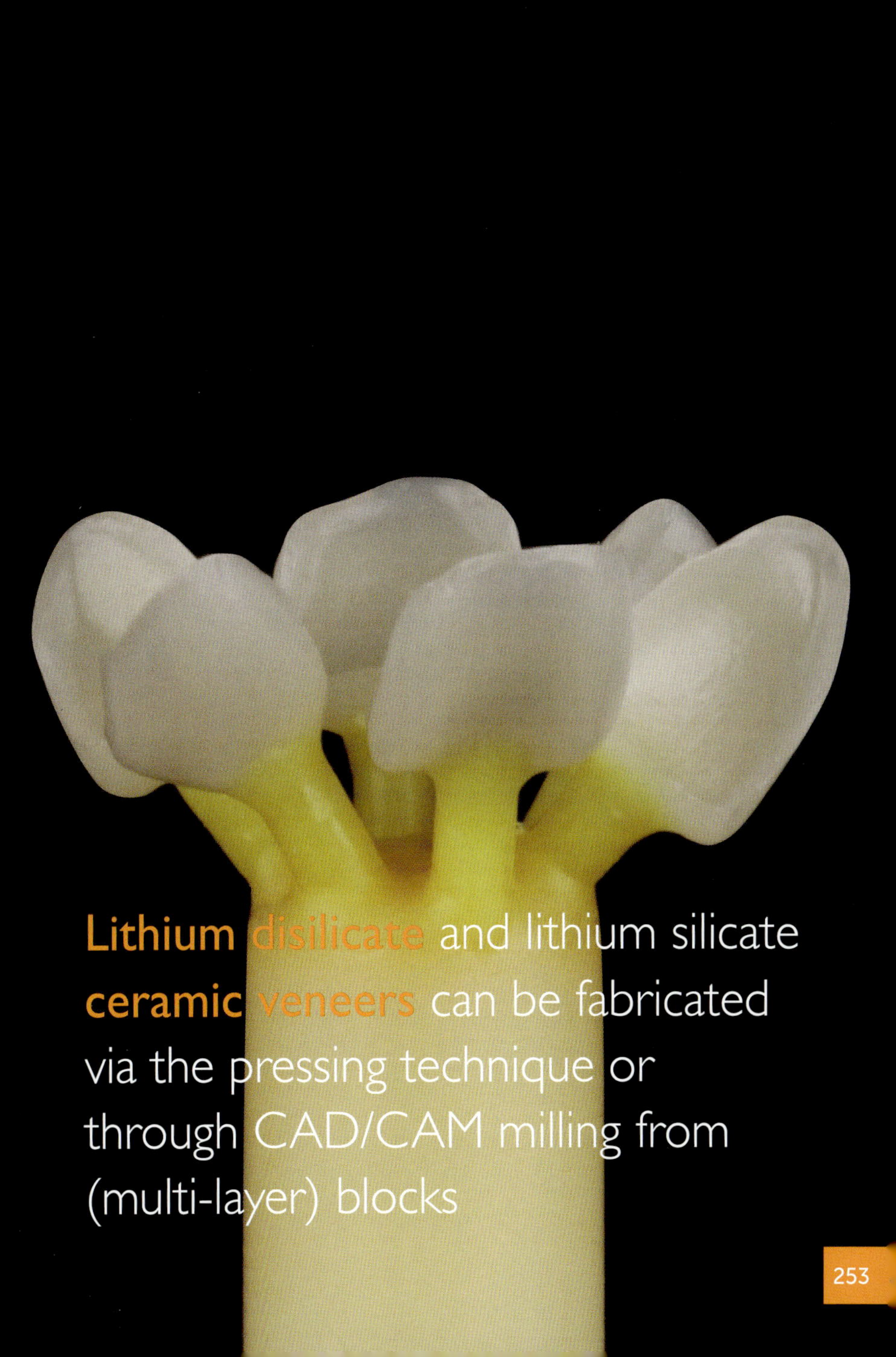

Lithium disilicate and lithium silicate **ceramic veneers** can be fabricated via the pressing technique or through CAD/CAM milling from (multi-layer) blocks

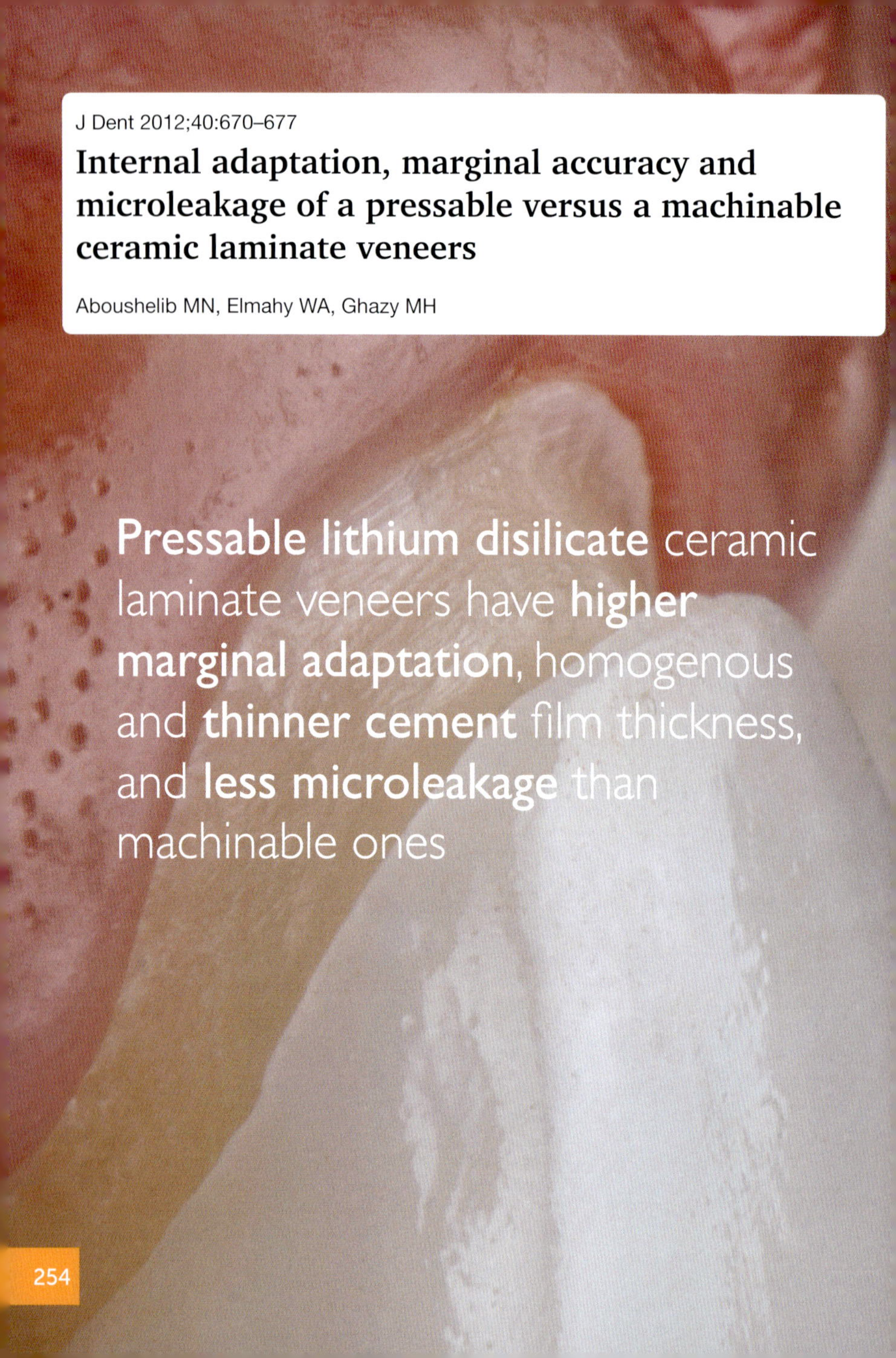

J Dent 2012;40:670–677

Internal adaptation, marginal accuracy and microleakage of a pressable versus a machinable ceramic laminate veneers

Aboushelib MN, Elmahy WA, Ghazy MH

Pressable lithium disilicate ceramic laminate veneers have **higher marginal adaptation**, homogenous and **thinner cement** film thickness, and **less microleakage** than machinable ones

J Prosthet Dent 2019;121:470–476

A comparison of the marginal and internal fit of porcelain laminate veneers fabricated by pressing and CAD-CAM milling and cemented with 2 different resin cements

Al-Dwairi ZN, Alkhatatbeh RM, Baba NZ, Goodacre CJ

Smaller marginal and **internal discrepancies** with **pressing** than with **milled lithium disilicate** laminate veneers

Larger **discrepancies incisally** than cervically

J Prosthodont 2019;28:504–510

Comparison of marginal and internal adaptation of heat-pressed and CAD/CAM porcelain laminate veneers and a 2-year follow-up

Yuce M, Ulusoy M, Turk AG

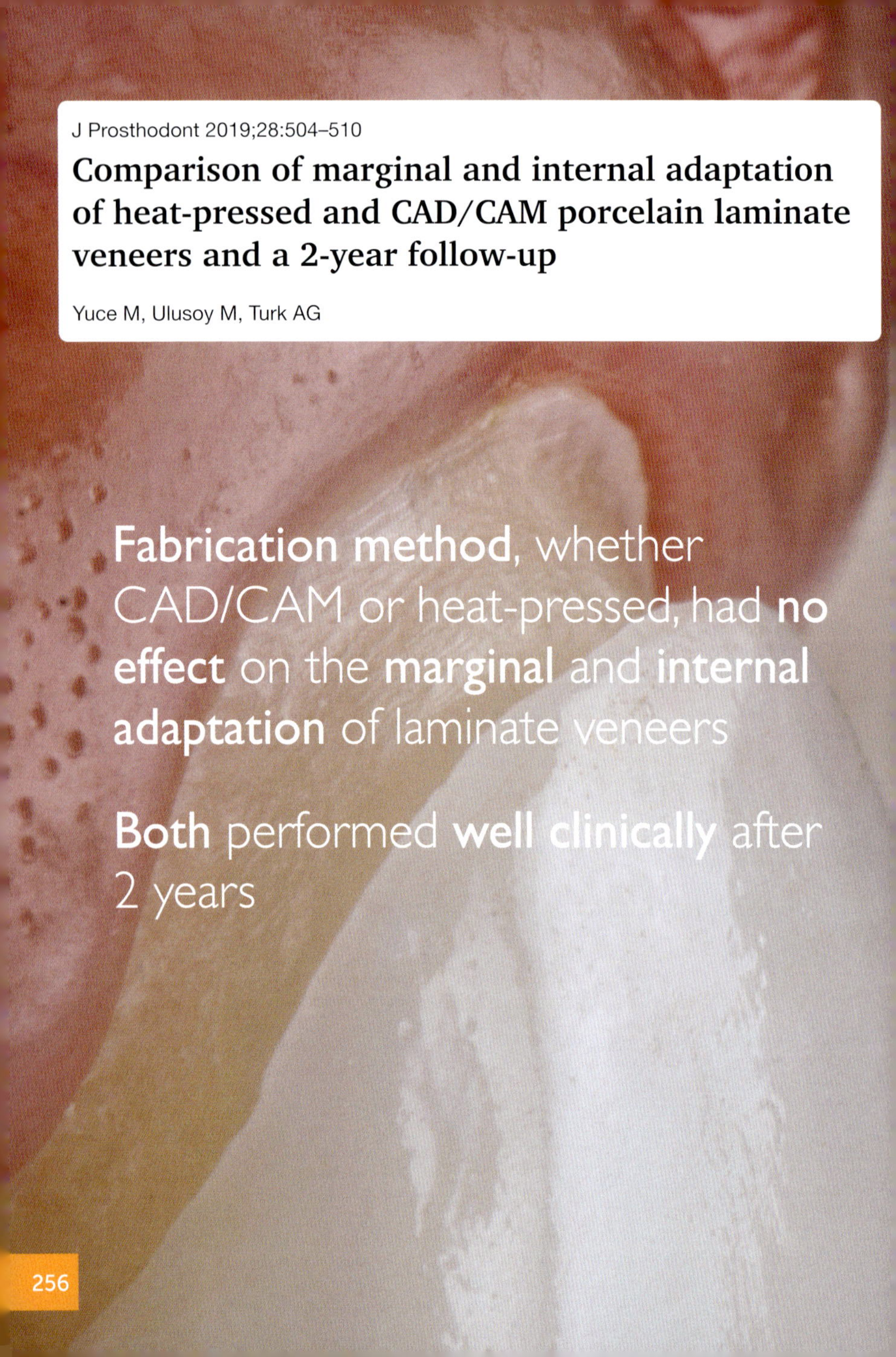

Fabrication method, whether CAD/CAM or heat-pressed, had **no effect** on the **marginal** and **internal adaptation** of laminate veneers

Both performed **well clinically** after 2 years

MY PERSONAL VIEW…

Pressing *may provide* ***better marginal fit*** *of laminate veneers than* ***milling****, since the fit is affected by the milling process, bur size, post-milling crystallization, among other things*

However, ***milling*** *has become* ***more popular*** *and* ***more accurate*** *as interesting new developments are being made in* ***3D printing*** *and* ***3D-printed materials***

Remember that ***better preparations*** *without sharp corners and rough surfaces lead to* ***better fit*** *of all, especially CAD/CAM, restorations*

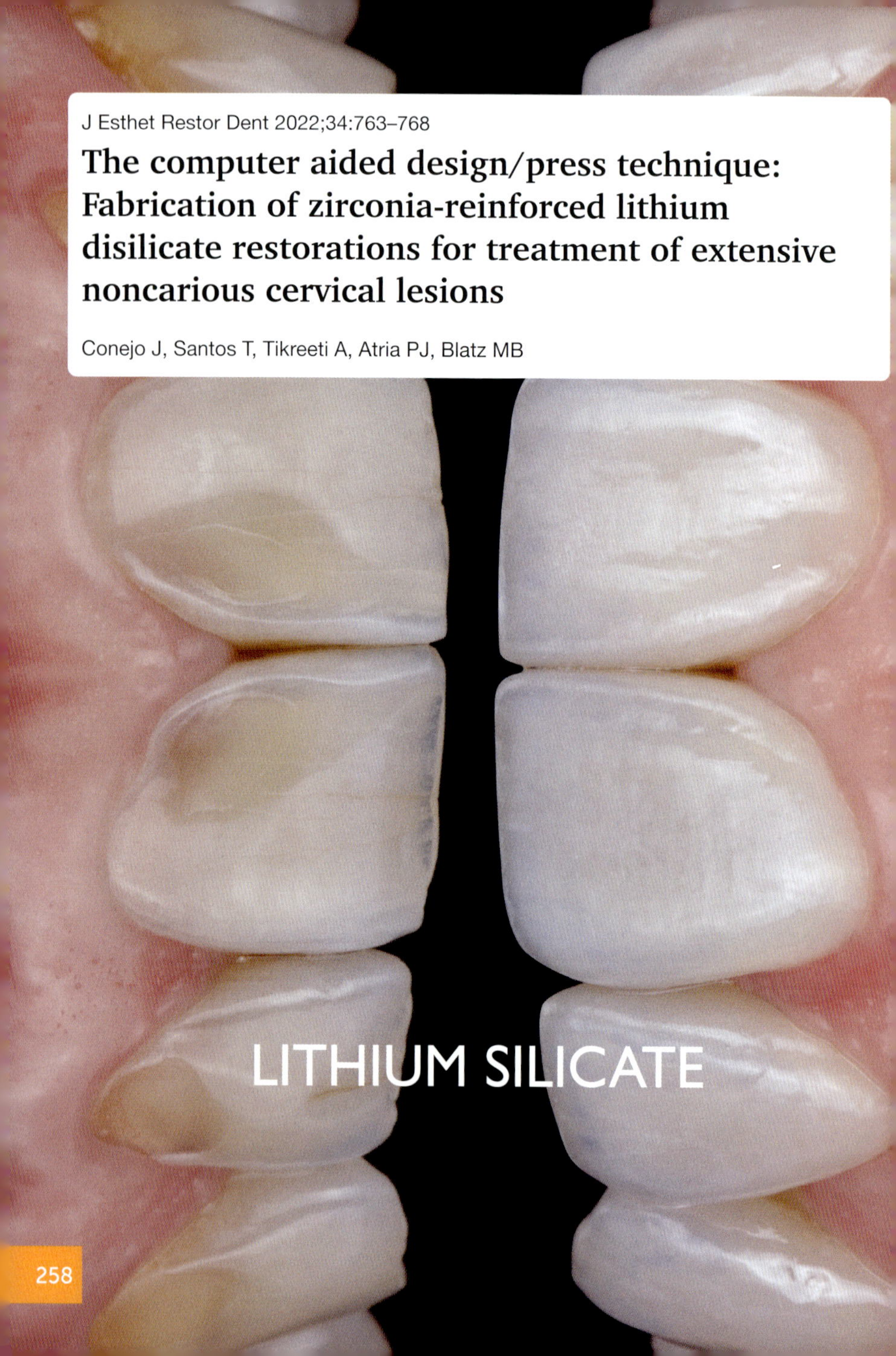

J Esthet Restor Dent 2022;34:763–768

The computer aided design/press technique: Fabrication of zirconia-reinforced lithium disilicate restorations for treatment of extensive noncarious cervical lesions

Conejo J, Santos T, Tikreeti A, Atria PJ, Blatz MB

LITHIUM SILICATE

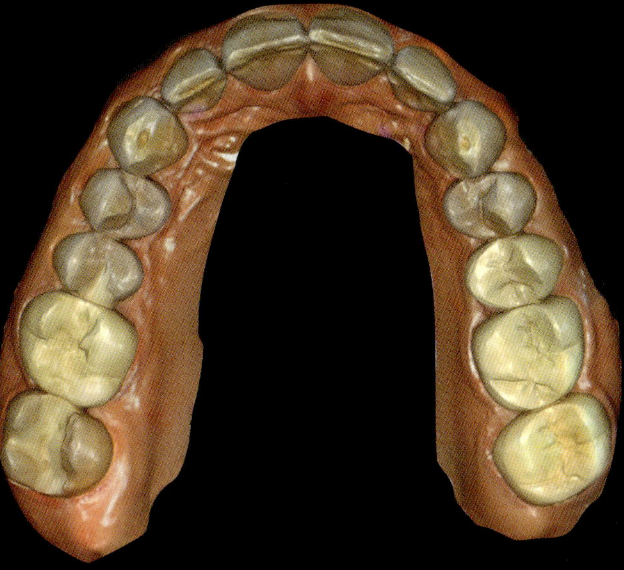

CAD/CAM design

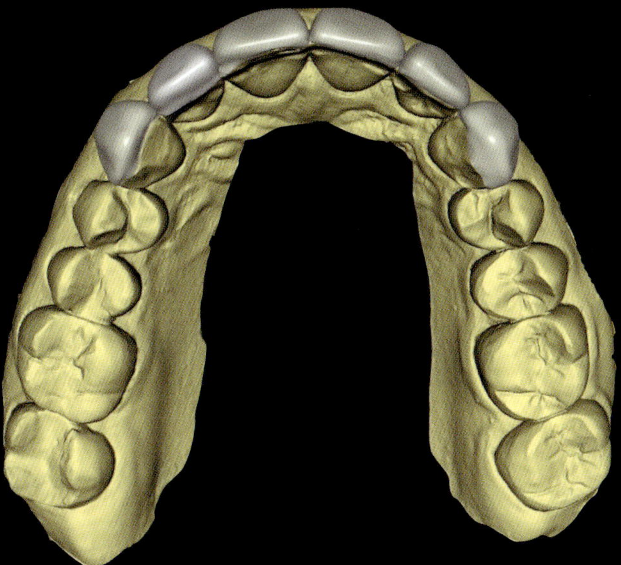

Conejo et al. J Esthet Restor Dent 2022;34:763–768

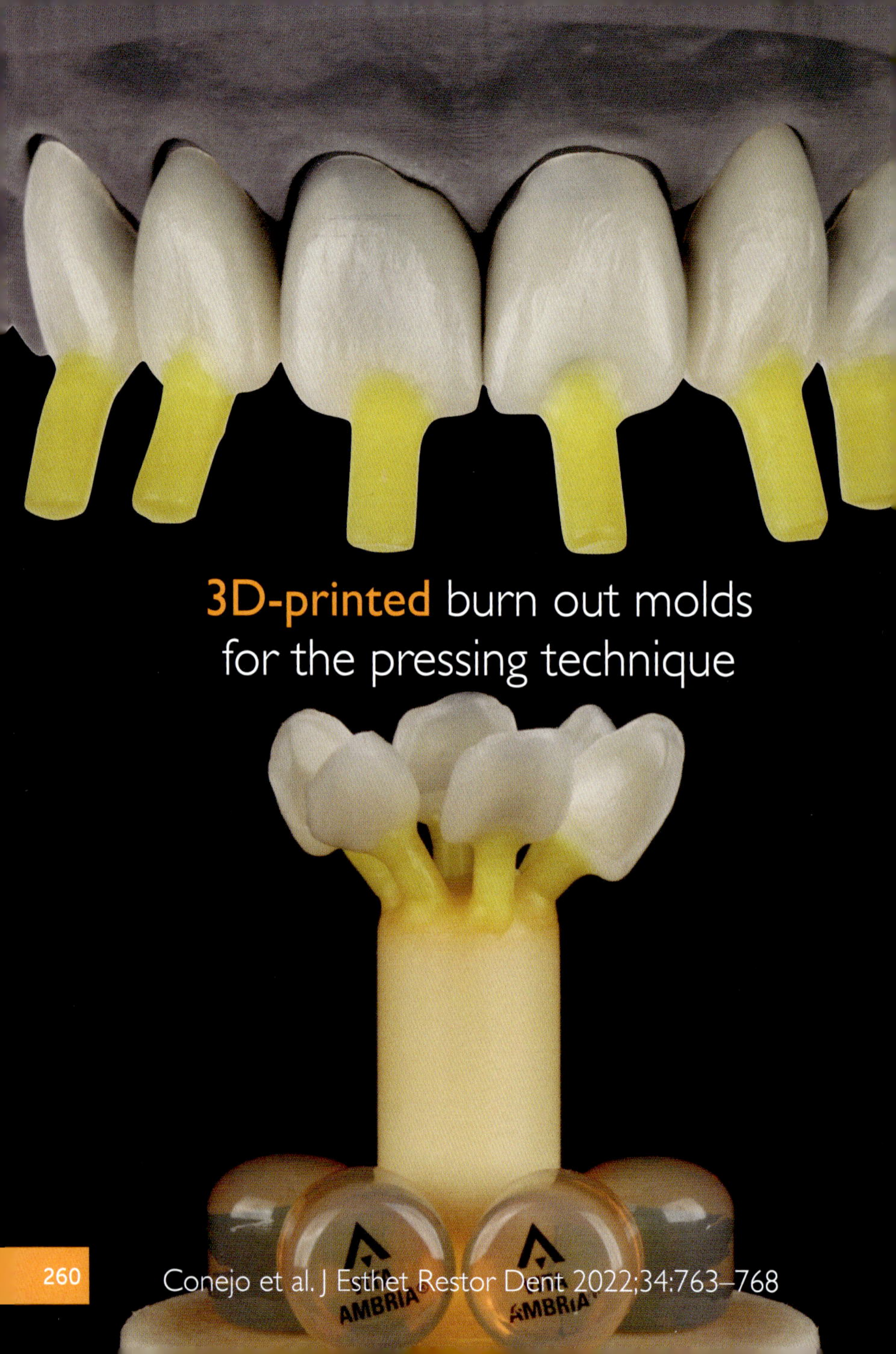

3D-printed burn out molds for the pressing technique

Conejo et al. J Esthet Restor Dent 2022;34:763–768

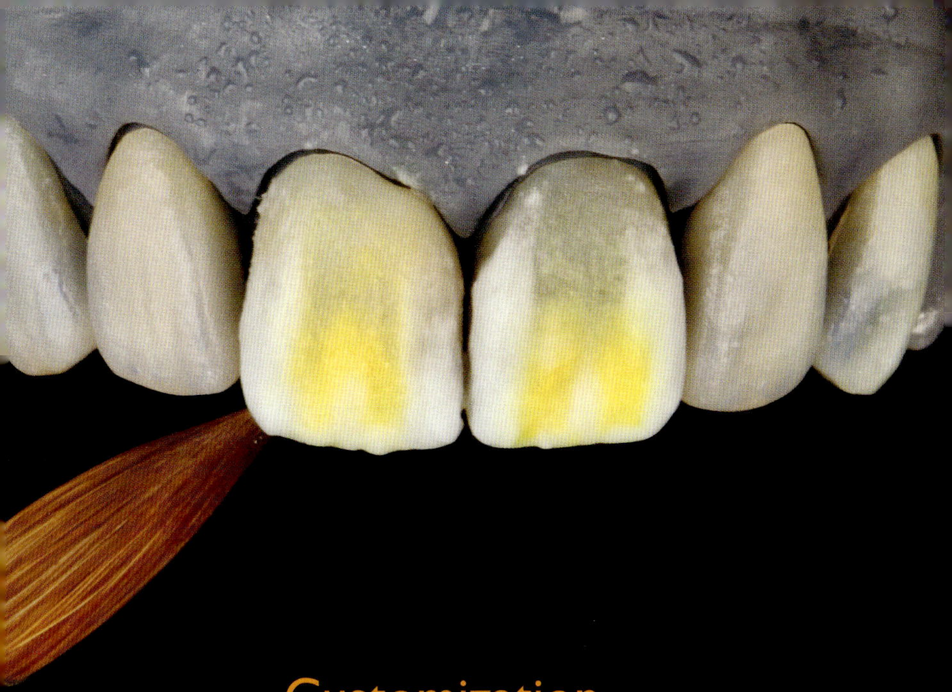

Customization
with layering porcelain

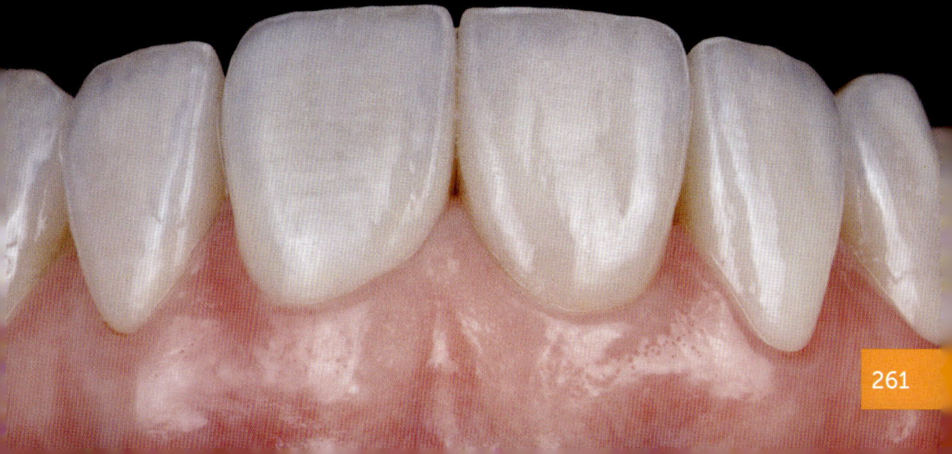

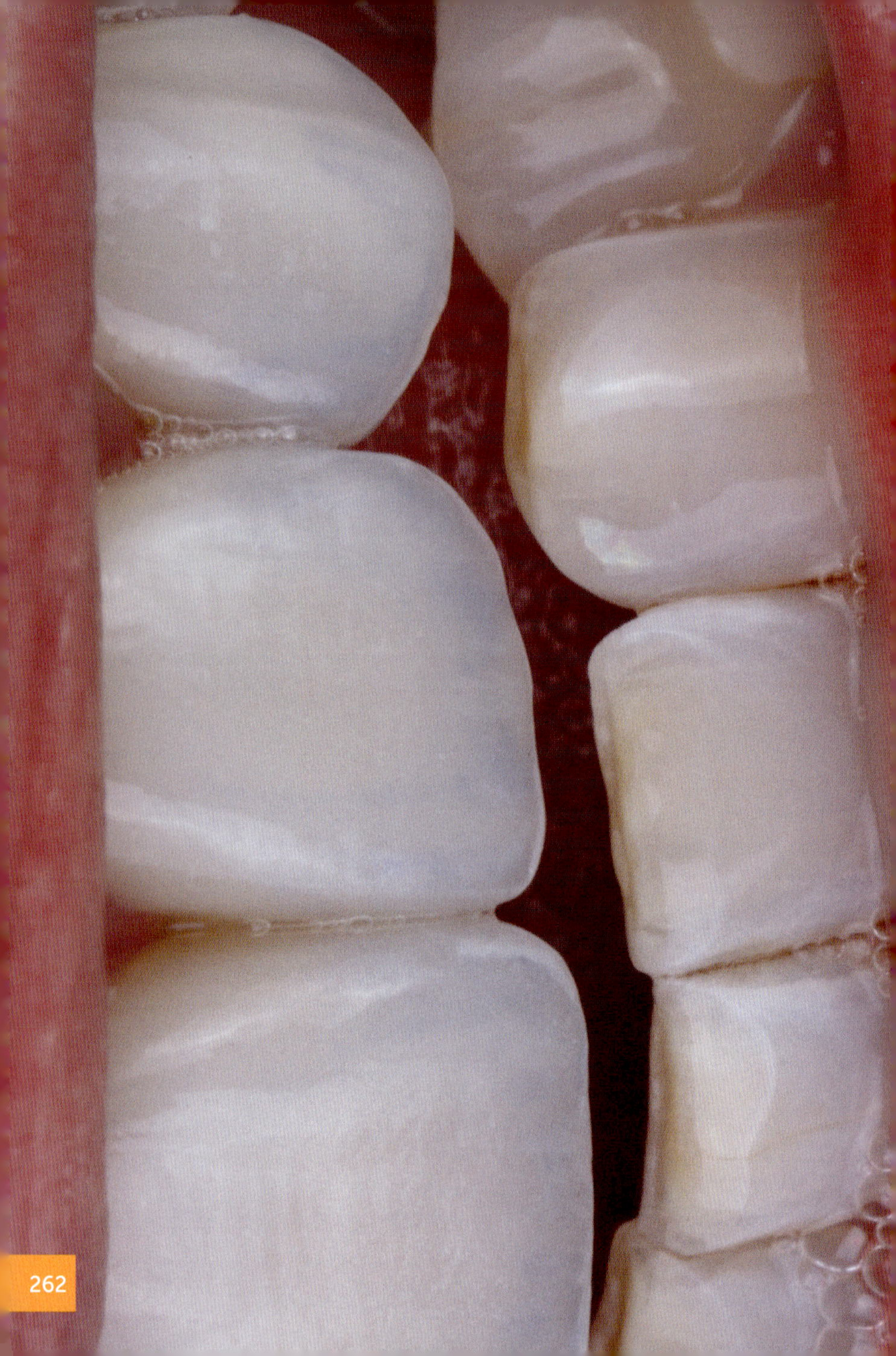

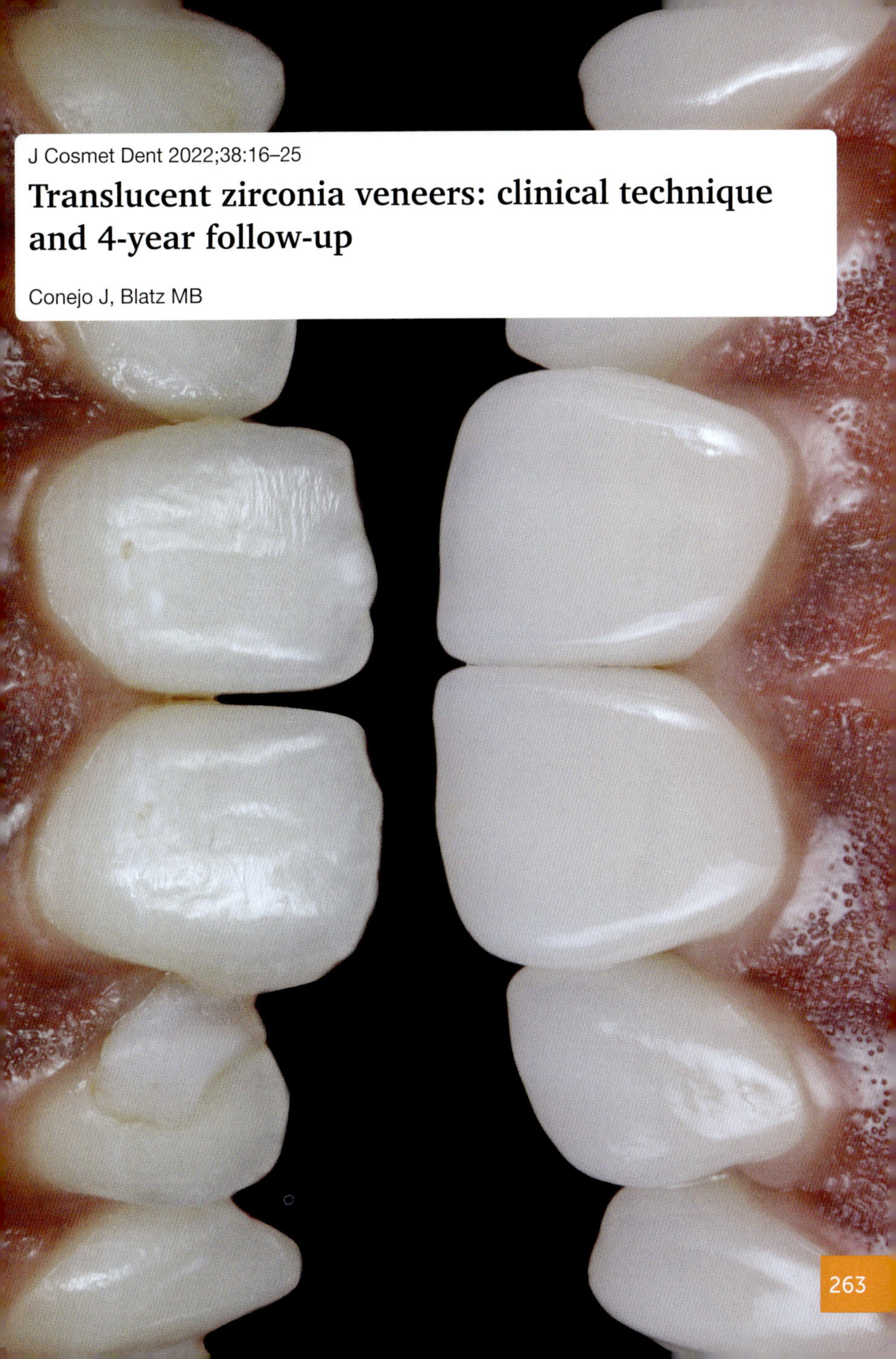

J Cosmet Dent 2022;38:16–25

Translucent zirconia veneers: clinical technique and 4-year follow-up

Conejo J, Blatz MB

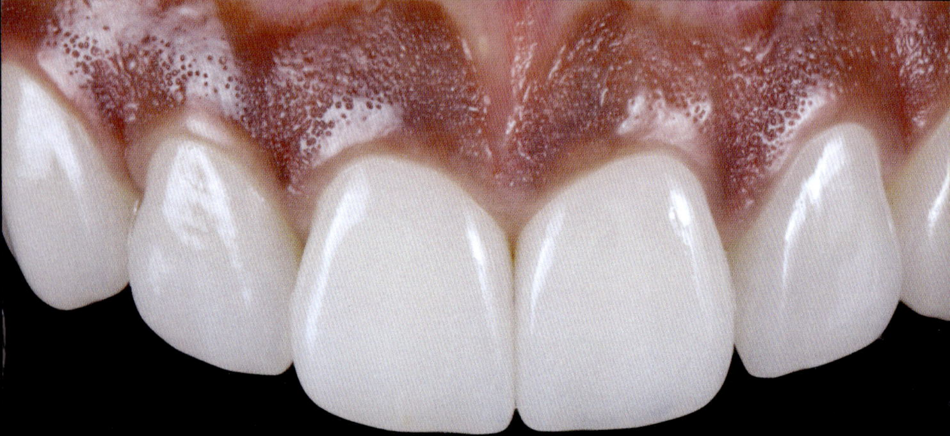

In select cases, especially when **high value** or **significant shade changes** are desired, **high-translucent zirconia** can be a viable option for veneers

Conejo and Blatz. J Cosmet Dent 2022;38:16–25

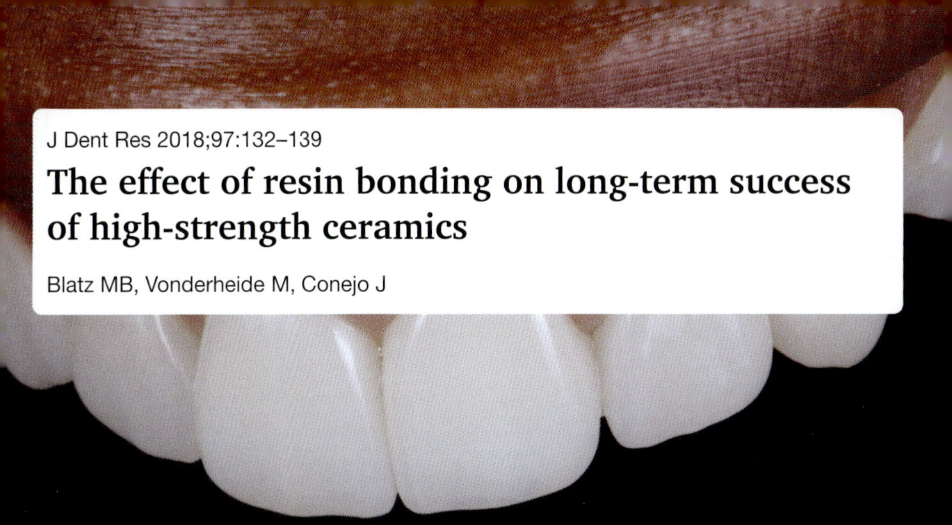

J Dent Res 2018;97:132–139

The effect of resin bonding on long-term success of high-strength ceramics

Blatz MB, Vonderheide M, Conejo J

Note that **bonding protocols** for **silica-based ceramics** are **not successful** for bonding **zirconia veneers**

The **APC zirconia bonding** concept is based on **over 25 years** of **clinical** and **laboratory research** and remains the **most effective**, **efficient**, and **long-term successful** protocol for bonding zirconia restorations to date

Compend Contin Educ Dent 2016;37:611–617

How to bond zirconia: The APC concept

Blatz MB, Alvarez M, Sawyer K, Brindis M

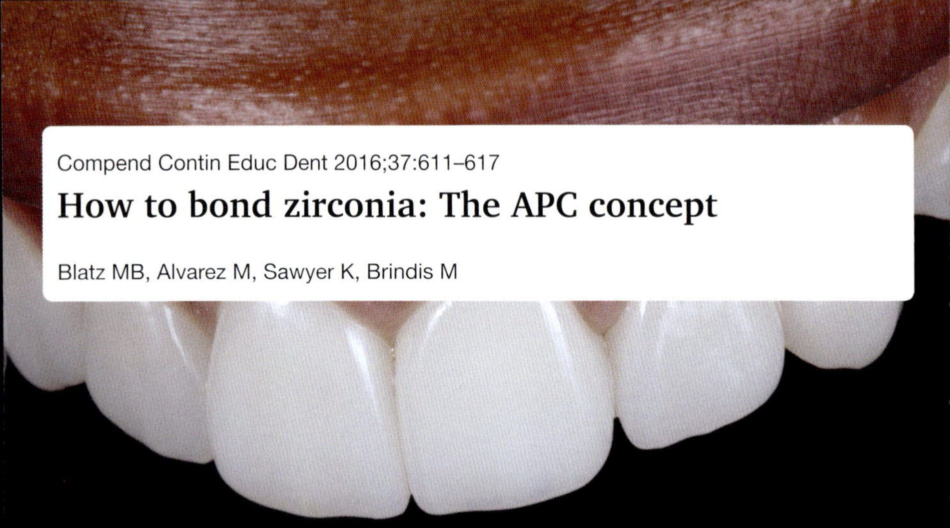

How to **bond zirconia veneers**

The APC Concept

Air-borne particle abrasion

Primer with special monomers

Composite cement

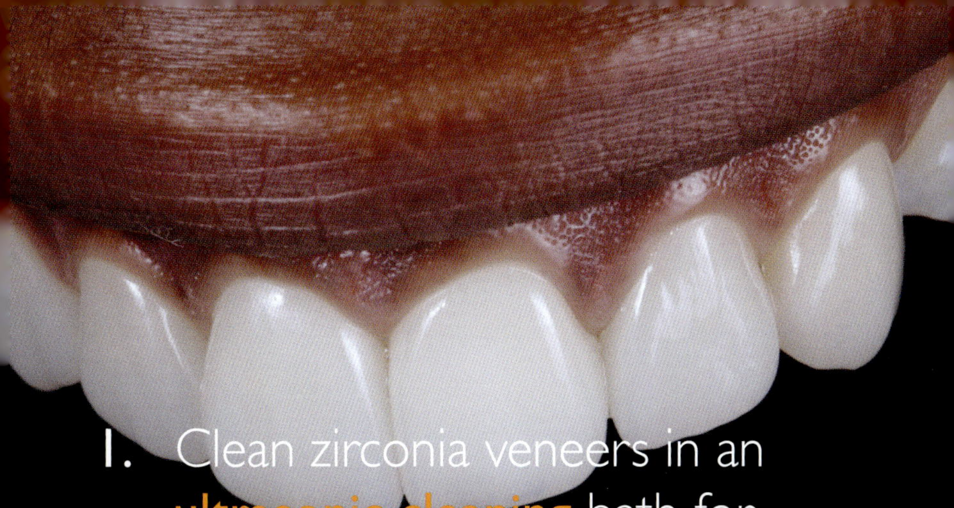

1. Clean zirconia veneers in an **ultrasonic cleaning** bath for for 2 to 5 min (alcohol) and dry
2. **Air-particle abrasion** (for example, 60-μm alumina particles at 2 bar for 10 s)
3. Apply special **zirconia primer** or bonding agent containing adhesive monomers that chemically bond to metal oxides (for example, MDP)
4. Insert restoration with dual- or self-cure **resin-based composite** cement

Blatz et al. Compend Contin Educ Dent 2016;37:611–617

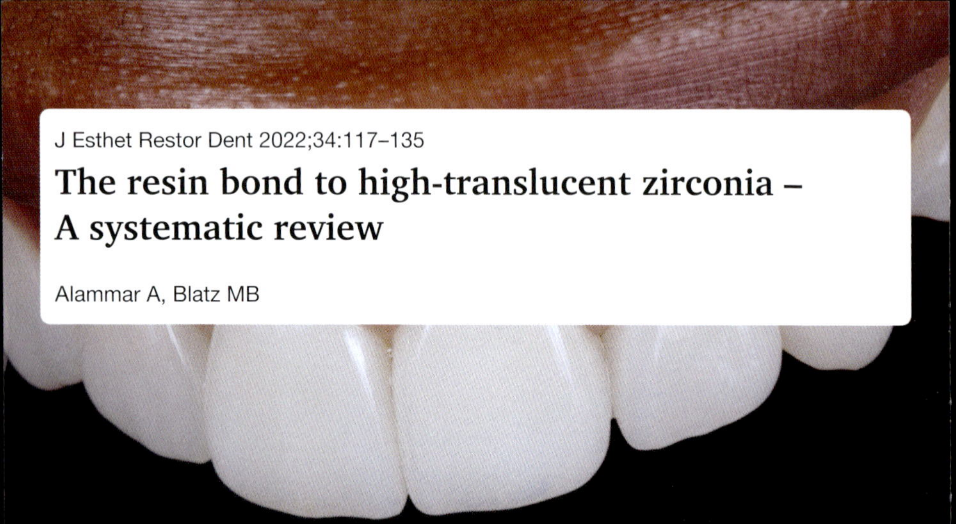

J Esthet Restor Dent 2022;34:117–135

The resin bond to high-translucent zirconia – A systematic review

Alammar A, Blatz MB

Bonding protocols are the **same** for **conventional** and **high-translucent zirconia**:

Airborne-particle abrasion, special phosphate monomer-containing **primers**, and **resin cements (APC)** provide long-term **durable resin bonds**

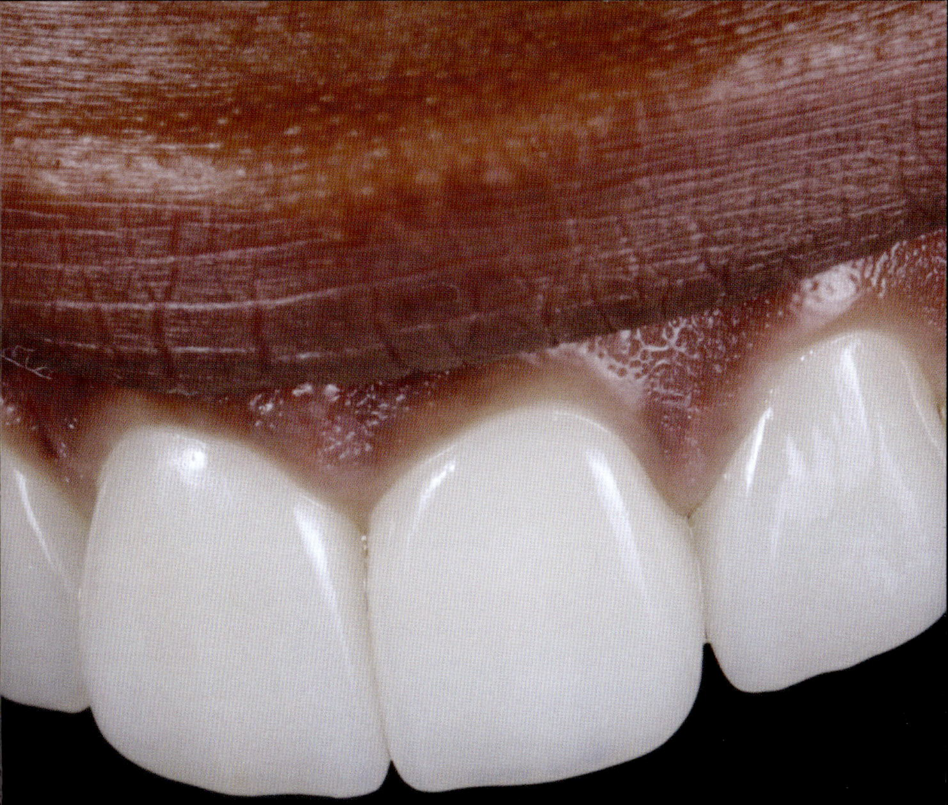

…**4-year** follow up

Conejo and Blatz. J Cosmet Dent 2022;38:16–25